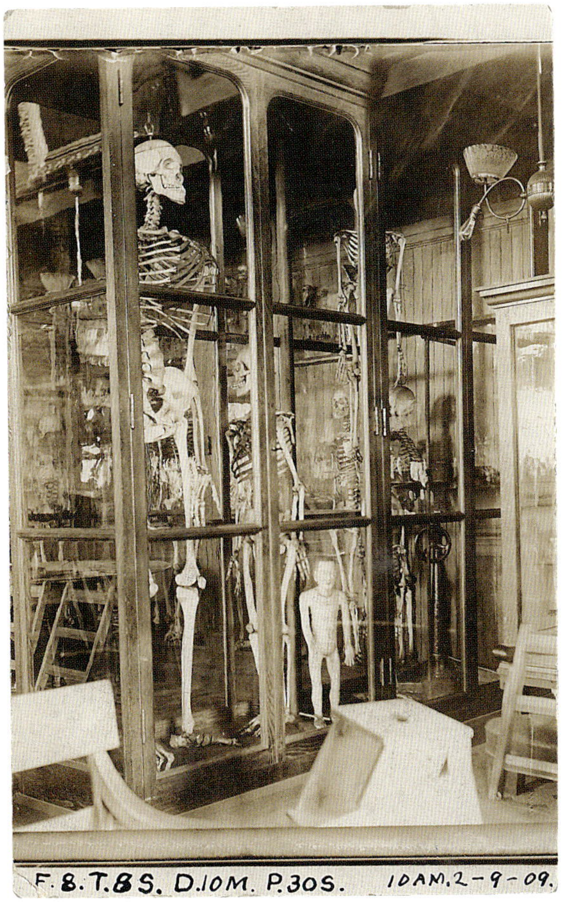
F. 8. T. 8 S. D. 10 M. P. 30 S.   10 AM. 2-9-09.

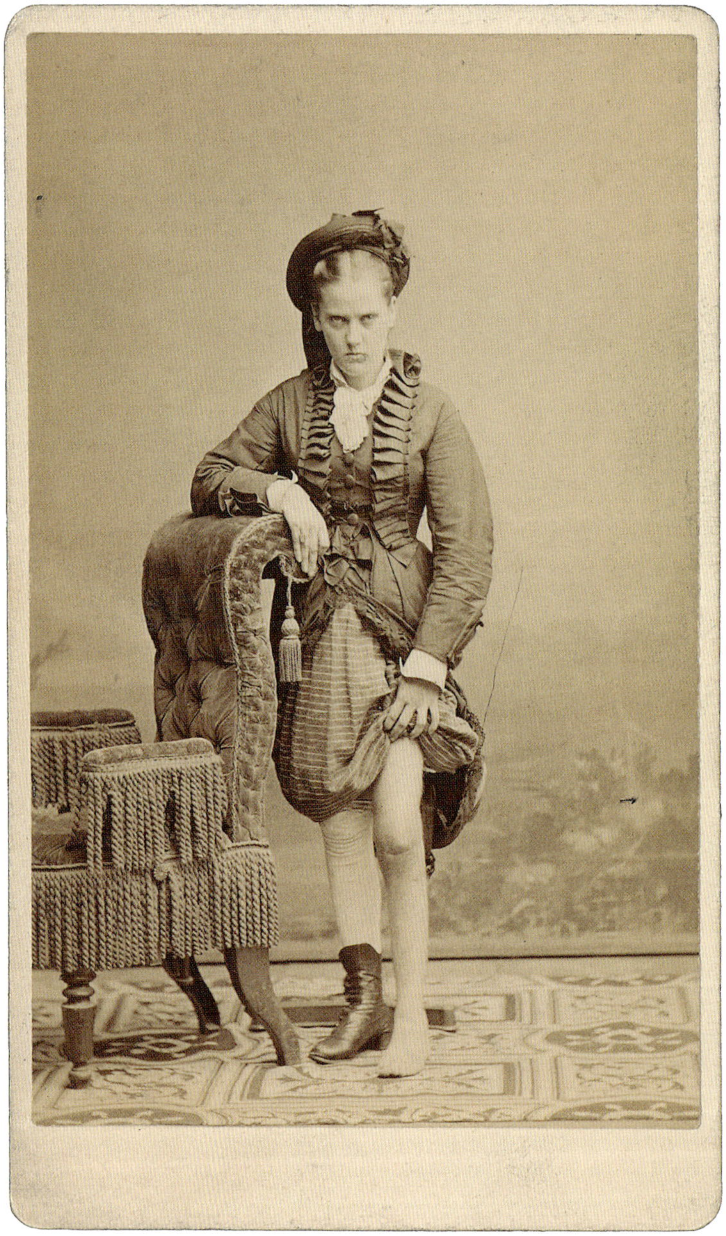

MÜTTER MUSEUM

HISTORIC MEDICAL PHOTOGRAPHS

THE COLLEGE OF PHYSICIANS OF PHILADELPHIA

Edited by Laura Lindgren

Introduction by Gretchen Worden

Foreword by Max Aguilera-Hellweg, M.D.

BLAST BOOKS · NEW YORK

For Gretchen

PAGE 1: Mütter Museum, February 9, 1909. Postcard, photographer unidentified.

PAGE 2: Tuberculosis of the joints. Photographed by William H. Rhoads, Philadelphia, undated, ca. 1866–98.

PAGE 5: Detail, lithographic plate by Armstrong & Co. Lith., Boston, from *Regional Anatomy*, 1892, showing a subject dissected, photographed, and colored from nature by George B. McClellan, M.D. (1849–1913).

PAGE 6: Cicatrices and tuberculosis affecting the arm, radius destroyed. Albumen print, photographer and date unidentified. Patient of DeForest Willard, M.D. (1846–1910).

Blast Books gratefully acknowledges the generous help of Max Aguilera-Hellweg, M.D., Anna Dhody, James Edmonson, Nava Hall, Donald Kennison, Andrea Kenyon, Margaret Lyman, Ken Siman, Kim Tieger, and James Wheeler, M.D.

Library of Congress Cataloging-in-Publication Data
Mütter Museum : historic medical photographs / The College of Physicians of Philadelphia ; edited by Laura Lindgren ; introduction by Gretchen Worden ; foreword by Max Aguilera-Hellweg. — 1st ed.
p. ; cm.
Includes index.
ISBN 978-0-922233-28-1 (alk. paper)
1. Medical photography—History. 2. Medicine—History—Pictorial works. 3. Mütter Museum—Photograph collections. 4. Photograph collections—Pennsylvania—Philadelphia. I. Lindgren, Laura. II. Mütter Museum. III. College of Physicians of Philadelphia.
[DNLM: 1. Mütter Museum. 2. Medicine—Pictorial Works. W 17 M992 2007]
TR708.M88 2007
779'.961—dc22 2007031924

Published by Blast Books, Inc.
P.O. Box 51, Cooper Station
New York, NY 10276-0051

Design and composition by Laura Lindgren

Printed in China
First Edition 2007
10 9 8 7 6 5 4 3 2 1

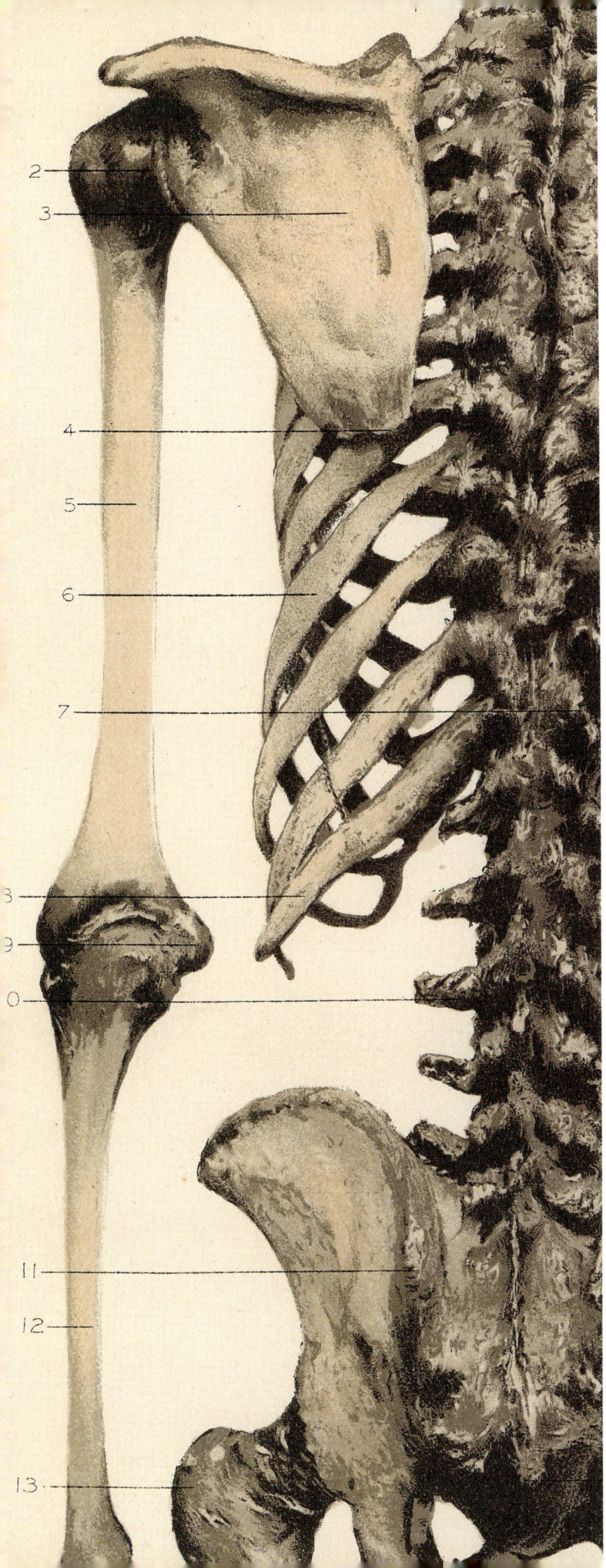

CONTENTS

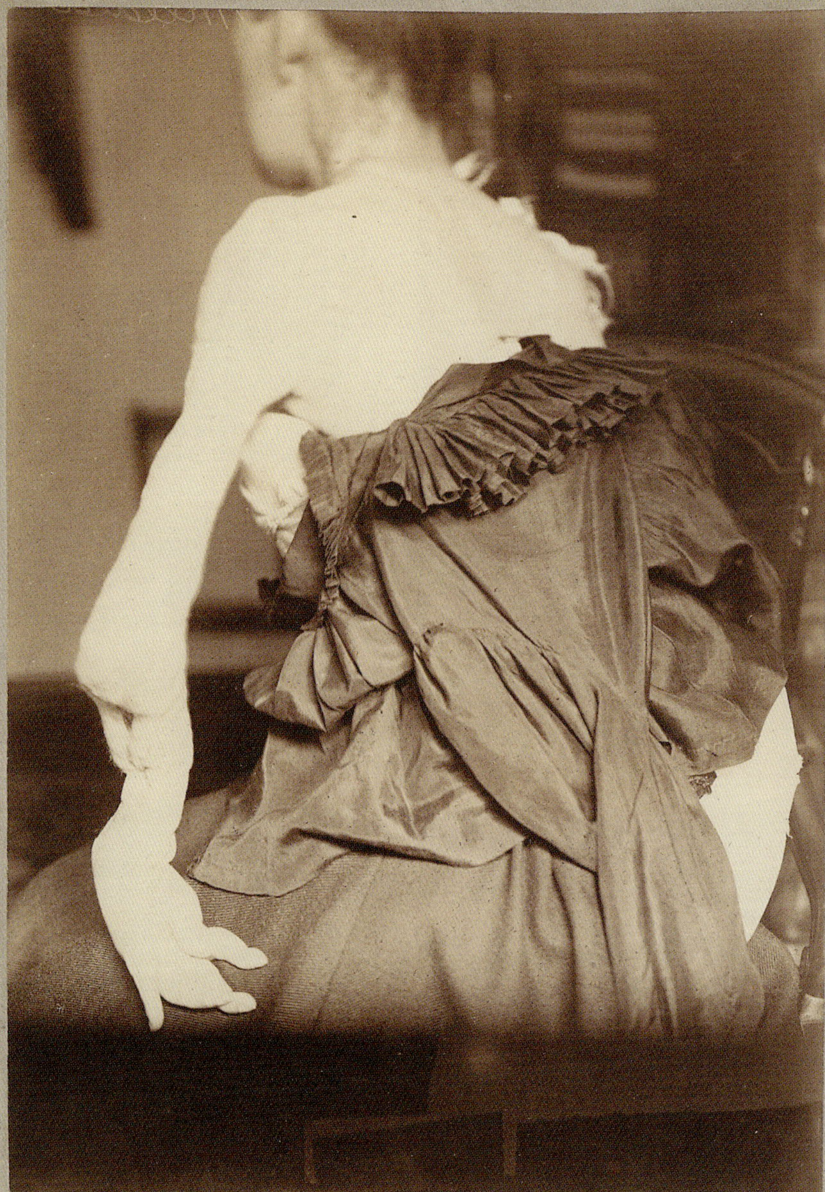

Cicatrices & Tuberculosis arm destroying radius.

Nature is nowhere accustomed more openly to display her secret mysteries than in cases where she shows traces of her workings apart from the beaten path; nor is there any better way to advance the proper practice of medicine than to give our minds to the discovery of the usual law of nature by the careful investigation of cases of rarer forms of disease. For it has been found in almost all things, that what they contain of useful or of applicable nature, is hardly perceived unless we are deprived of them, or they become deranged in some way.

—William Harvey, M.D. (1578–1657)

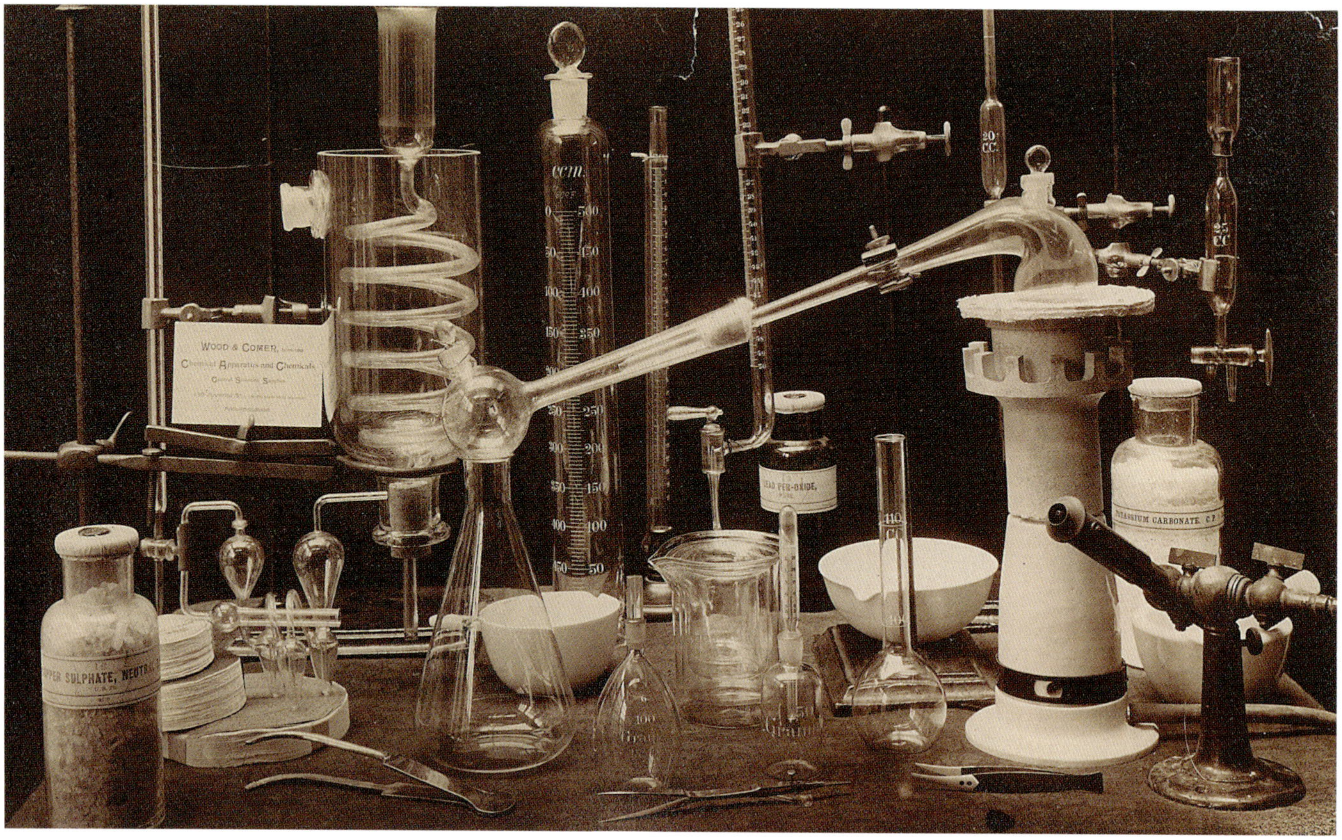
WOOD & COMER,
Chemical Apparatus and Chemicals
LEAD PER-OXIDE,
CARBONATE. C.P.
SULPHATE, NEUTR

FOREWORD

It is the care and concern. The use of a chair. Or a table. The refined borders or an elaborate signature on the print. An oval matte. A sheet of velvet. The pedestal. A painted backdrop. The button-down shirt. The care to wax or grease and part the subject's hair. The classic pose, the sitter staring off, not into camera but beyond, as if staring into the future, his or her destiny, the very future that is now as we stare back agape, wondering what the hell went wrong here. Something horrible has happened. Birth, war. Or maybe just cancer. The photographer was there. The first photographers.

When I was a premed, I was required to attend a semester of English composition and one of art history. As a photographer for twenty-odd years, thinking I knew everything, nothing was more revelatory as I learned the classics of Western civilization than my introduction to British poet and artist William Blake. What really struck me about Blake was that in the 1700s he had laid words to paper that were as contemporary as anything I had ever read. It is with this same wonderment that I view the historic photograph collection of the Mütter Museum. Today there are photographers who knowingly or unwittingly pay homage in their own work to these early Mütter masters and in so doing expose the ultimate truth in art: everything has been done before.

It was painting that provided the before for photography. And photography stole heavily in its ardent pursuit to distinguish itself from mere copying or documentation. William Henry Fox Talbot, the inventor of the modern photographic process of a negative and positive, the calotype, may have been the first to identify painting as a source in his photography. On exhibition of his photographs at the Royal Institution in London in 1839, he wrote that the pictures

Wood & Comer, Limited. Chemical Apparatus and Chemicals. General Surgical Supplies, 130 Juvenal St., Philadelphia. Photograph by James F. Wood, from the album of photographs by Wood presented to the Mütter Museum in 1898.

he had made using a camera obscura in the summer of 1835 of his house in the country were "the first instance on record, of a house having painted its own portrait." And forever the two mediums were entwined.

Early photography consisted largely of portraits and landscapes, long the terrain of painting. Yet it was the composition, the framing, the use of perspective in painting from which early photography borrowed most. But the early photographers were as much scientists as they were painters and illustrators with their cameras, applying scientific formulas and chemistry to the rules of painting and the power and limitations of light. That physicians and surgeons might bring their brethren scientists into their world to record their discoveries of human anatomy both ordinary and gone wrong, laying bare in two dimensions human suffering, seems only natural. Medical doctors were in fact the first serious amateurs with the time and money to invest in the art.

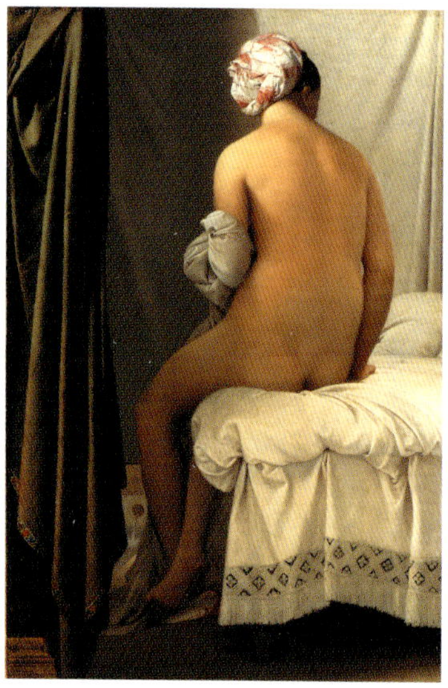

Jean-Auguste-Dominique Ingres (1780–1867), *La Baigneuse de Valpinçon* (*The Bather of Valpinçon*), 1808. Oil on canvas, 57½ x 38 3/16 in. (146 x 97 cm). Louvre, Paris. Réunion des Musées Nationaux/Art Resource, NY

Looking at the Mütter collection, I see two paintings, *La Baigneuse de Valpinçon* and *La Grande Odalisque*, both by Jean-Auguste-Dominique Ingres, and both in the collection of the Louvre, painted just before the dawn of photography. It is *La Odalisque* I recognize in Blanche Dumas as photographed in Paris by Pierre Petit circa 1880 (page 101). Were it not for her congenital third leg, dressed in sock and shoe, one might recognize the left lateral Sims position (hips resting on the edge of the bed, knees flexed, chest downward, left arm extended behind), developed by James Marion Sims, a general practitioner and surgeon, who circa 1845 performed surgical experiments in a small hospital he built on his own property for slave women suffering with vesicovaginal fistulas. The contrivances of *La Baigneuse* can be found throughout the book: drapery gracing the backdrop, if only from the side; a point of view at level with the subject; and the central act of *La Baigneuse*, the simple but erotic presentation of a woman's back—she looks away from the observer, her hair confined in a wrap. There she is in the photograph on page 6, of cicatrices and tuberculosis destroying the radius, and again on page 106, in the case of paralytic deformity before and after treatment with artificial limb, and then again on page 160 in Dr. Stelwagon's case of mycosis fungicides. We find it once more in a photograph on page 164, surface wounds and the word MAY scratched into the dermis of a woman's back, urticaria dermographia erupting, an allergic rash in response to lesions to the skin. There are at least two more examples of *La Baigneuse*, but I'll let you find them.

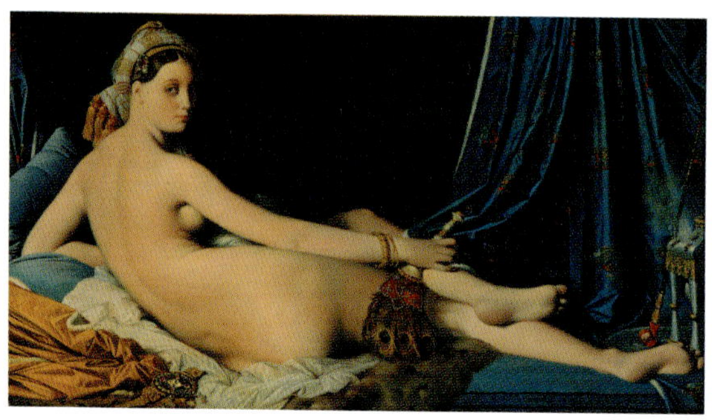

Jean-Auguste-Dominique Ingres, *La Grande Odalisque* (*The Great Odalisque*), 1808. Oil on canvas, 35 13/16 x 63¾ in. (91 x 162 cm). Louvre, Paris. Réunion des Musées Nationaux/Art Resource, NY

It is said that Thomas Eakins's best-known work, *The Gross Clinic* (1875), was influenced by Rembrandt's *Anatomy Lecture of Dr. Nicolaes Tulp* (1632). Would it be far-fetched to suggest that the photograph on page 221 of Dr. William Osler and students in the pathology dissecting laboratory of Philadelphia General Hospital, 1884, was influenced by either of these two? Or that my contemporaries Gwen Akin and Allan Ludwig might have been inspired by the laterally conjoined twins (ectopagus) on page 209? On page 29 the caption for the photograph showing an abdominal wound from the Civil War notes that "mirrors were sometimes used to provide a rear view of a patient's wound or disorder." But look at the photograph closely—what other convention is used? The man is a soldier in uniform; he stands with an object in his right hand. A cane? A telescope? A sword? Whatever this object, his pose, his demeanor, the air with which he stands with the thing indicates it must be his weapon. But why the mirror? Why not just a close-up showing the wound? Because the mirror reveals that the wound goes from front to back. This isn't just a medical photograph. Someone, the photographer maybe, was interested in something more. And he used the conventions of the time, the pose, the uniform, the artifice of a weapon; if not the photographer, I hear the subject speak, "This is Captain John Doe, a soldier who received a proud wound in battle." The photograph transcends mere documentation and tells much more.

The photographs in the Mütter collection were taken in the era when photography was considered a mechanical exercise rather than an art such as painting or sculpture. To make their case, to prove that photography was indeed an art, photographers got a foothold imitating the painting of the time. A great effort was under way by the picture takers known as pictorialists to do more with an image; some such as Julia Margaret Cameron went so far as to blur their photographs. Muybridge studied movement and, as chronicled in the pages of this very book, was commissioned to create a set of images depicting neurologic disorders. And like the great photographers of this era, Mathew Brady, Fox Talbot, Daguerre, and others, these early medical photographers whose works have survived in the Mütter Museum's collection made a grand contribution. If their works were not considered art in their lifetimes, they now can be recognized as such today. The proof is here.

Max Aguilera-Hellweg, M.D.

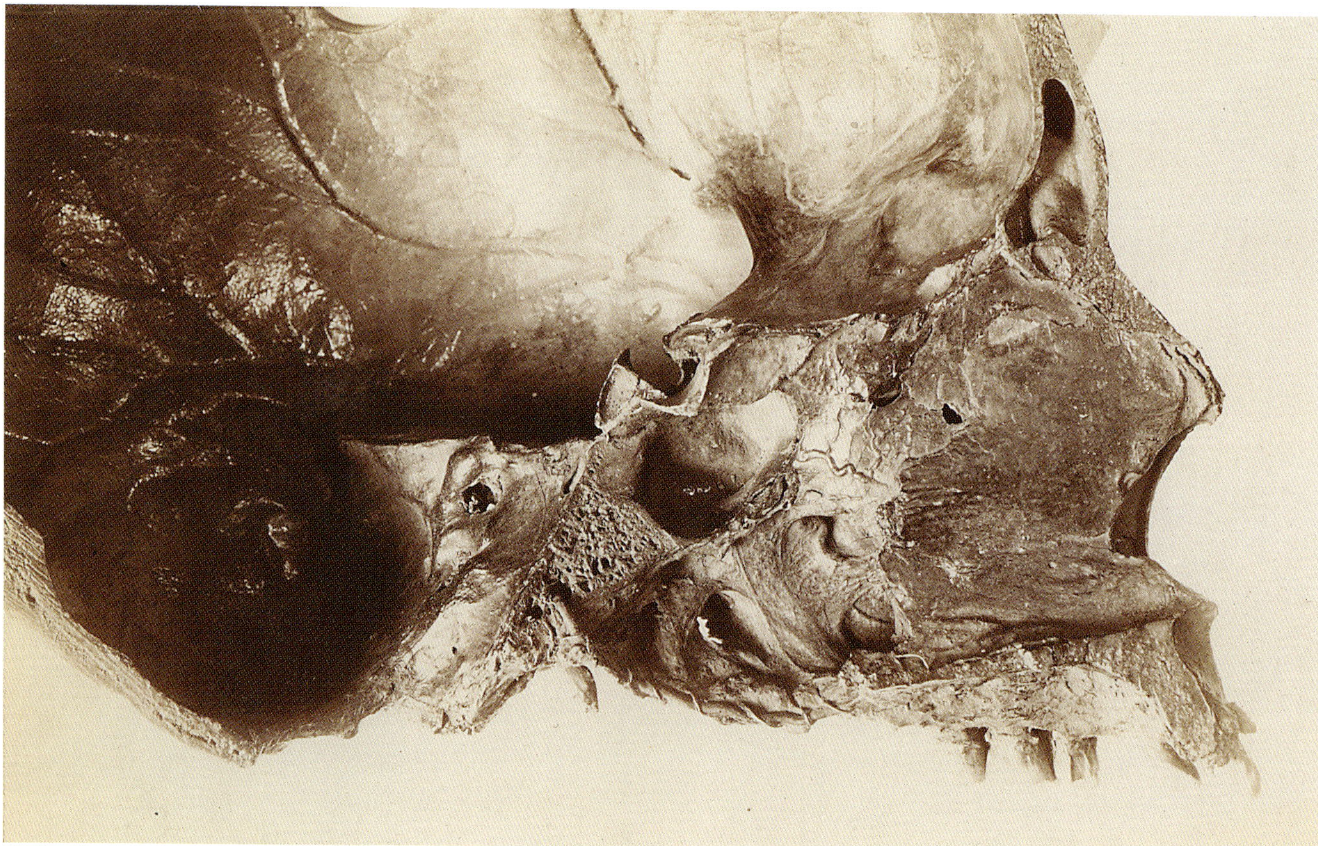

PREFACE

Soon after my first visit in autumn 1986 to the Mütter Museum, Gretchen Worden (1947–2004) and I began to talk about how to introduce the museum's collections to an audience beyond museum visitors. Gretchen, a person of extraordinary intelligence, humor, and dedication, had worked at the Mütter Museum since 1975, becoming its director in 1988. We eventually settled on the publication of a wall calendar, and in 1993 I produced the first of seven calendars for the museum presenting the museum's collection through photographs by contemporary fine-art photographers. Over the years I also curated several exhibitions of Mütter Museum photographs and objects held in galleries and museums in Los Angeles, New Orleans, New York City, and elsewhere. In 2002 I published the first Mütter Museum book, the culmination of the preceding years' work with the museum. Even before that book was completed, Gretchen and I had planned to publish a companion book of historic medical photographs from the museum's archives. Gretchen passed away in August 2004, and in honor of her unflagging devotion to the Mütter Museum I have edited and published the book we envisioned creating together.

One of the last medical museums from the nineteenth century, the Mütter Museum serves not only the medical community but the public at large. From the mid-1980s the annual visitorship to the museum has grown from roughly five thousand to more than sixty thousand.

A detailed history of the Mütter Museum appears in the 2002 book, so I'll include only a brief outline here. The foundation of the Mütter Museum dates to 1856, when Dr. Thomas Dent Mütter (1811–1859) wrote to the College of Physicians of Philadelphia that ill health was forcing him to resign his post as professor of surgery at Jefferson Medical College and that

Human skull, age and identity unknown. Photograph by James F. Wood for Dr. Laurence Turnbull (1821–1900), from the album of photographs by Wood presented to the Mütter Museum in 1898.

he wished to offer the College guardianship of the anatomic and pathological materials he had collected for his own personal "museum." The College, a private medical society of which Mütter was a member, was founded in 1787 and is the oldest private medical society in continuous existence in the United States. The College of Physicians of Philadelphia signed the agreement with Mütter in 1858, and in 1863 the museum moved into its first home (since demolished) at Thirteenth and Locust streets near the center of downtown Philadelphia. In 1910 the museum moved to its present building at 19 South 22nd Street. Since its inception, with 1,344 items from Dr. Mütter joining 92 specimens at the College, the collection has grown to include more than twenty thousand objects, including fluid-preserved anatomical and pathological specimens, air-dried, varnished anatomic specimens, wax and papier-mâché models, oil and watercolor paintings, medical instruments, items of memorabilia of famous scientists and physicians, and medical illustrations. The Mütter Museum's collection also includes an archive of some three thousand historic medical photographs from which I have selected nearly two hundred images, spanning the period between 1852 and the 1940s, for inclusion in this book.

In 1510 Leonardo da Vinci (1452–1519) wrote, "Dispel from your mind the thought that an understanding of the human body in every aspect of its structure can be given in words; for the more thoroughly you describe, the more you will confuse: it is therefore necessary to draw as well as to describe." Yet even in the late 1700s Scottish anatomist John Bell (1763–1820) identified a "continual struggle between the anatomist and the painter, one striving for elegance of form, the other insisting upon accuracy of representation." With the advent of photography, a new method of depiction became possible, and in the mid-1850s photography became a preferred way to illustrate pathological conditions. As Dr. Heimann Wolff Berend (1809–1873) in Berlin noted, photography was better able to achieve accurate representations of patients than drawings. Whereas John Bell was able to make his own illustrations, many physicians lacked that ability and encountered difficulty in training artists to copy from nature rather than idealize what they saw. Thus photography became medicine's ally in the quest for accurate documentation and for comprehension of physiological conditions.

The medical photographs at the Mütter Museum were donated to the museum throughout its long history by College Fellows, physicians, institutions, and by the photographers who made them. The subject matter of the photographs is as broad as medicine itself. Their purpose was to document cases and to disseminate information; occasionally a photograph is inscribed "Compliments" (as on page 31), indicating that the picture was given by one physician to another. A number of the photographs in the collection have appeared from 1892 onward in issues of the *Transactions & Studies of The College of Physicians of Philadelphia*.

I selected many of the photographs for inclusion in this book for their skillful presentation of situations breathtaking and poignant. The artistry of the photographer shines through his documentation of the stark reality of the pathological condition before him, and each resulting photograph far exceeds its fundamental purpose. Curiously, the imprint of a painter's palette adorns photographs by Henry C. Phillips and by Herman H. Henrici as a part of these photographers' signatures (pages 87, 93, and 143), surely an indication that they viewed their work as art.

As do the museum's exhibits, many of these photographs document unusual, sometimes nearly unimaginable, challenges of disorder, disease, and injury. A great many of these photographs are disquieting, yet they are equally moving in their portrayal of how these people endured their fate. A few photographs demonstrate the limited relief that medical science at the time was able to offer and thus show how very far medicine has advanced.

By bringing the museum's historic photography collection to view, this book serves to enrich our experience of the Mütter Museum and its extraordinary collections. Like the museum itself, this book challenges our concepts of humanity, of beauty, of science and art. It presents the stories of those who came before us and shows us what a puzzle life can be.

LAURA LINDGREN

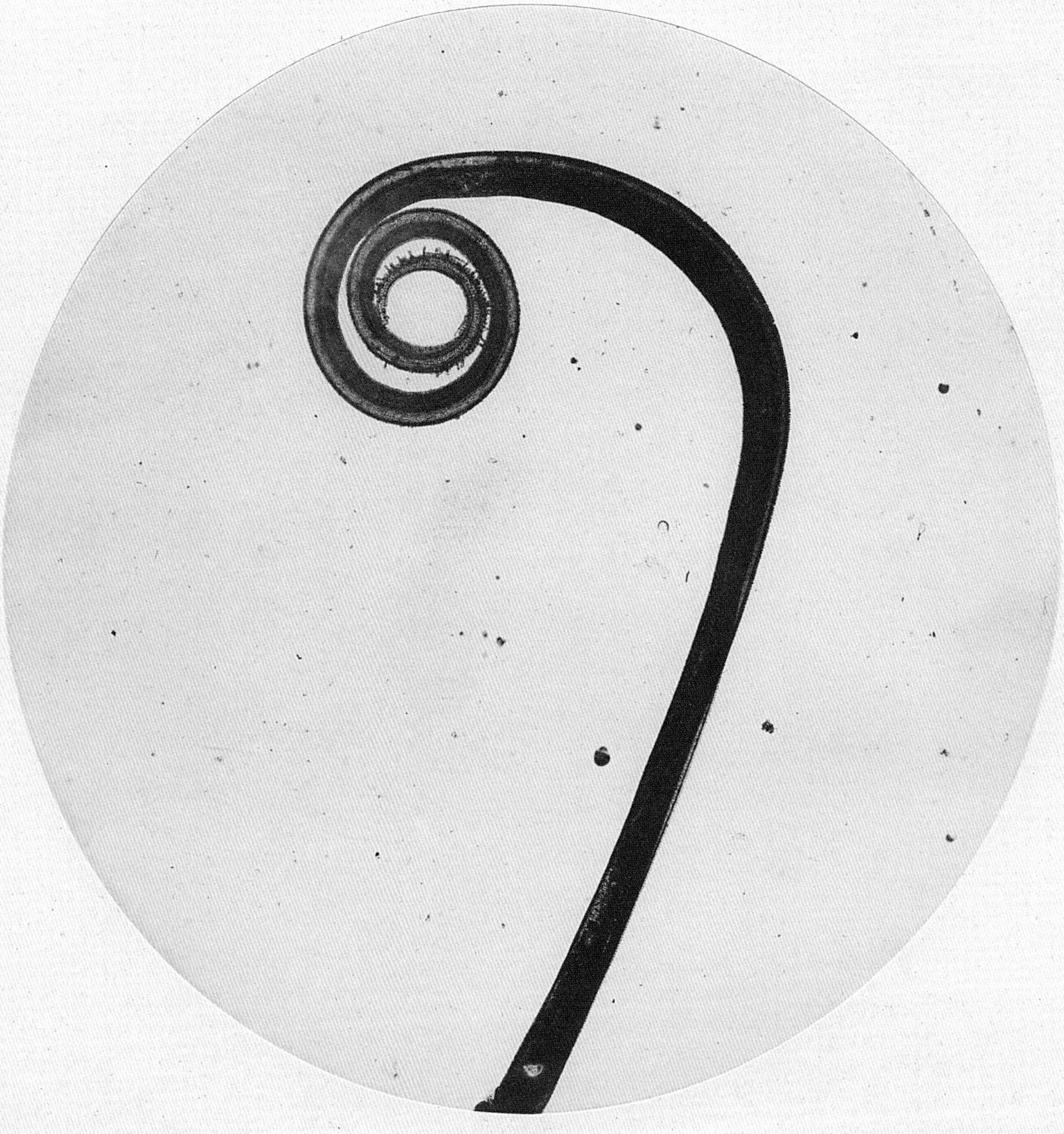

WAR DEPARTMENT,

Surgeon General's Office, Army Medical Museum.

PROBOSCIS OF BUTTERFLY.

Magnified 40 diameters. Objective used, 1½ inch (Wales).

(Negative No. 316. Microscopical Series.)

Photographed by Brevet Major Edward Curtis, Asst. Surg., U. S. A.

By Order of the Surgeon General:

J. J. WOODWARD,

Bvt. Lt. Col. and Asst. Surg., U. S. A.

INTRODUCTION

> In Microscopy, Natural History, Physiological and Pathological research, what an invaluable agent will Photographic art prove . . . for truthfulness is insured. To the physician it offers a means in many cases of conveying to the student an idea of the "Physiognomy of Disease" . . . whilst in the accident ward, or the operating theatre, exact delineation of many a curious and interesting case might, in a few seconds, be added to the records of the hospital, when time and the restlessness of the sufferer would not permit a draftsman to exercise his art.
>
> Samuel Highley, 1853

Medical photography beginning in the early to mid-nineteenth century served as a new form of communication between physicians and their professional colleagues and students to convey facts about patients and disease. But many of the photographs in the collection of the Mütter Museum of the College of Physicians of Philadelphia have an aesthetic value as well.

Some represent the earliest uses of medical photography in documentation and publication and demonstrate a variety of photographic processes, as well as techniques combining the camera with other technologies such as microscopy and radiology. Most of the photographs in the museum's archives were taken in Philadelphia, but others were sent to Philadelphians by their professional colleagues around the world. Philadelphia was a major center of medical education and publishing during the second half of the nineteenth and into the twentieth centuries, and these activities are reflected in the photographic collection at the Mütter Museum.

Proboscis of butterfly, magnified 40 diameters, photographed by Brevet Major Edward Curtis (1838–1912) by order of Surgeon General Joseph Janvier Woodward (1833–1884), for the War Department of the Army Medical Museum, undated.

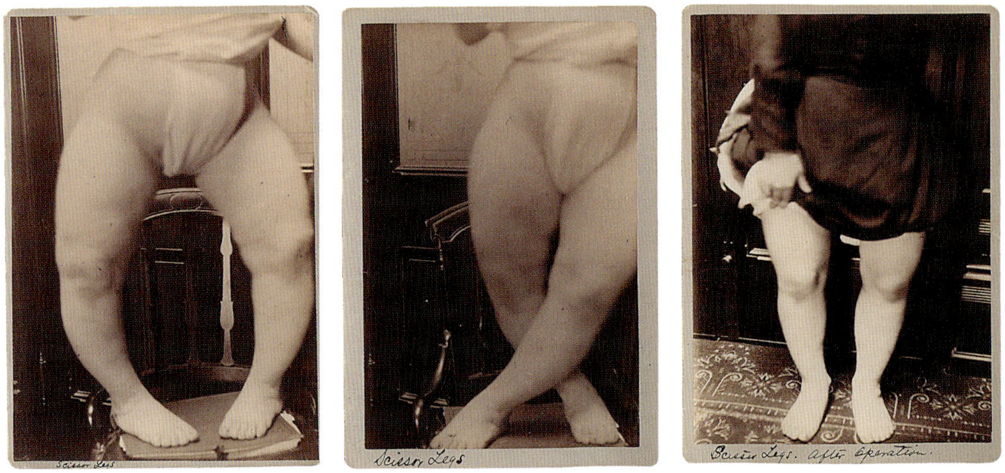

Scissor legs (spastic diplegia), before and after corrective surgery. Photographed for Dr. DeForest Willard (1846–1910). Photographer and date unidentified.

The usefulness of photography as a visual document was exploited in almost every area of medical science, but certain applications were discovered to be particularly appropriate. Heimann Wolff Berend (1809–1873), an orthopedic surgeon in Berlin, is credited with being the first to present pre- and postoperative views of patients (1853). The original Berend collection numbered more than a thousand photographs; long thought to be lost, more than a hundred from the collection were located in 2001 in the Wellcome Library in London. Plastic surgical procedures were also among the earliest medical images, which is hardly surprising, since appearance is a major element in judging the success of both types of operations.

Dermatologists also found photography invaluable in showing the superficial lesions that characterize their specialty. They provided much of the impetus for improving the technology of color reproduction, since that was so essential to the correct identification of skin diseases.

Enormous tumors and congenital abnormalities were perpetually popular subjects for the camera, especially the remarkable examples found in places such as China, which had only recently been exposed to Western medicine. These photographs demonstrate the transition of the images from objects of amazement to records of progress in surgical technique.

Photographic Methods

Before the dry plate process was perfected in 1878, the photographer using the wet plate technique had to use large, heavy cameras on tripods and have an elaborate setup to prepare and

OPPOSITE: Successful excision at hip joint for gunshot wound, performed thirty-seven days after injury. Charles B. Scott, seaman of the U.S. Navy, age thirty-four, wounded by a rifle ball in an attack on a piratical vessel in Teacapan River, Mexico, June 17, 1870. On July 25 Scott was chloroformed and Surgeon W. E. Taylor sawed off the fractured bone and removed fragments, resulting in the limb being about three and a half inches shorter than its fellow. On September 7 patient was able to sit up and, with assistance, to walk with crutches on September 18. On January 20 a prosthetic apparatus was adjusted. Photographed at the Army Medical Museum under the supervision of Assistant Surgeon George A. Otis (1830–1881), undated.

develop his plates while they were still wet, usually within fifteen minutes of their exposure. This limited the photographer's mobility, thus it was easier for the physician to take his patient, if ambulatory, to the photographer's studio. The dry plate process, which allowed plates to be made ahead of time and stored, opened up the field to amateur photographers who could now have their plates developed by others. George Eastman's introduction of the Kodak camera in 1888 further popularized photography and made it even easier to take pictures in the hospital ward, doctor's office, or patient's home. Hospitals began routinely taking admission or preoperative shots, either in an area set aside for photography or in the wards with makeshift backdrops.

Clinical Photographic Conventions

From the 1840s to the 1890s most clinical photographs looked like traditional portraiture, with patients dressed in regular clothing, showing either the head, bust, or full body. The similarity to portraiture was heightened by the fact that many of these photographs were taken in professional photographic studios, using the same props and backgrounds as in formal portraits.

Many of the patients in these photographs display an unself-consciousness often found in those accustomed to being the objects of medical interest. This was fortunate, since the physician was primarily concerned with making sure that the pathology was clearly visible and would undrape the patient to whatever extent was necessary. However, there was a definite tendency, especially noticeable in the photographs taken of officers and enlisted soldiers during the Civil War, to allow more modesty in those of higher social rank. Sometimes, though, the privates were allowed to cover up their privates, be it only with a leaf from the paulownia tree outside.

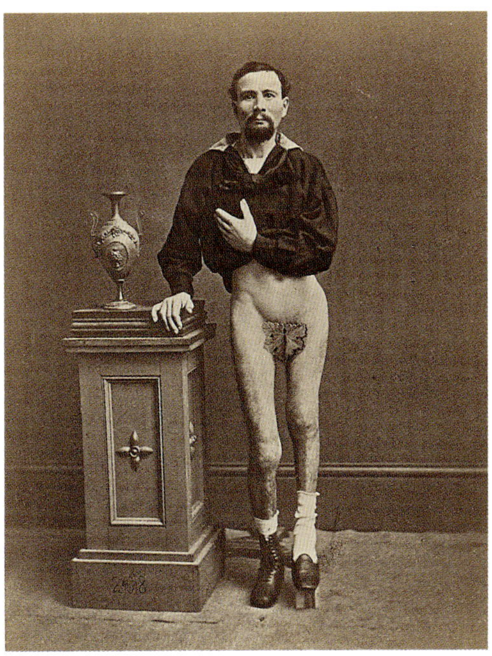

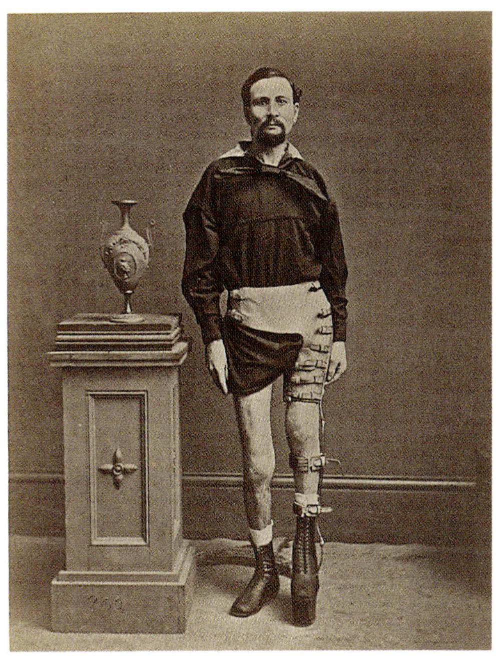

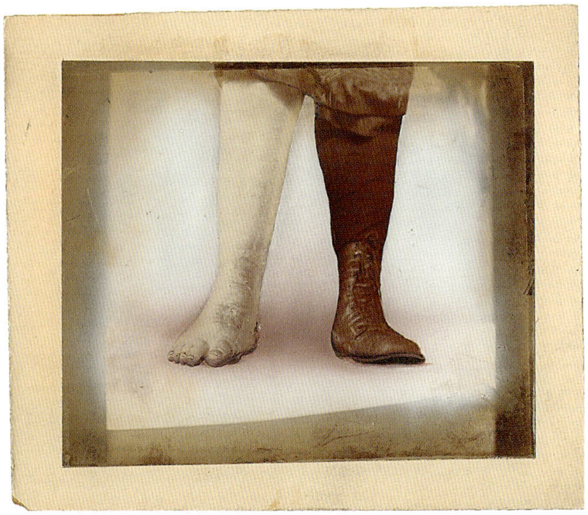

Mary Murphy, age twenty, after transplant of extensor hallucis longus to tuberosity of fifth metatarsal for infant palsy. Equino varus. Case of Dr. Astley Paston Cooper Ashhurst (1876–1932), photographer unidentified, 1906.

By the 1890s, with the influence of the pathology laboratory changing the perception of the patient from an individual to a disease entity, certain conventions were established, which included making the patients anonymous by blacking out their eyes, photographing them naked against plain backgrounds, and eliminating irrelevant parts of the body from the print.

As the physician's knowledge of disease progressed from the gross pathological to the cellular level toward the end of the nineteenth century, the camera likewise began focusing on the affected part rather than on the individual bearing it.

In some cases, the individuals associated with a patient are as interesting as the condition being represented, as in the case of Theodore Scrivener, a boy afflicted with precocious sexual development (page 77).

Eventually the patient was reduced to the image of a histological slide or X-ray, and, with the modern concept of molecular biology, illustrative material in many slide lectures consists of only text and graphs.

Photomicrography

From the very beginning, the camera was combined with other technologies to record images never before seen by the naked eye. The first medical photographs of any kind were microscopic daguerreotypes made by Alfred Donné, M.D., of Paris in 1839. However, no major advances in the technique were made until Joseph Janvier Woodward, a Philadelphia-trained physician and assistant surgeon and brevet major, U.S.A., began his work at the Army Medical Museum in preparing the medical history of the Civil War.

Woodward's microscopical studies grew out of an attempt to investigate the nature and causes of camp diseases. He regarded photographic reproduction as the best means of making the study results more widely available to the medical profession. Acting on practical suggestions from another photomicrographic experimenter, Mr. Lewis Rutherfurd of New York, Woodward and Assistant Surgeon Edward Curtis produced an outstanding series of photomicrographs.

Unlike earlier researchers, Woodward did not connect the microscope to a camera but found a dark room most convenient. Sunlight admitted through a small hole in the shuttered window was directed through the microscope and specimen slide and focused on the photosensitive plate. The dimness of the room required the photographer to time the exposure with a metronome set to strike at second intervals.

The seven-inch-square glass negatives produced by the wet collodion process were printed as glass positives for a study collection, but producing publishable illustrations directly from the photographs was a problem until the introduction of photomechanical printing processes in the 1870s. For illustrations published during the 1860s, Woodward relied on the skill of Philadelphia engraver Hermann Faber, who also made many of the illustrations for the *Medical and Surgical History of the War of the Rebellion* (see page 23). Beginning in 1870, Woodward issued a number of reports of his photomicrographic experiments illustrated with albumen prints, and a special edition of his work was prepared for the 1876 Centennial Exposition in Philadelphia.

In addition to his innovative work in photomicrography, Woodward made a major contribution to pathology in 1864 as the first American to use aniline dyes in staining tissues for microscopical research. In 1865 he and Edward Curtis collaborated in another historical event—the autopsy of President Abraham Lincoln.

In November 1869 Woodward began experimenting with artificial light sources in an attempt to overcome the limitations imposed by unreliable weather conditions (he attributed the Europeans' lack of progress in photomicrography to their even more variable weather). Woodward concluded that artificial light produced successful photomicrographs at higher powers, and that the electric light was superior to all other sources.

Though his experiments with artificial light were successful, Woodward wrote "so many cloudless days are offered to the photographer in Washington that I could not but regret their results." He found that by passing the sun's rays through an achromatic condensing glass instead of the piece of ground glass generally used, he could get rid of the diffraction and interference phenomena, reduce exposure time, and produce pictures with greater sharpness and definition. He reported to the surgeon general in 1871 that with this improved method he "arrived at results which must materially modify the conclusions of my former reports."

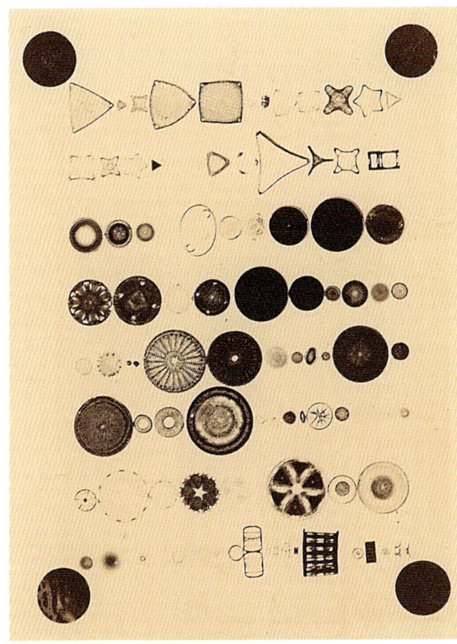

Albumen photograph, the sixth square of a Möller's type-plate of the diatomaceæ, taken by electric light, by Brevet Lieutenant Colonel Joseph Janvier Woodward for the War Department of the Army Medical Museum, ca. 1865–70.

X-rays

Photography was directly linked to the discovery of X-rays. In 1879 British chemist Sir William Crookes unwittingly produced the rays when the vacuum of the glass tubes with which he was experimenting was high enough to give off a pale green fluorescence. He often found that photographic plates stored near his worktable were fogged (obviously these were dry plates). He complained to the manufacturer and returned the defective plates. Arthur W. Goodspeed at the University of Pennsylvania produced the first American X-ray picture in 1890 (again without understanding its significance) when he observed that the image of a colleague's Woodland Avenue trolley fare, left on top of an unexposed photo-sensitive plate during an experiment with an electrified vacuum tube, was unmistakably preserved as a number of dark, round images.

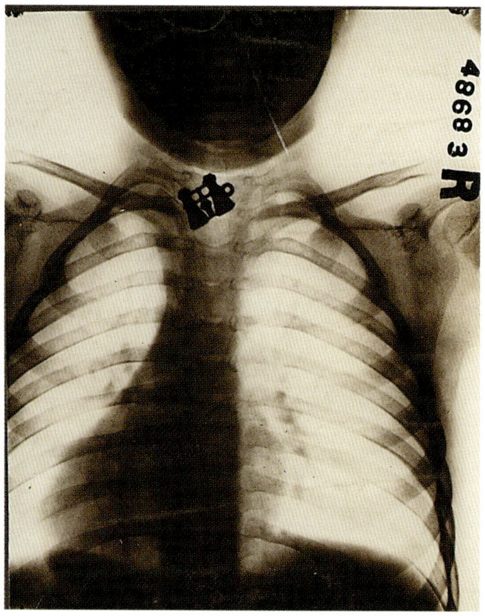

Pair of toy opera glasses in esophagus. E. Richmond Steel, age four. Radiograph by Dr. Willis F. Manges (1876–1936), July 30, 1921, from the Dr. Chevalier Jackson (1865–1958) collection of foreign bodies removed from the throats and airways of patients by pioneer bronchoesophagologist Jackson and his colleagues.

However, Wilhelm Conrad Roentgen of Germany is rightly credited with the discovery, since he recognized the nature of the rays and published the fact in November 1895. The new science of radiology also paralleled photography in the speed with which it was adopted around the world. The first American reports of successful X-ray photographs were published within two months of Roentgen's announcement.

One of Roentgen's first images, the bones of his wife's hand with her rings, pointed the way to the use of X-ray photographs (or skiagraphs, as they were often called at first, from the Greek) in diagnosing skeletal problems and locating metallic objects hidden from view beneath the skin, information of great practical use to the surgeon.

Clinical Photographic Publications

It was commonplace during the nineteenth century to bring patients before medical students or professional societies for a discussion of their cases. Gradually the photographic print or lantern slide took the place of the actual patient. Because they could be published or sent through the mails, photographs permitted the dissemination of clinical information without limitations of time or space, thus serving the purposes of both education and consultation.

Photographic Review of Medicine and Surgery

One of the most remarkable publications of the period was the *Photographic Review of Medicine and Surgery*, a bimonthly illustrated periodical of interesting cases, accompanied by notes, edited by Francis Fontaine Maury, M.D. (1840–1879), and Louis A. Duhring, M.D. (1845–1913), of which only two volumes were published, by J. B. Lippincott & Co. in Philadelphia, 1870–72. The editors were both Philadelphians: Duhring was a dermatologist and Maury was a surgeon.

In the preface to volume one, Maury and Duhring state:

> The object of the publication has been to bring together some of the rare and interesting examples of disease occurring in our country, with a view of ultimately forming a valuable collection of photographs and records. The superiority of photography to other means for the portrayal of morbid structure is too well known to require any comment; while for the success which our undertaking has attained, the present volume must answer for itself.
>
> It has been our aim to select the most striking and remarkable from the cases offered, especially those whose interesting points would admit of clear representation.

Publication of this journal was suspended after two years and forty-eight albumen prints, but the cases illustrated were such classic or extreme examples that the photographs were reproduced for many years in textbooks and articles.

The Army Medical Museum Photographic Series

In 1862, the surgeon general of the U.S. Army, William A. Hammond, made two decisions that created a continuing medical and photographic legacy of the Civil War. He announced his intention to publish a medical and surgical history of the Civil War so that the vast amount of information on surgical techniques and medical treatment provided by the experiences of army medical officers could be used to improve future military and civilian medical practice. He also established the Army Medical Museum to collect specimens of war wounds and camp diseases for the immediate purpose of providing study material to the inexperienced surgeons being confronted with unprecedented numbers of sick and wounded.

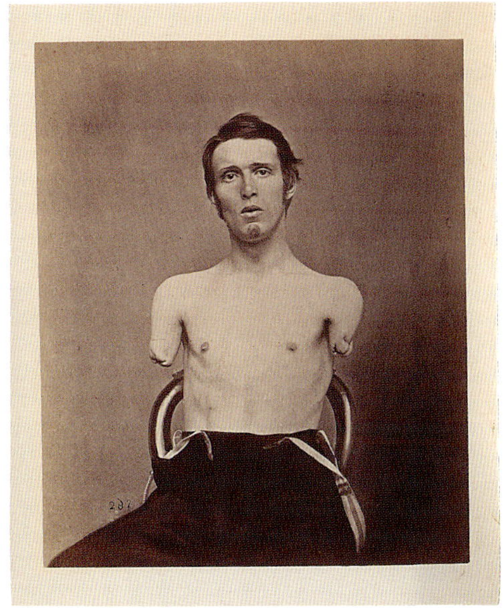

Double amputation of the arms at the upper thirds. Private A. Stratton, Co. G. 147th New York, had both arms carried away by a solid cannon shot on June 18, 1864. Cordials were given and immediate amputation performed by Surgeon A. S. Coe. Stratton was subsequently supplied with artificial arms of Grinnell's make. Photographed at the Army Medical Museum December 24, 1869, by order of Surgeon General George A. Otis.

For the photographic series Hammond assigned the medical portion of the history to Joseph Janvier Woodward, M.D. The surgical portion was committed to fellow Philadelphian John Hill Brinton, M.D., also named as curator of the museum. He was succeeded by George A. Otis, M.D., in 1864.

Photography played a major role in recording and disseminating the information provided by the specimens and written reports sent to the museum by medical officers. In 1864 a photograph gallery was established, and photographs of museum specimens and surgical cases with their histories were sent out to medical directors for the instruction of the physicians serving under them. They were also used by artists to engrave illustrations for various catalogues of the museum and other publications issued by the surgeon general's office.

Photography at the museum continued after the war and included records of interesting civilian cases. William Bell of Philadelphia was the chief photographer at the museum from 1865 to 1869, taking pictures of the many soldiers coming to Washington to visit the pension offices for their disability claims. These postwar follow-up pictures were an excellent source of information about the long-term results of various medical and surgical treatments.

Each of the eight volumes published between 1867 and 1882 as *Photographs of Surgical Cases and Specimens* had fifty albumen prints made from 10 x 12" negatives, mounted on 12 x 14" cards with histories printed on the back. Volume six was ready for the 1876 Centennial International Exposition in Philadelphia. In the form of engravings, these photographs served to illustrate the six-volume *Medical and Surgical History of the War of the Rebellion*, printed between 1870 and 1888.

According to Otis's introduction to the *Medical and Surgical History*, Surgery Volume, Part I, 1870, "Sets of these volumes have been distributed to the principal medical colleges and learned societies of the country." The College of Physicians of Philadelphia received the first four volumes in 1869, sent by Otis at the request of the surgeon general.

The Army Medical Museum developed into the Armed Forces Institute of Pathology, a major referral center for pathologic diagnosis worldwide. The museum collections, located within the AFIP and now called the National Museum of Health and Medicine, continue to play an important educational role in contemporary and historical medicine.

. . .

In the majority of the historic photographs in the collection of the Mütter Museum of the College of Physicians of Philadelphia, the health professional is an implied but rarely glimpsed presence. The overwhelming impression left on the viewer is that of an emotional empathy with these people of a century past. As no graphic illustration could, the camera confronts us with the fact that these are human beings living with the horrendous ravages of injury, disfiguring and deadly disease, or congenital deformities, in most cases without the hope of cure or alleviation offered by modern medicine. One is grateful for the few before-and-after images, knowing that for those individuals, at least, something was done to help.

Gretchen Worden (1947–2004)

Trauma

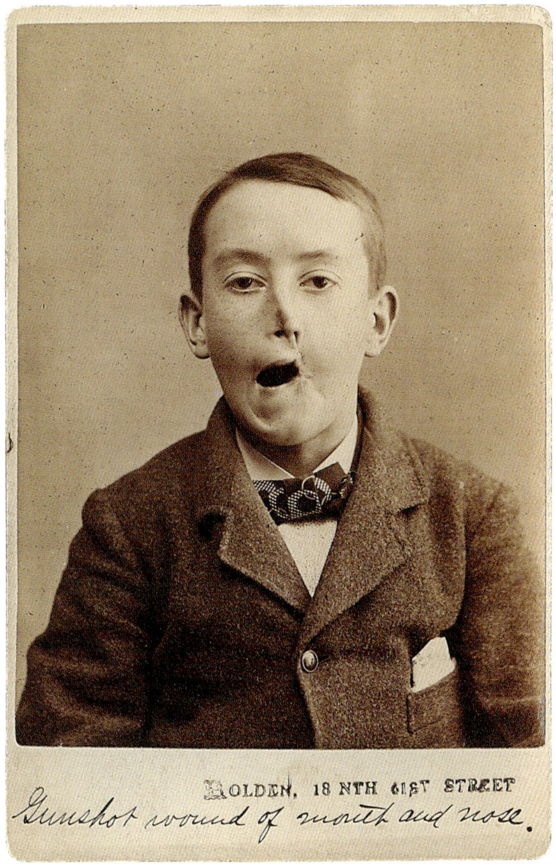

Gunshot wound of mouth and nose. Photographed by Alfred Holden for Dr. DeForest Willard (1846–1910), undated, ca. 1895–1900.

Recovery after excision of humerus for gunshot injury. Private James P. Kegerreis, wounded at age nineteen at the battle at Petersburg, Virginia, June 17, 1864, by a conoidal ball that entered three-fourths of an inch below the thyroid cartilage just to the left of the trachea, passed a little downward and to the right under the jugular vein, carrying away one of the wings of the trachea, and emerging half an inch above the clavicle, three inches from point of entrance, was deflected in its course by hitting the butt of the musket, and again entered in front of the right clavicle two inches from the acromial end, passing through the surgical neck of the humerus, and emerging near the center of the deltoid muscle. He was taken to the field hospital and marked for an amputation on the following day, but tearing off the label, he crawled away among the "slightly wounded." Over the next several months a number of spiculæ of bone were removed. In December 1867 a sequestrum six inches long was removed; his wounds healed and never reopened. Employed in 1870 as a clerk in the Pension Office, Kegerreis was reported to be able to lift about 135 pounds with the injured limb. Photographed at the Army Medical Museum by order of Surgeon General George A. Otis, undated.

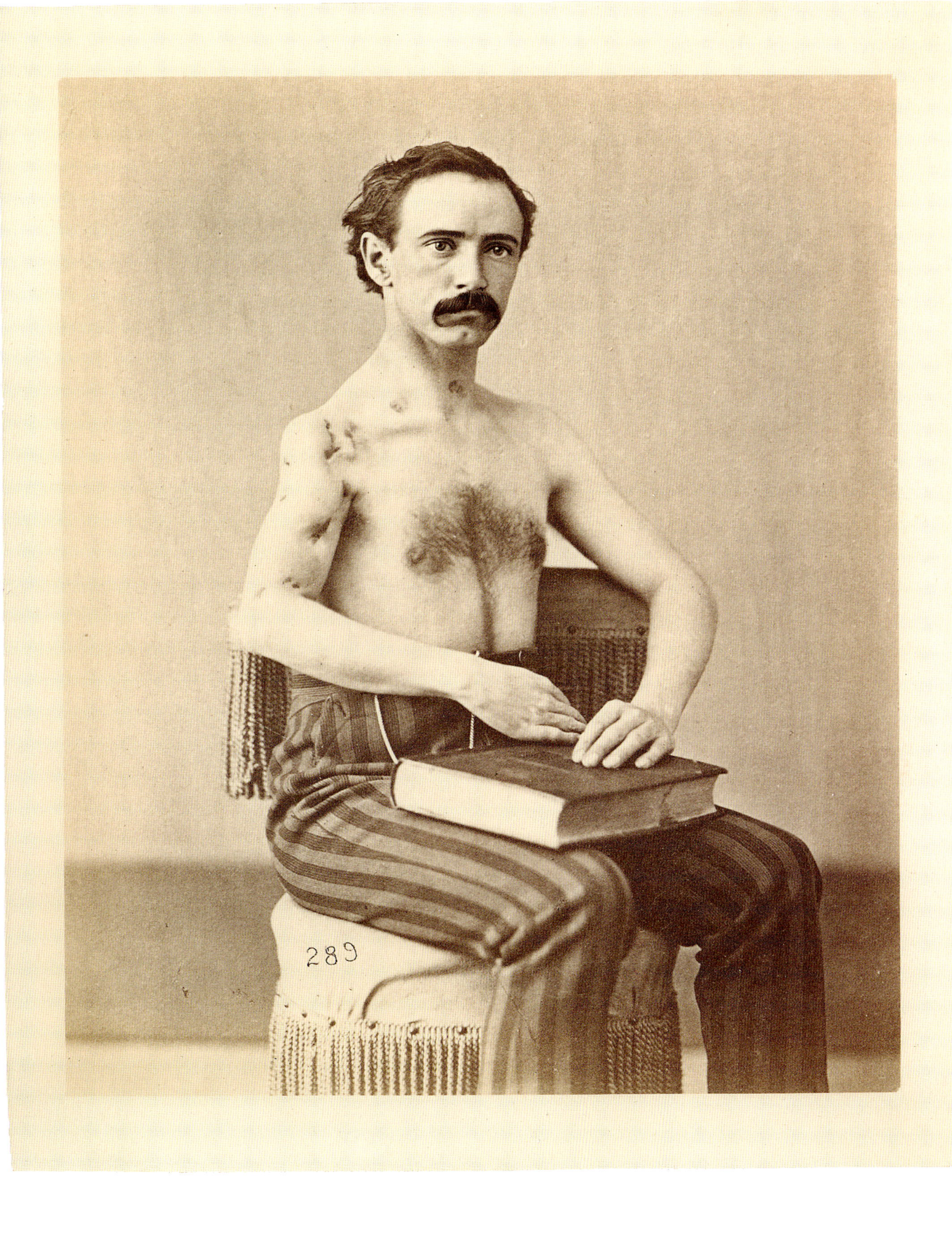
289

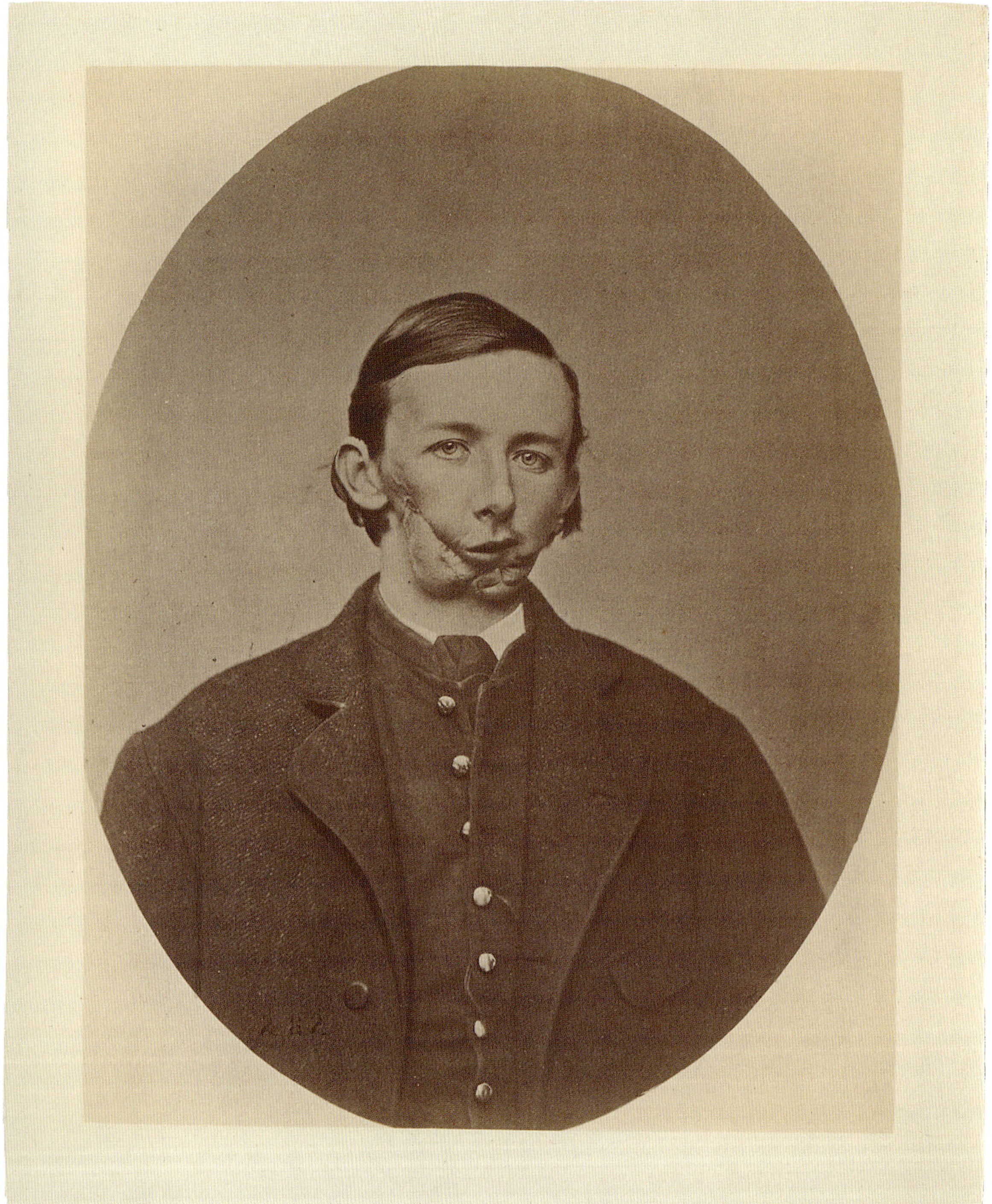

Result of a plastic operation for relief of a deformity caused by a gunshot wound of the face. Elbert Hewitt, a private of Co. C, 6th Vermont Volunteers, was wounded at age twenty-one on September 19, 1864, at Winchester, Virginia, when a fragment of shell carried away a large portion of the superior and inferior maxillæ. Surgery was performed on February 28, 1865, by Dr. Gordon Buck (1807–1877). Previous to the operation the mouth could be neither freely opened nor entirely closed. The right half of the lower lip and the symmetry of the lips have been in a great measure restored, though the mouth is much drawn to the right side. Photographed at the Army Medical Museum by order of Surgeon General George A. Otis, undated.

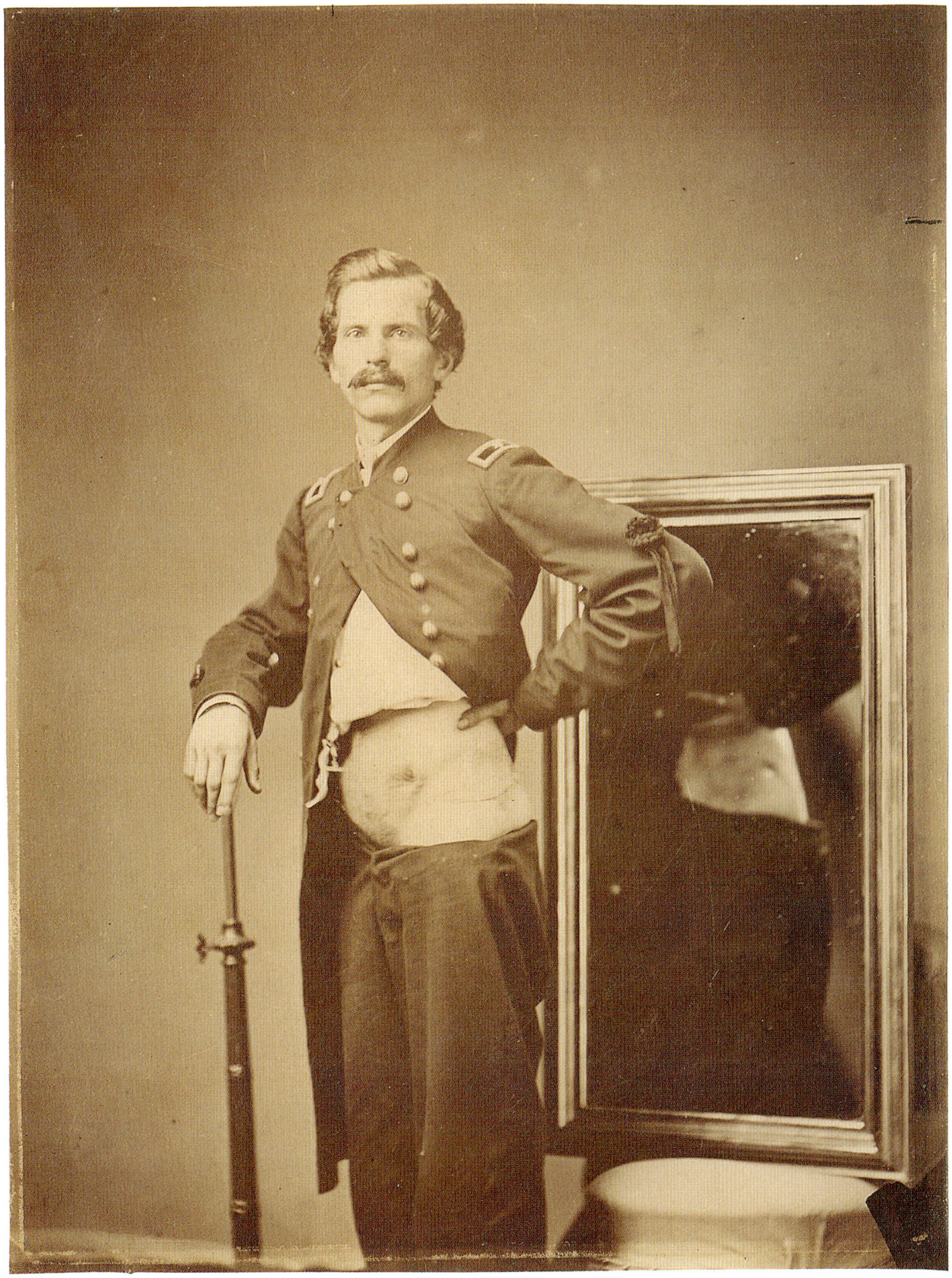

Abdominal wound, Civil War. Mirrors were sometimes used to provide a rear view of a patient's wound or disorder. Probably taken by Surgeon General George A. Otis, ca. 1875.

Stab wound of Tom Barry at thorax and abdomen, nineteen inches in length. Complete sections of fourth, fifth, sixth, seventh, eighth, and ninth cartilages and intestinal evisceration. Recovery complete. Patient of Augustus Van Liew Brokaw, M.D., St. Louis, Missouri (1863–1907). Photographer and date unidentified. Donor: Dr. Joseph Price (1853–1911).

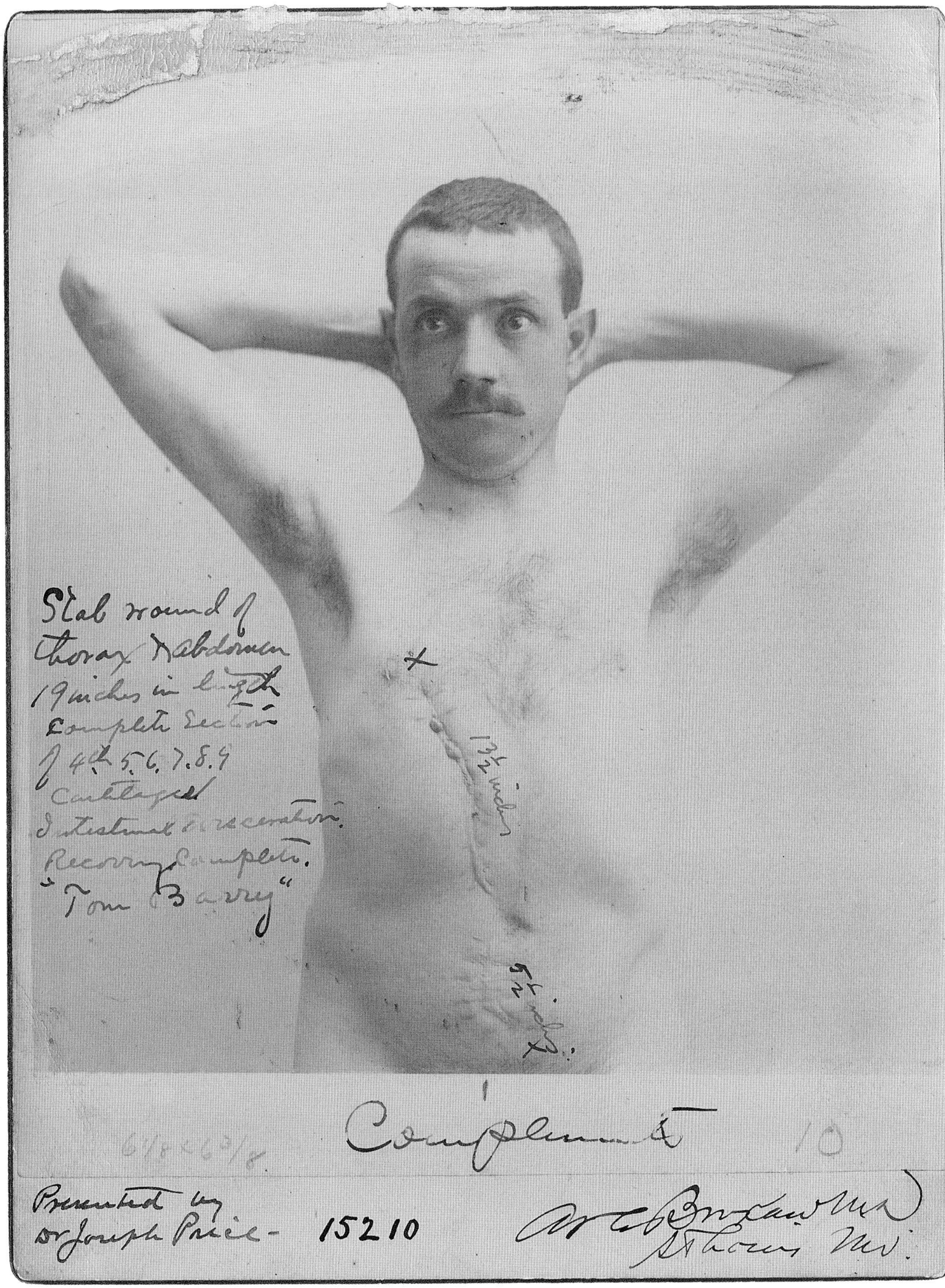
Stab wound of
thorax & abdomen
19 inches in length
Complete section
of 4th. 5. 6. 7. 8. 9
cartilages
Intestinal evisceration.
Recovery complete.
"Tom Barry"
13½ inches
5½ inches
Compliments
10
Presented by
Dr Joseph Price -
15210
St Louis Mo.

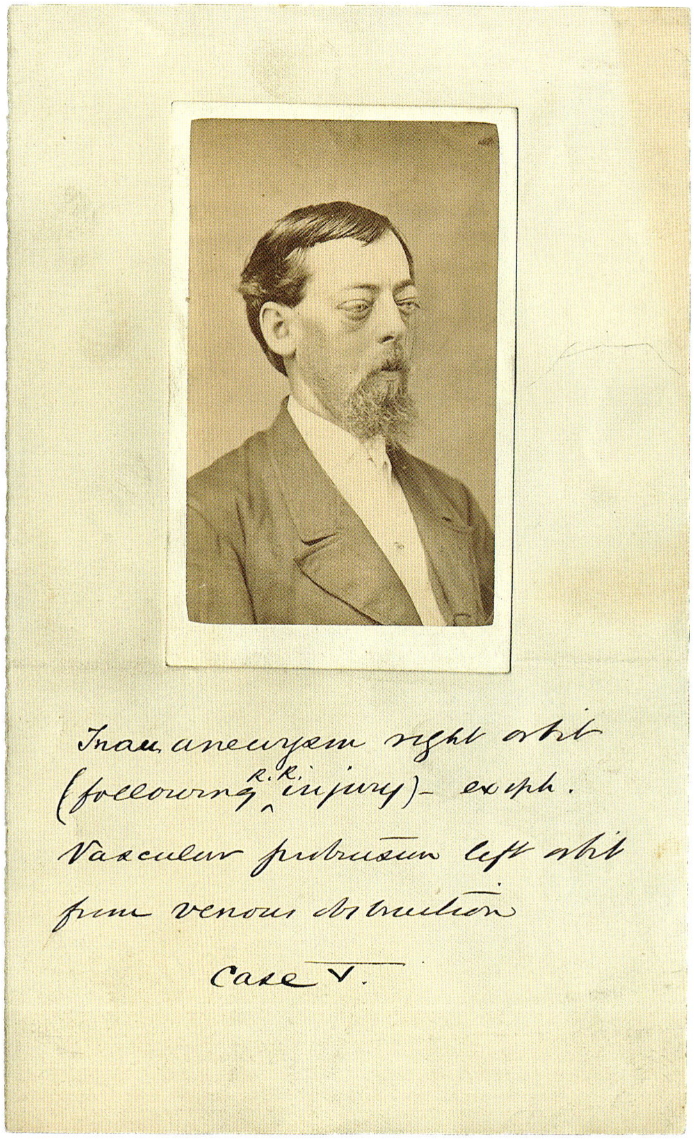

Traumatic aneurysm, right orbit, following railroad injury; vascular protrusion of the left orbit from venous obstruction. Photographer and date unidentified.

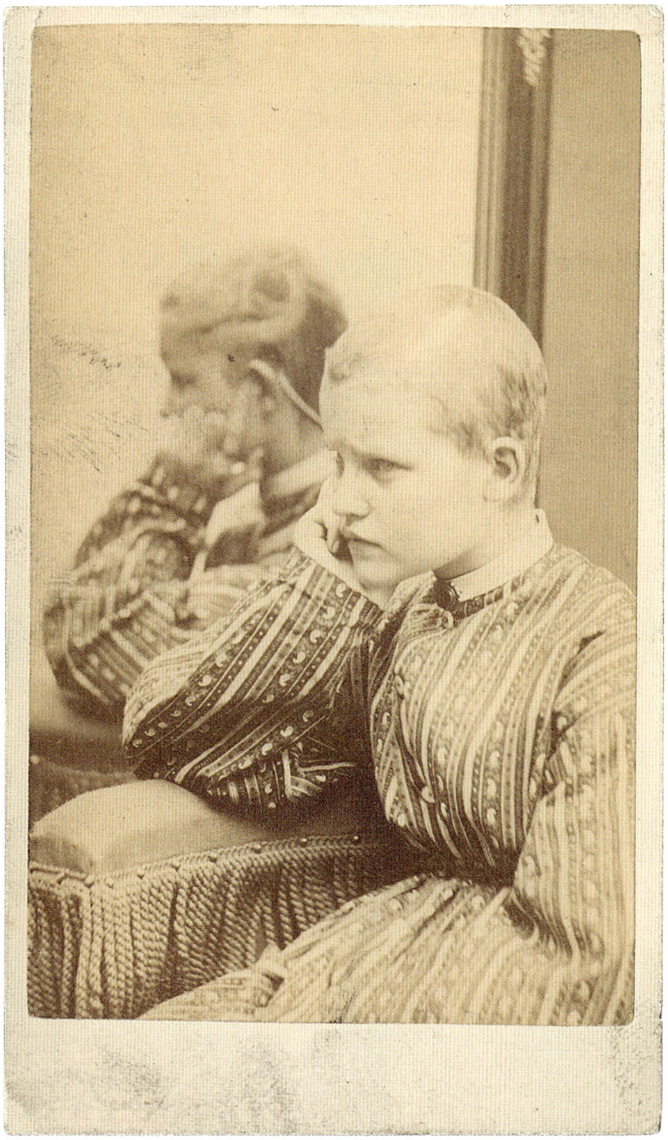

Head injury. Linear extent of wound fourteen inches; undivided base of flap four inches. Photograph by William H. Rhoads, Philadelphia, ca. 1866–98.

Rupture of the heart from fall on bicycle handlebar. On September 19, 1898, F. M., age twenty-eight, was thrown from his bicycle when he collided with a hydrant hose lying across the road as it filled a water car. The post of the handlebar struck his chest with great force, and he died of cardiac rupture an hour and a half after the fall. Rupture of the heart from contusion without penetration of the chest wall is a rare accident. Case of Richard Cole Newton, M.D. (1851–1919), reported in *Transactions of American Climatological Association*, 1899. Photograph by Dr. Henry Power, 1898. Donor: Dr. Guy Hinsdale (1858–1948).

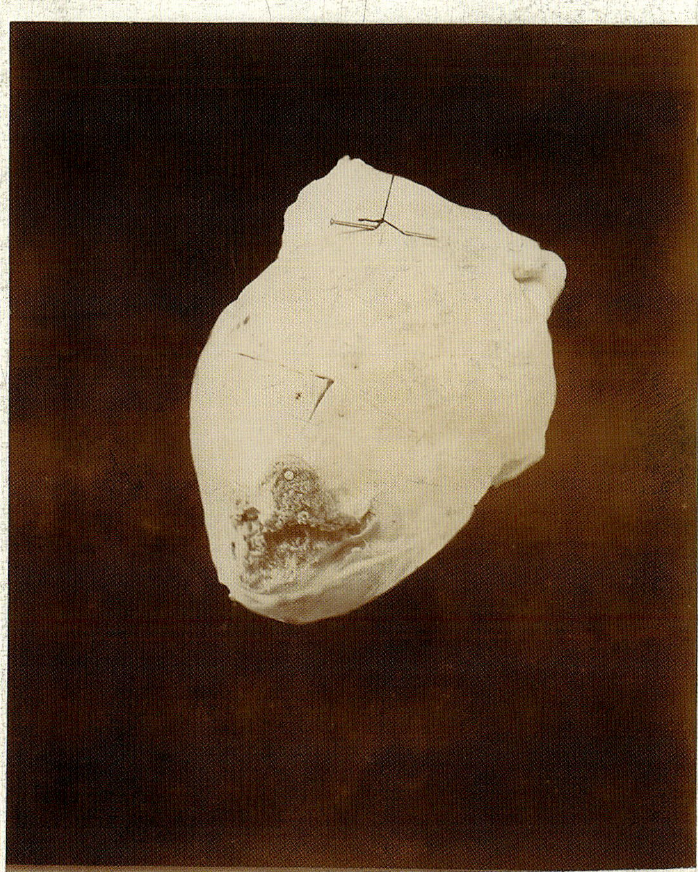

Rupture of the Heart from fall on bicycle Handle-bar.

15701

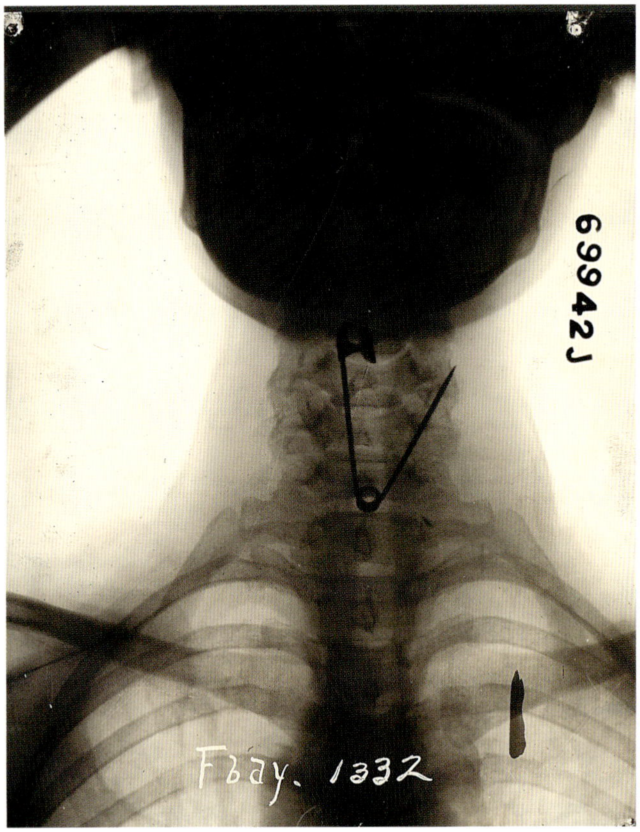

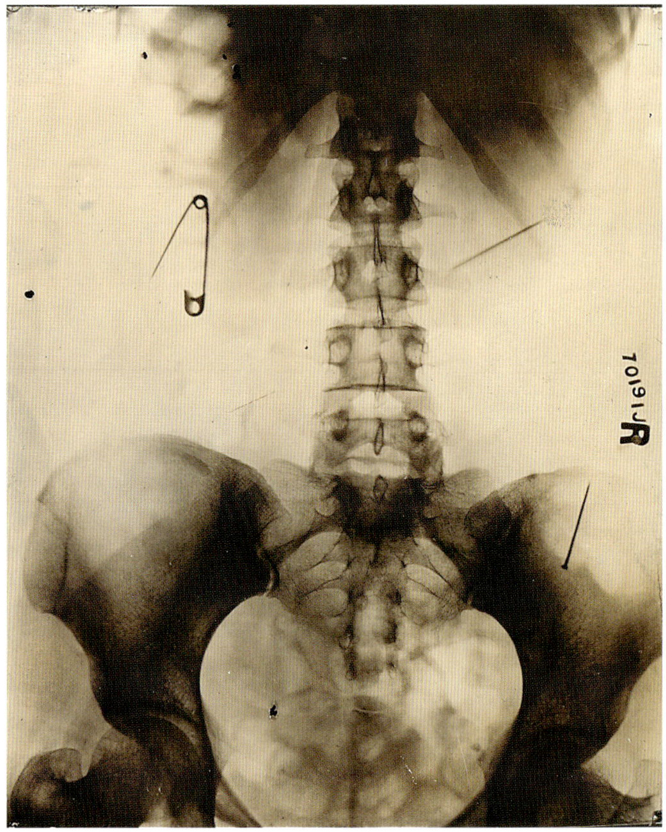

ABOVE AND OPPOSITE: Skiagraphs (radiographs) from the Dr. Chevalier Jackson (1865–1958) collection of foreign bodies removed from the throats and airways of patients by pioneer bronchoesophagologist Jackson and his colleagues. Dr. Jackson presented his collection of swallowed objects to the Mütter Museum in 1924.

ABOVE, LEFT AND RIGHT: Open safety pin in esophagus and multiple foreign bodies in alimentary tract. Mrs. B. Lightfoot, age thirty-six. Radiograph by Dr. Willis F. Manges (1876–1936), June 13, 1924.

OPPOSITE: Toy dog in esophagus. Anna Zurawinski, age three. Radiograph by Dr. Willis F. Manges, February 28, 1919.

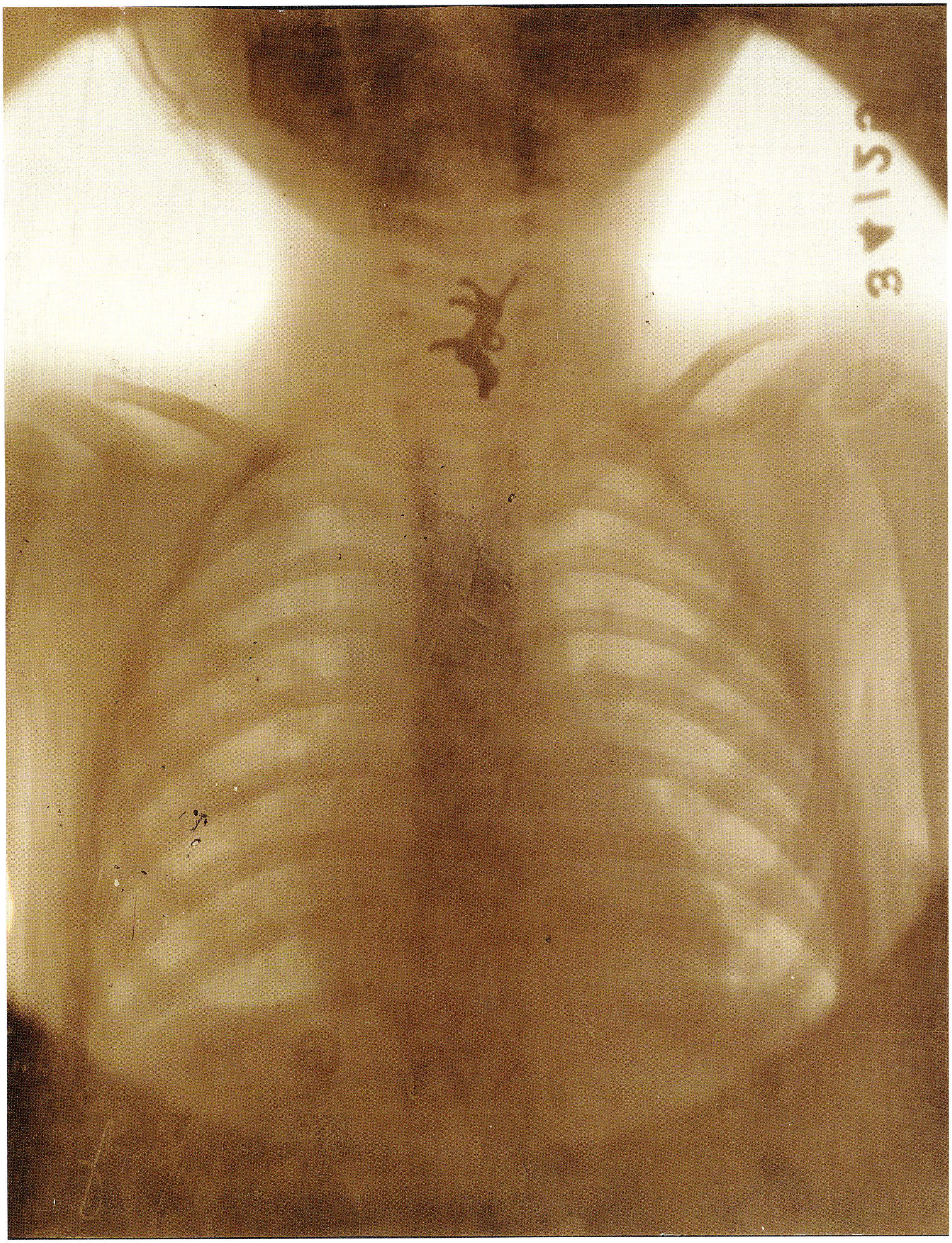

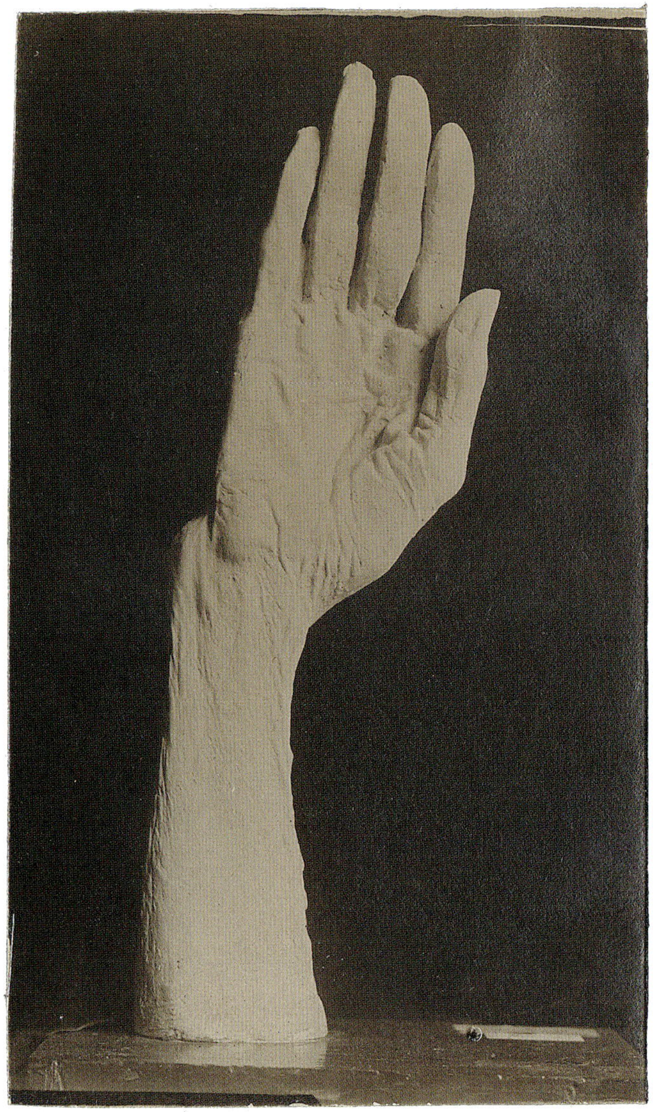

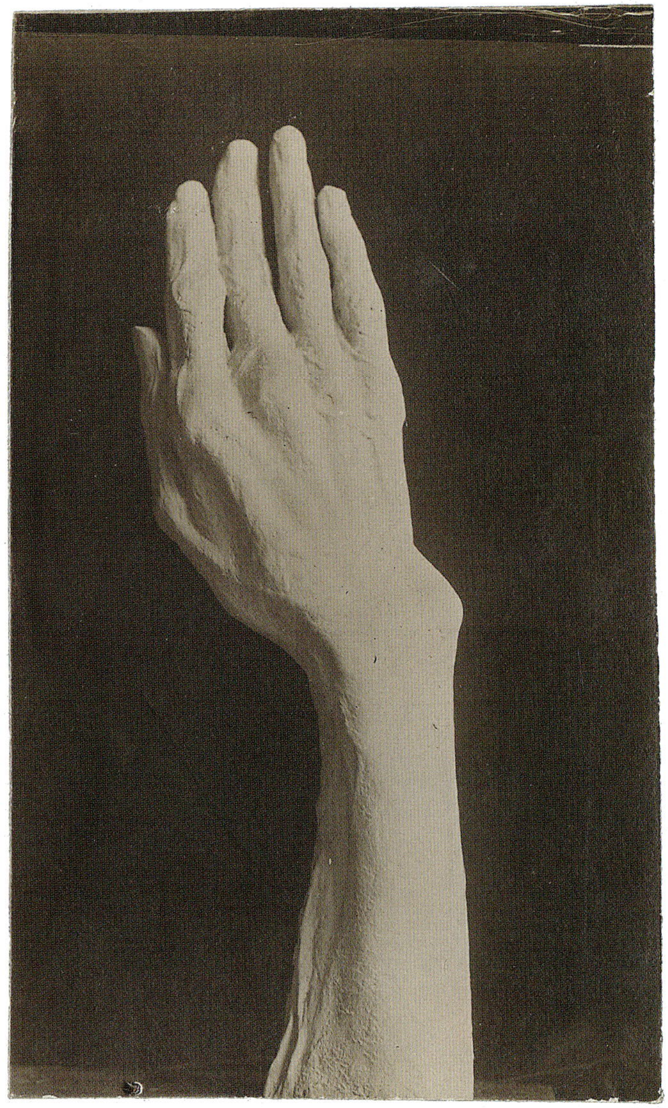

ABOVE: Two views of a fractured lower end of radius with forward displacement. Photograph of specimen in the Museum of the Royal College of Surgeons, Edinburgh, Scotland. *Transactions of American Surgical Association*, 1896. Received from J. Alfred Scott, April 6, 1896. Donor: Dr. John B. Roberts (1852–1924), 1901.

OPPOSITE: Skiagraph of old fracture of lower end of radius with forward displacement ("Smith's Fracture"). Woman forty-six years. About one year after injury. Patient of Dr. George Thomas Beatson (1848–1933) of Glasgow, Scotland, who saw woman first one year after fall. Cast accompanies skiagraph. Donor: Dr. John B. Roberts, 1901.

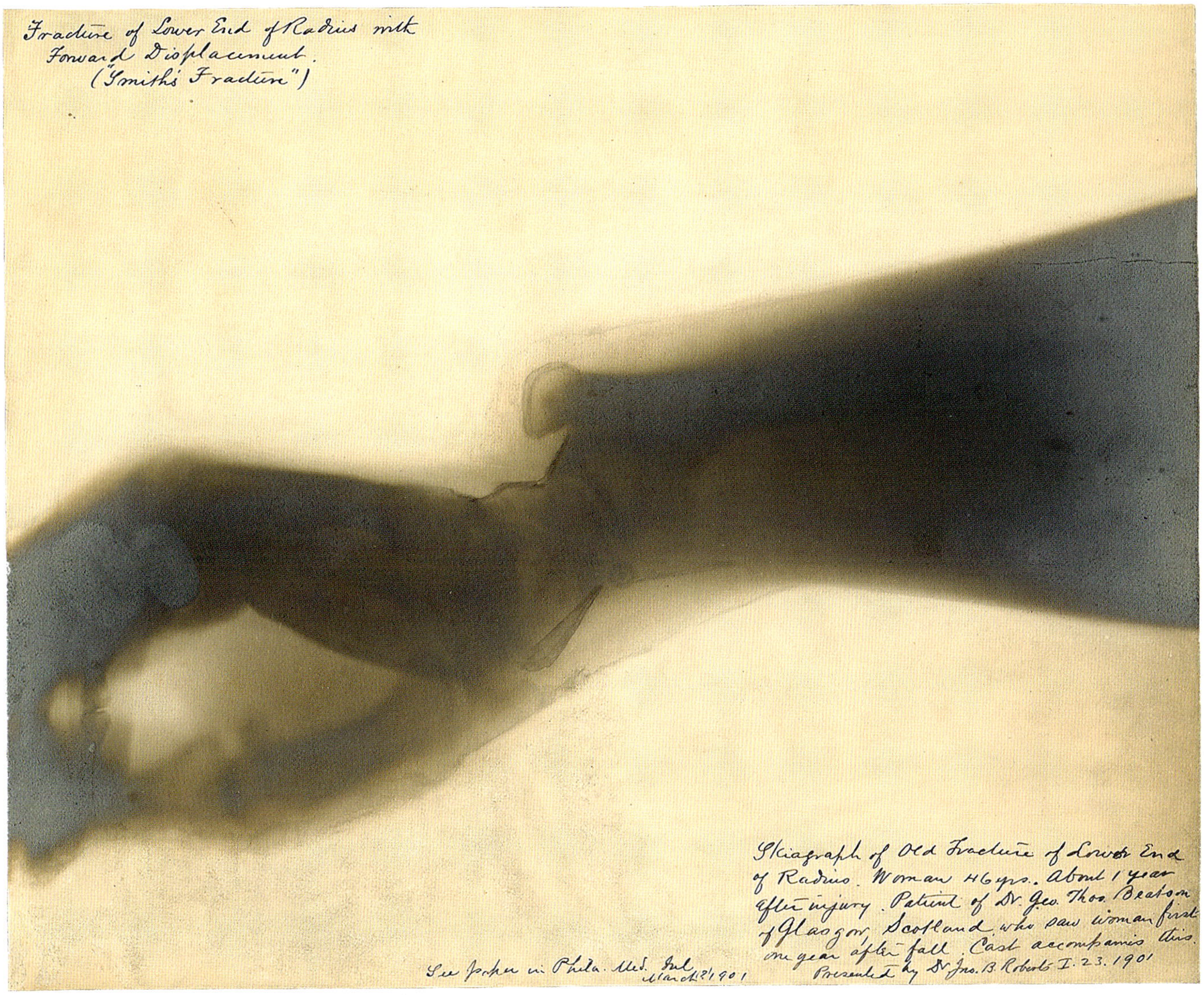
Fracture of Lower End of Radius with
Forward Displacement.
("Smith's Fracture")
Skiagraph of Old Fracture of Lower End
of Radius. Woman 46 yrs. About 1 year
after injury. Patient of Dr. Geo. Thos. Beatson
of Glasgow, Scotland who saw woman first
one year after fall. Cast accompanies this.
Presented by Dr. Jno. B. Roberts I. 23. 1901
See paper in Phila. Med. Jnl. March 2, 1901

Shark bite. Patient of Dr. Richard Hickman Harte (1855–1925). Photographs by William H. Rhoads, Philadelphia, ca. 1866–98.

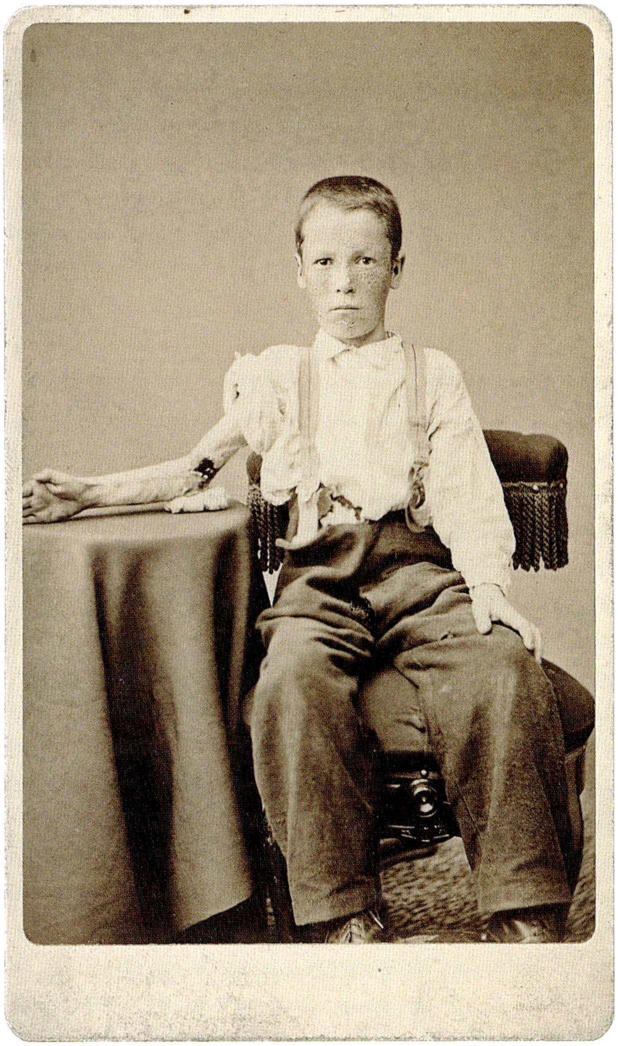

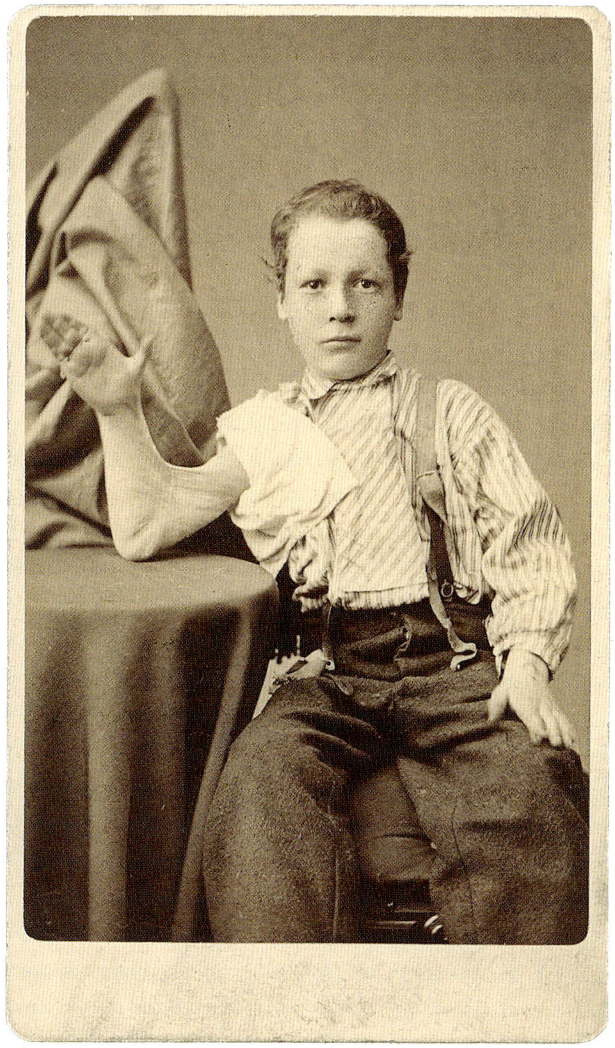

Fibrous pads from pressure of chair poles. Surgically removed. From an album by John Glasgow Kerr, M.D. (1824–1901), of photographs of his practice in Canton, China. After graduating from Jefferson Medical College Kerr went to China in 1853 as a medical missionary with the Presbyterian church. He performed nearly fifty thousand surgeries during his lifetime and in 1898 founded the Canton Refuge for the Insane.

Litters, also known as sedan chairs, were a precursor to the rickshaw and used for centuries as a form of transportation for the elite. The seat of the litter is suspended by two poles, one on each side, and carried by hand by four men. The *jianyu* is a litter whose poles are supported on the shoulders rather than carried by hand.

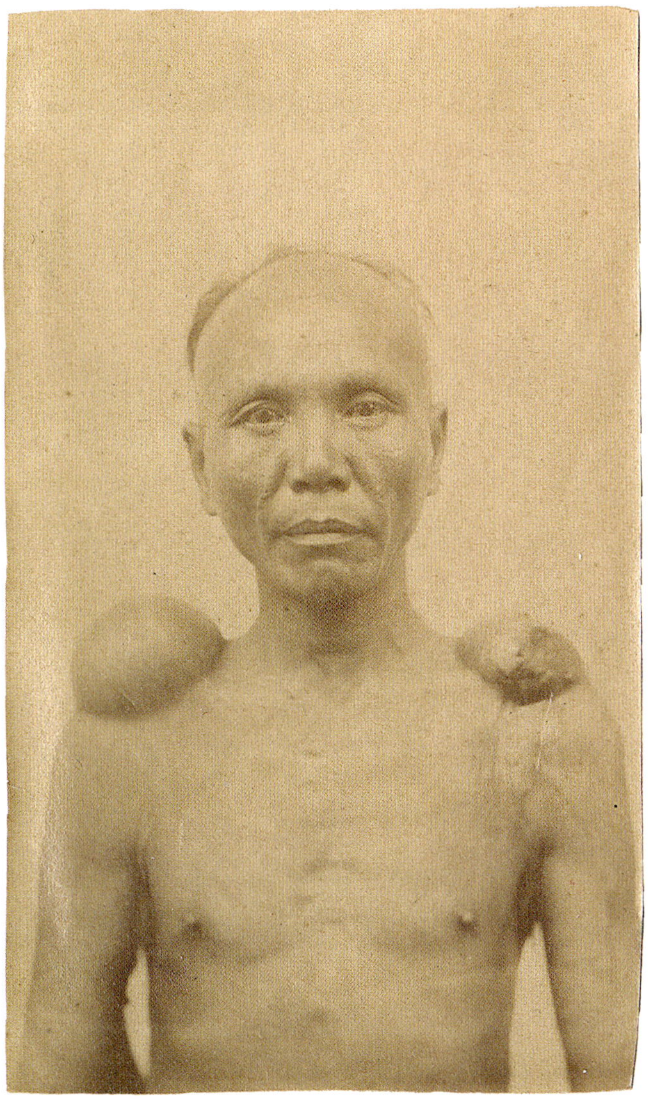

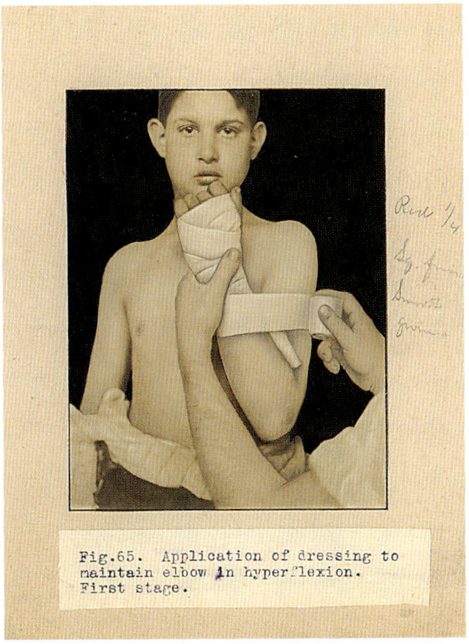

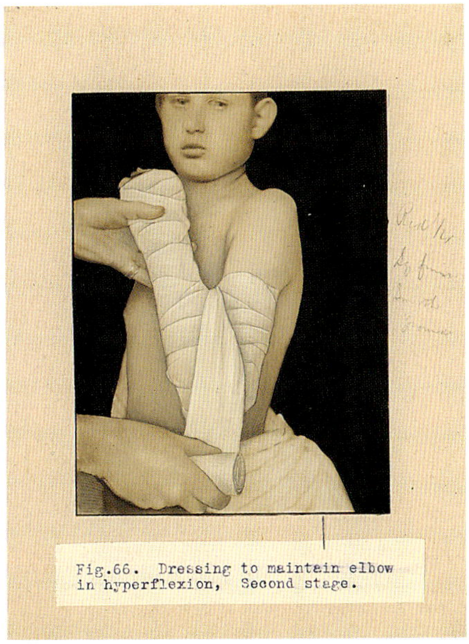

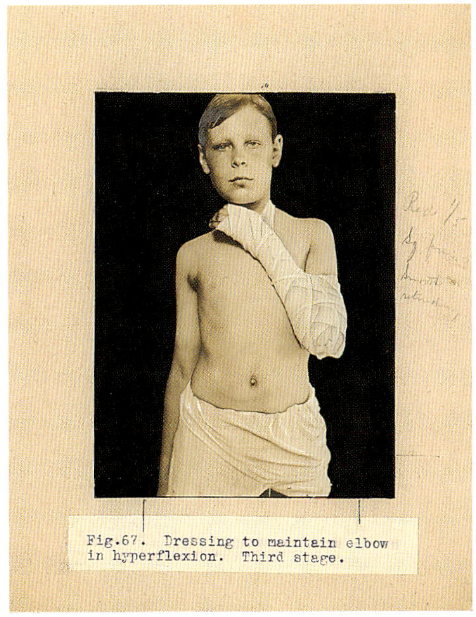

Sequential photographs showing application of dressing for fracture of elbow to maintain elbow in position of hyperflexion. Silver gelatin print with graphite and india ink opaquing. Photographer and date unidentified.

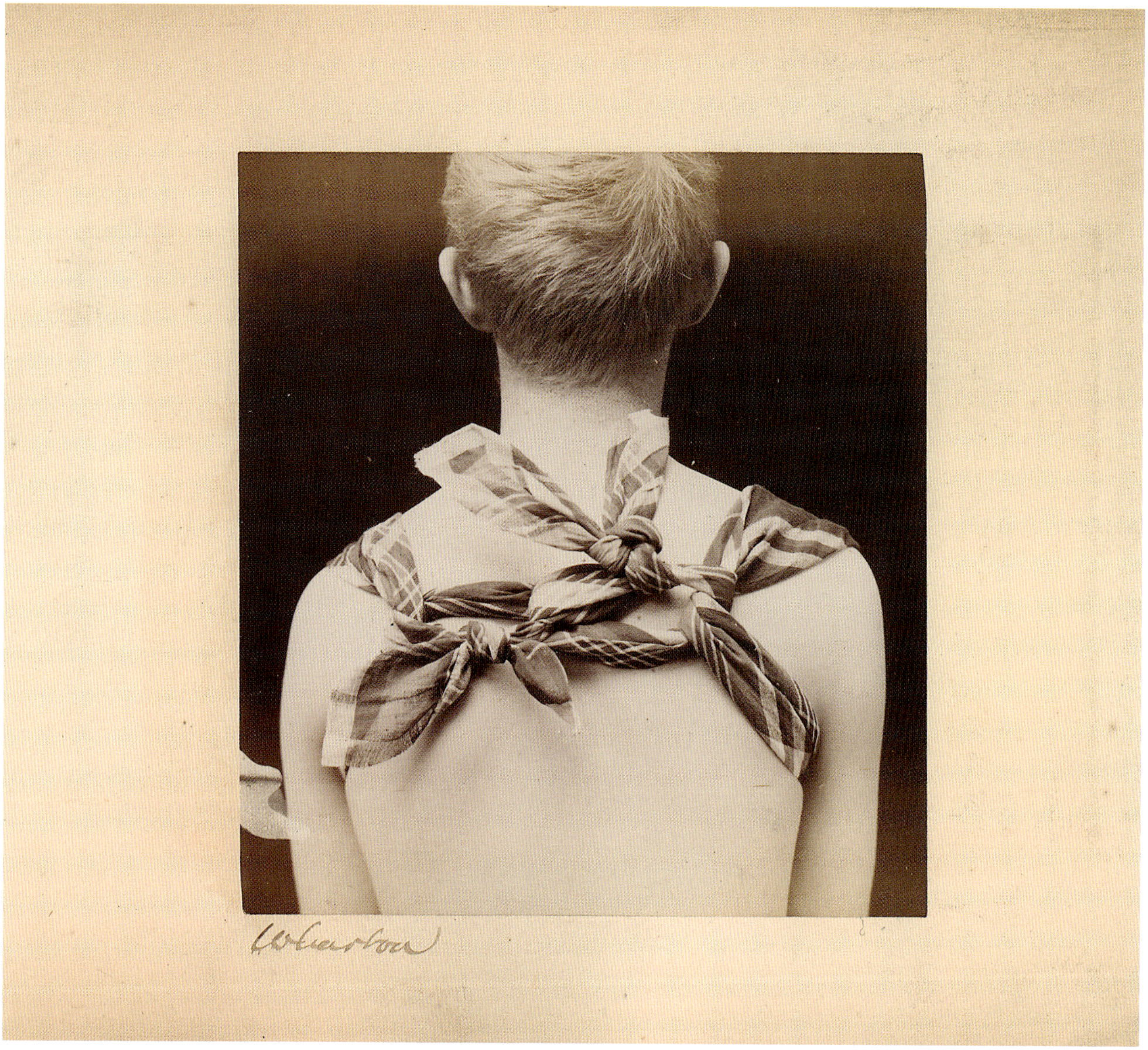

ABOVE AND OPPOSITE: Bandaging techniques photographed for Dr. Henry Redwood Wharton (1853–1925), author of *Minor Surgery and Bandaging* (1899) and others. Photograph by James F. Wood, from the album of photographs by Wood presented to the Mütter Museum in 1898.

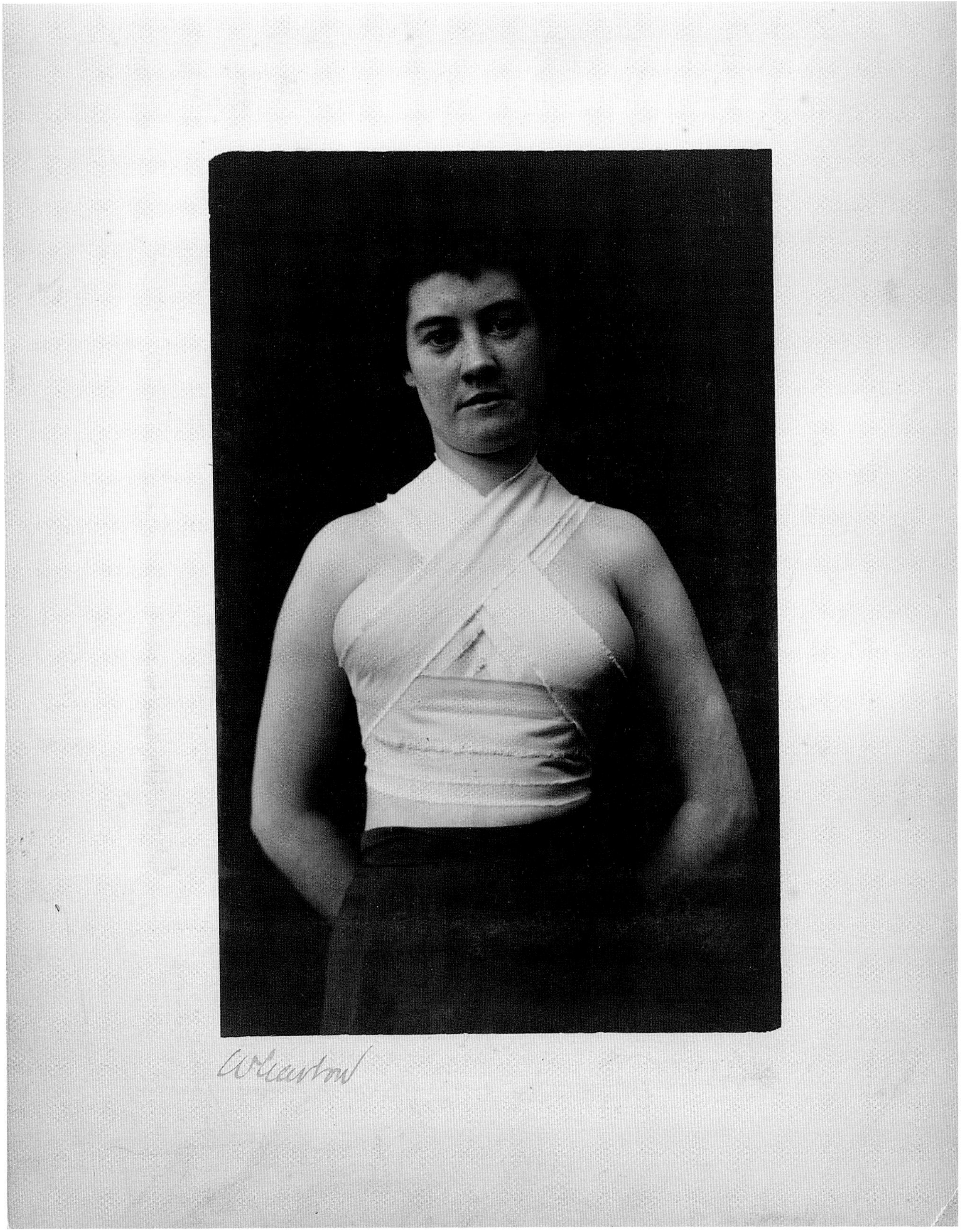

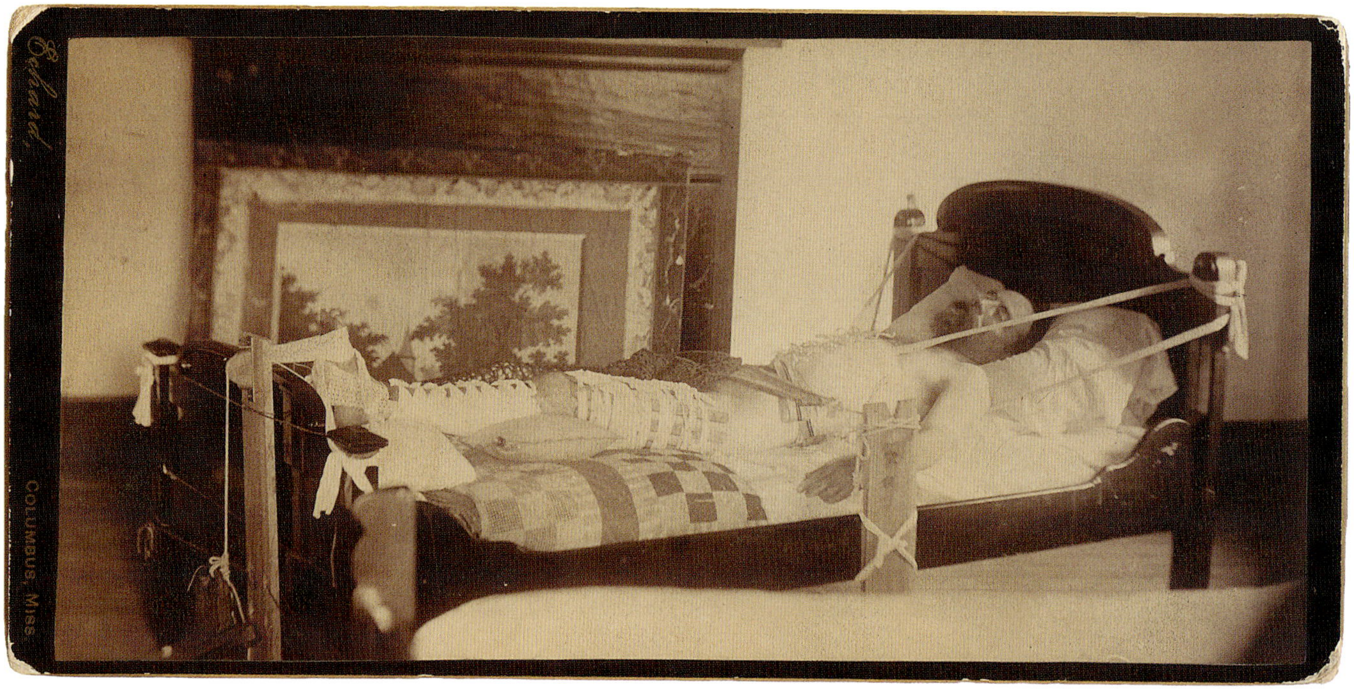

ABOVE: Dr. Brownrigg's extension apparatus for the treatment of gunshot and other fractures of the femur. Published in *Transactions of the Mississippi State Medical Association*, 1885. John Brownrigg, M.D. (1832–1902), of Columbus, Mississippi, a former surgeon in the Confederate Army, devised this apparatus based on his Civil War experiences, which employed a counter-extension jacket, Buck's extension, coaptation splints, and an air pillow to elevate the knee so the wound could be cleaned or dressed. It prevented ankylosis and shortening of the limb and could be applied in any farmhouse or army camp with the materials at hand. Albumen print, photograph by Echard, Columbus, Mississippi, ca. 1885. Donor: John Hooker Packard, M.D. (1832–1907).

OPPOSITE: Flexion in hip disease causing lordosis (concave curvature of the lumbar and cervical spine). Photographer and date unidentified. Donor: Dr. Edson, 1897.

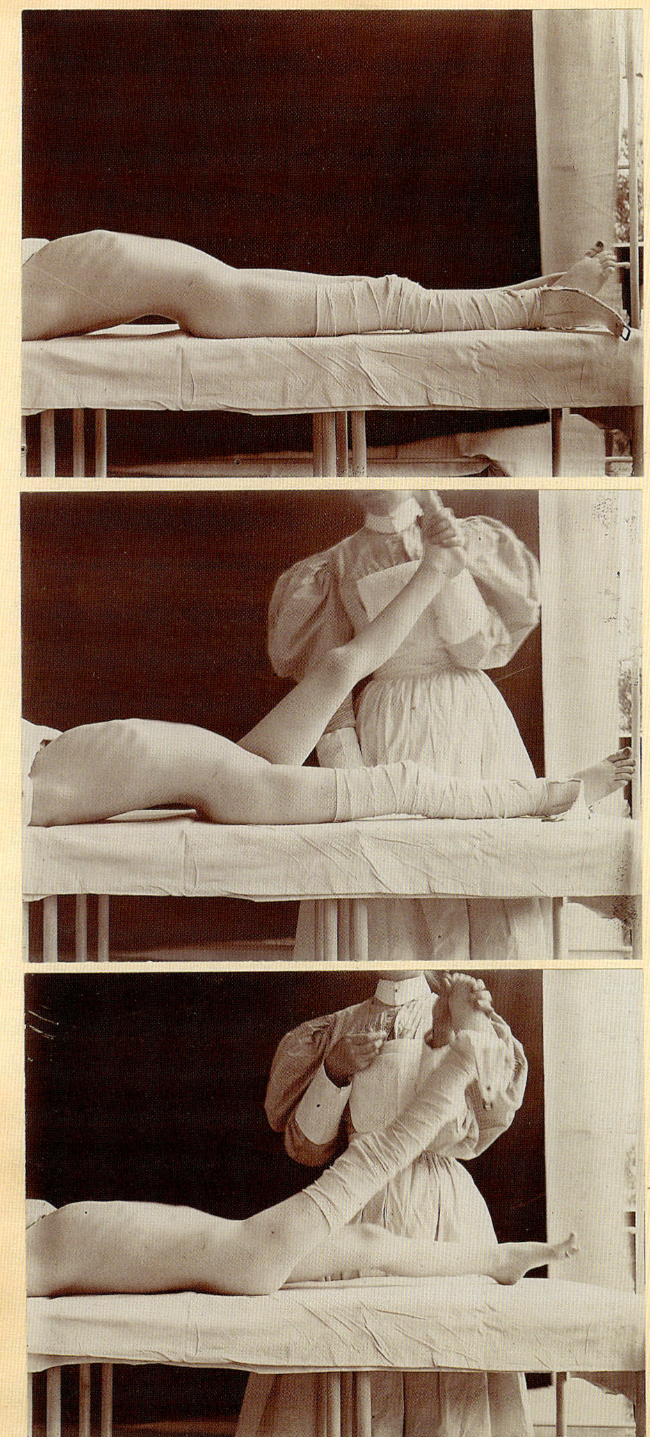

Flexion in hip-disease causing Lordosis.

(From D. Edson. Aug. 22. 1897.)

Splint for wrist drop devised by Lieutenant R. C. Buerki, M.D. (1892–1991), World War I. Thumb is held extended in a plane with the rest of the fingers. Distal two phalanges are left free so as to permit normal movement. No bandages necessary to hold splint in place. Photographer and date unidentified, ca. 1914–18. Donor: John H. Arnett, M.D. (1889–1981) .

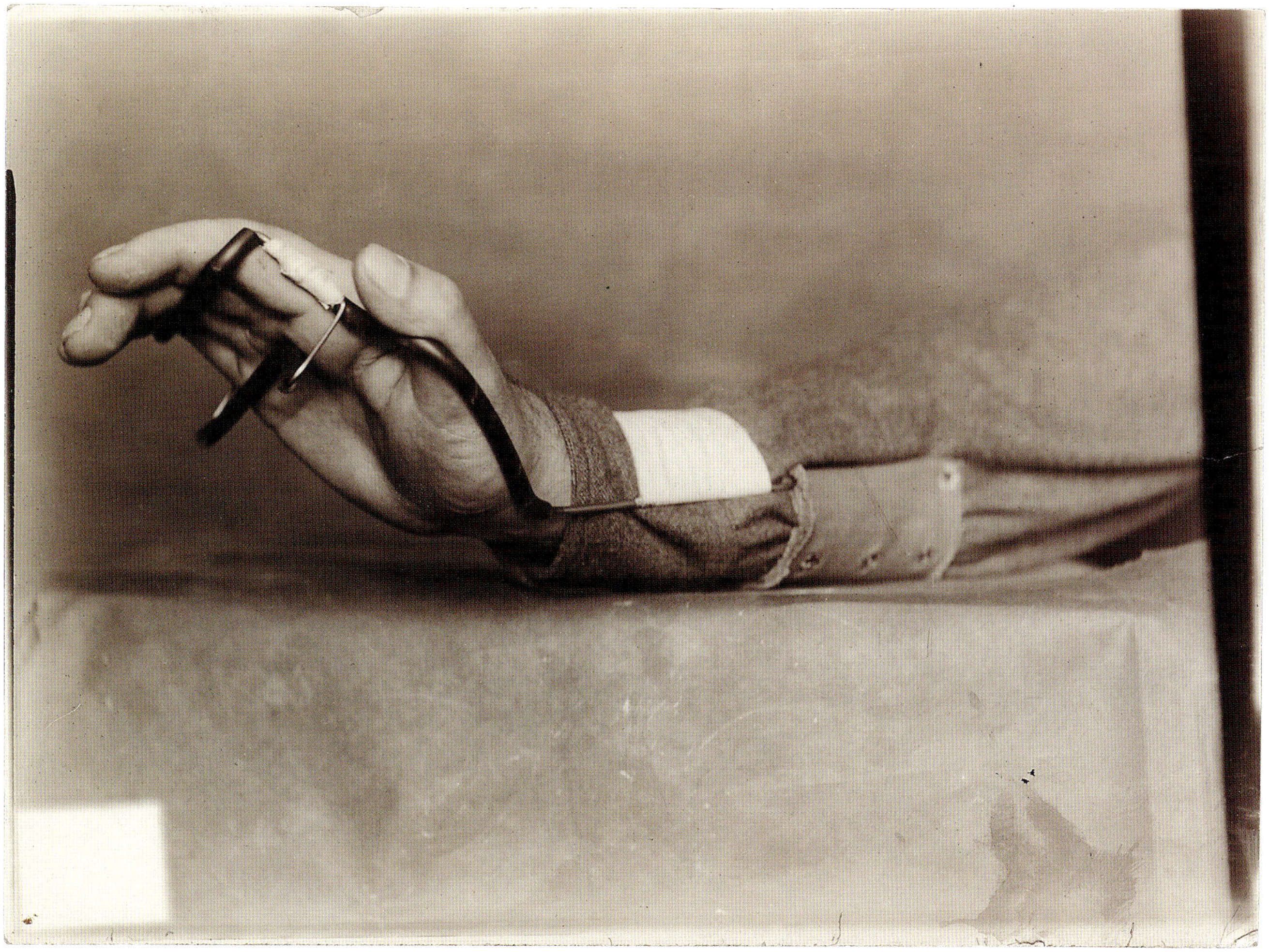

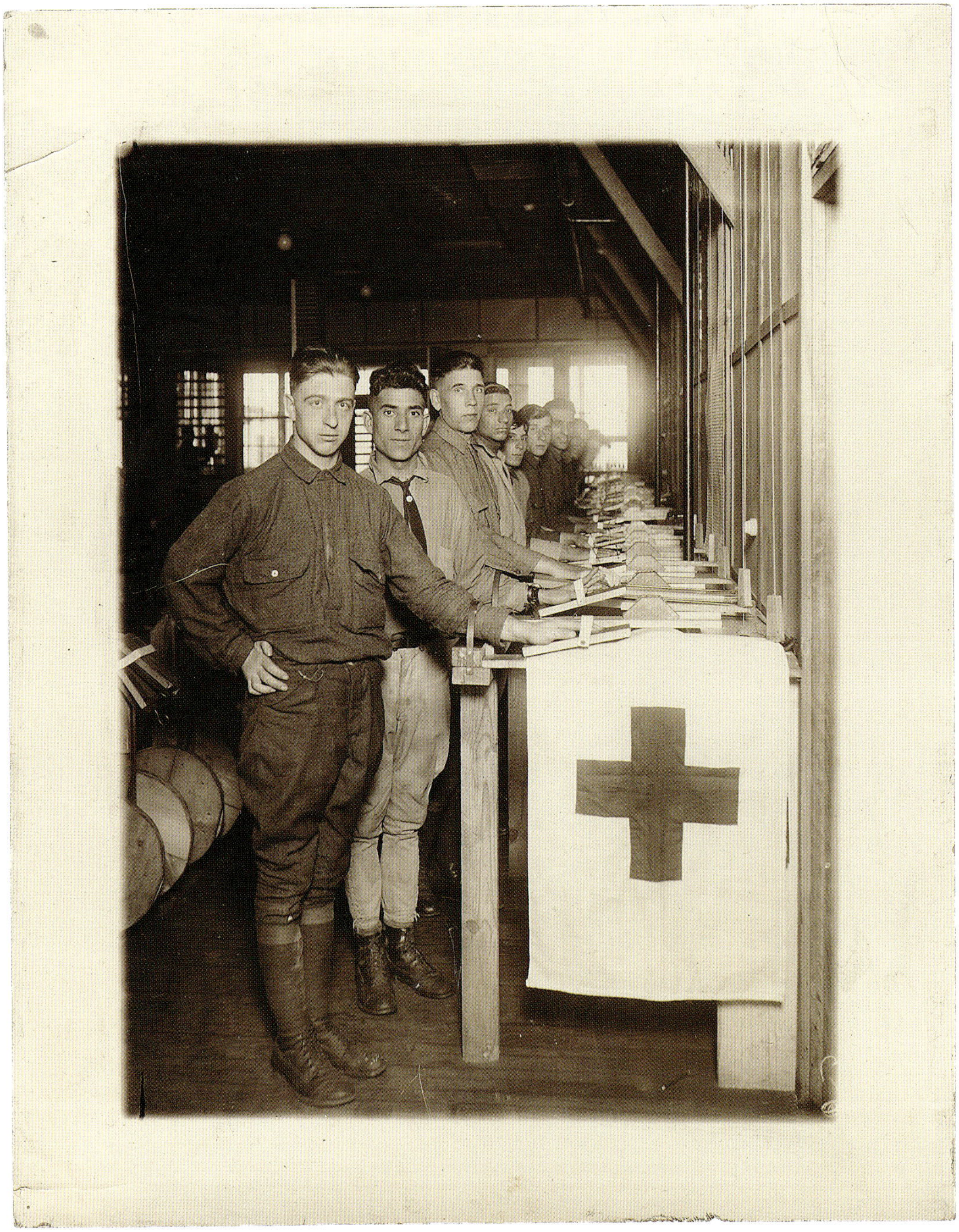

ABOVE AND OPPOSITE: Apparati designed by John H. Arnett, M.D. (1889–1981), first lieutenant, Medical Corps, while on duty on the neurosurgical staff of U.S.A. General Hospital No. 41, Staten Island, New York, World War I.

ABOVE: Apparatus for active flexion and extension of the wrist joint, to prevent or overcome fibrosis of the wrist joint and to maintain nutrition of the muscles producing flexion and extension of the wrist, to aid in its reeducation when function is returning after paralysis. Photographer and date unidentified, ca. 1914–18.

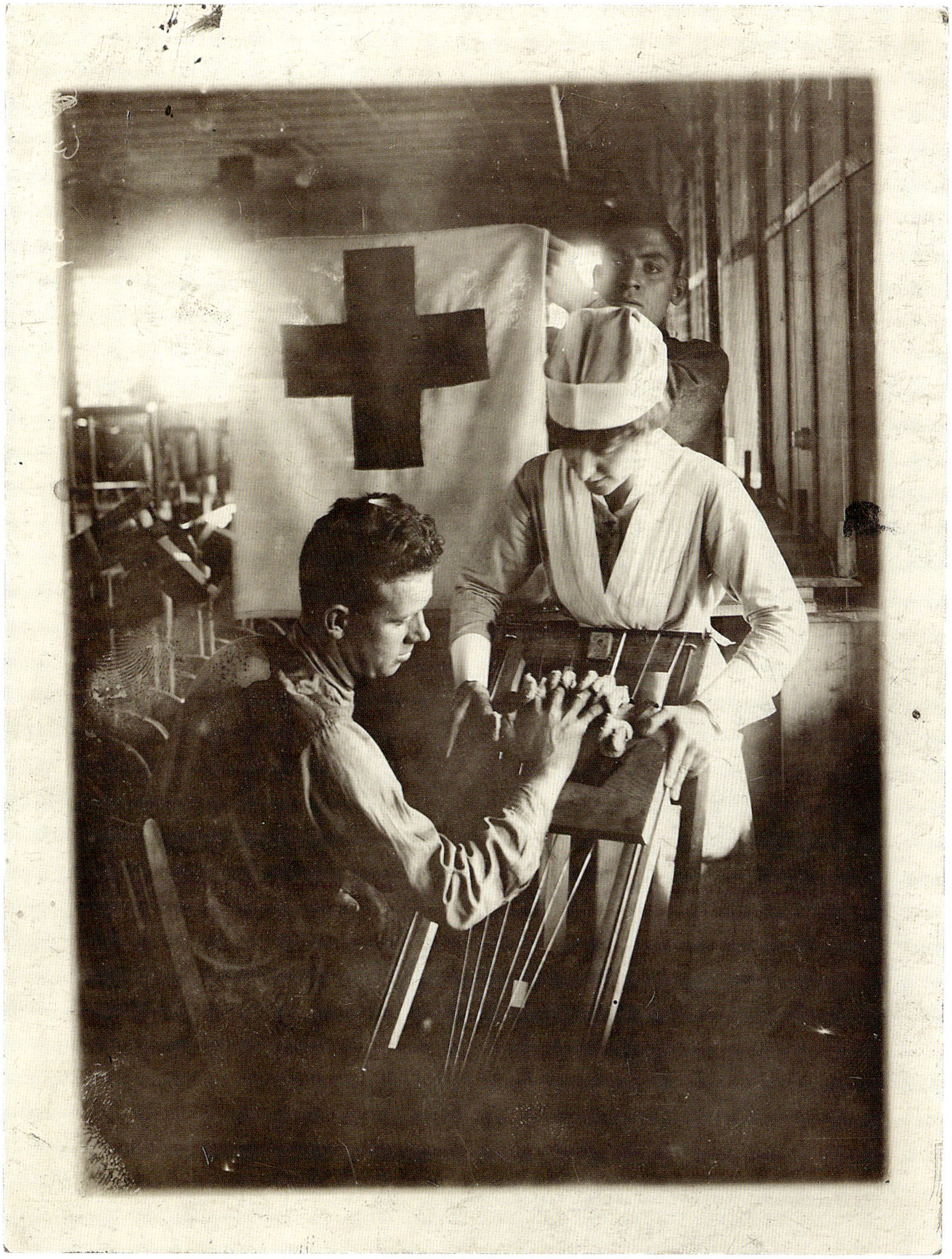

Apparatus for passive abduction and adduction of the fingers and thumb, to prevent or overcome fibrosis in the metacarpo-phalangeal joints and secure passive movement for the muscles of abduction and adduction of the fingers and thumb. Photographer and date unidentified, ca. 1914–18. Apparatus in Mütter Museum collection.

Amputation

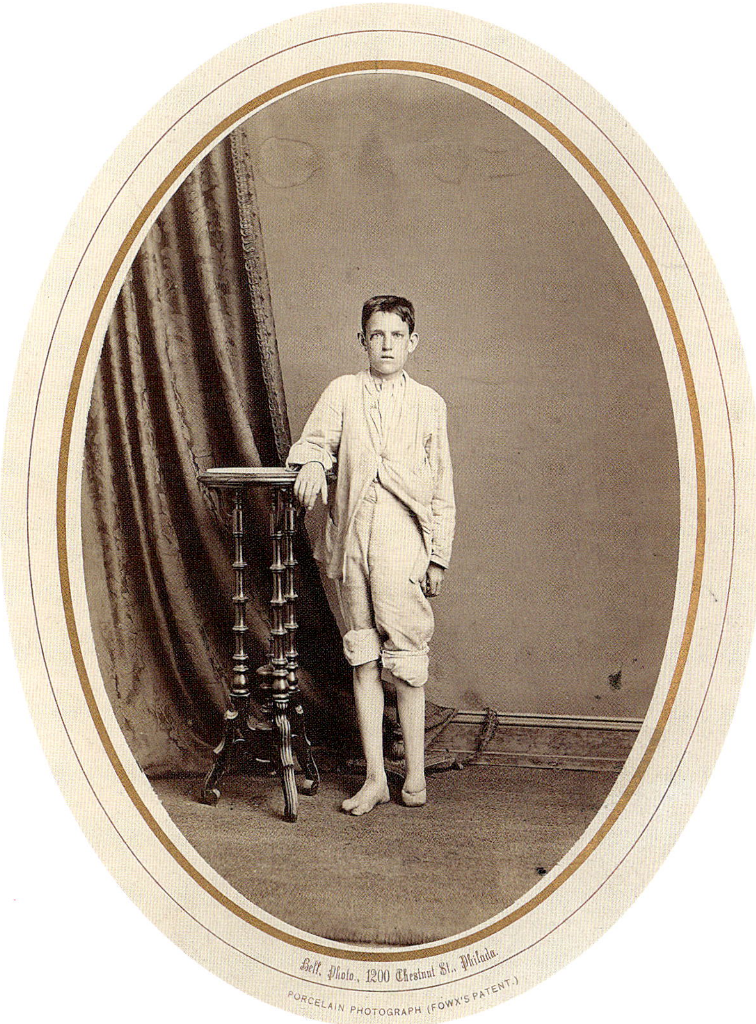

Pirogoff amputation (same subject, page 57). Developed by Nikolai Ivanovich Pirogov (1810–1881) during the Crimean War, Pirogoff amputation is the osteoplastic amputation of the foot at the ankle, with part of the heel bone being left in the stump for added support. Performed by Dr. Thomas George Morton (1835–1903), a founder of and surgeon at the Orthopedic Hospital, Philadelphia. Porcelain photograph (Fowx's patent) by William Bell, Philadelphia, ca. 1869–74.

Pirogoff amputation (see also page 55) by Dr. Thomas George Morton (1835–1903). Photographer and date unidentified.

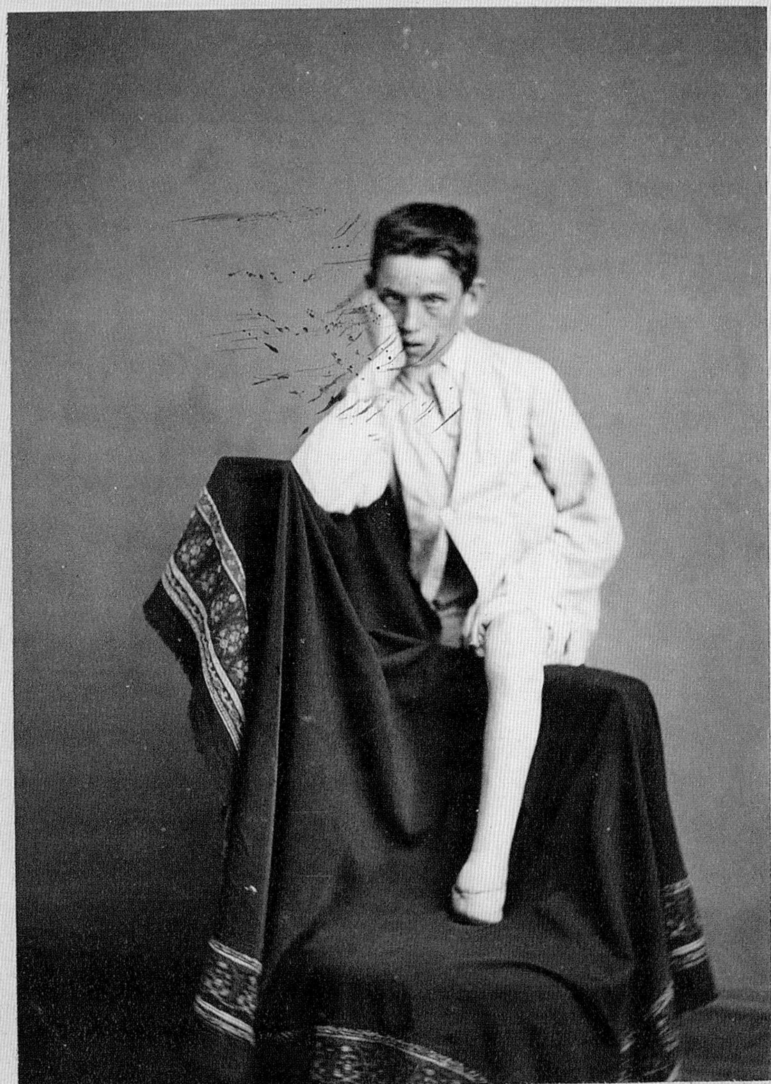

Pirögoff amputation
by Dr Morton -

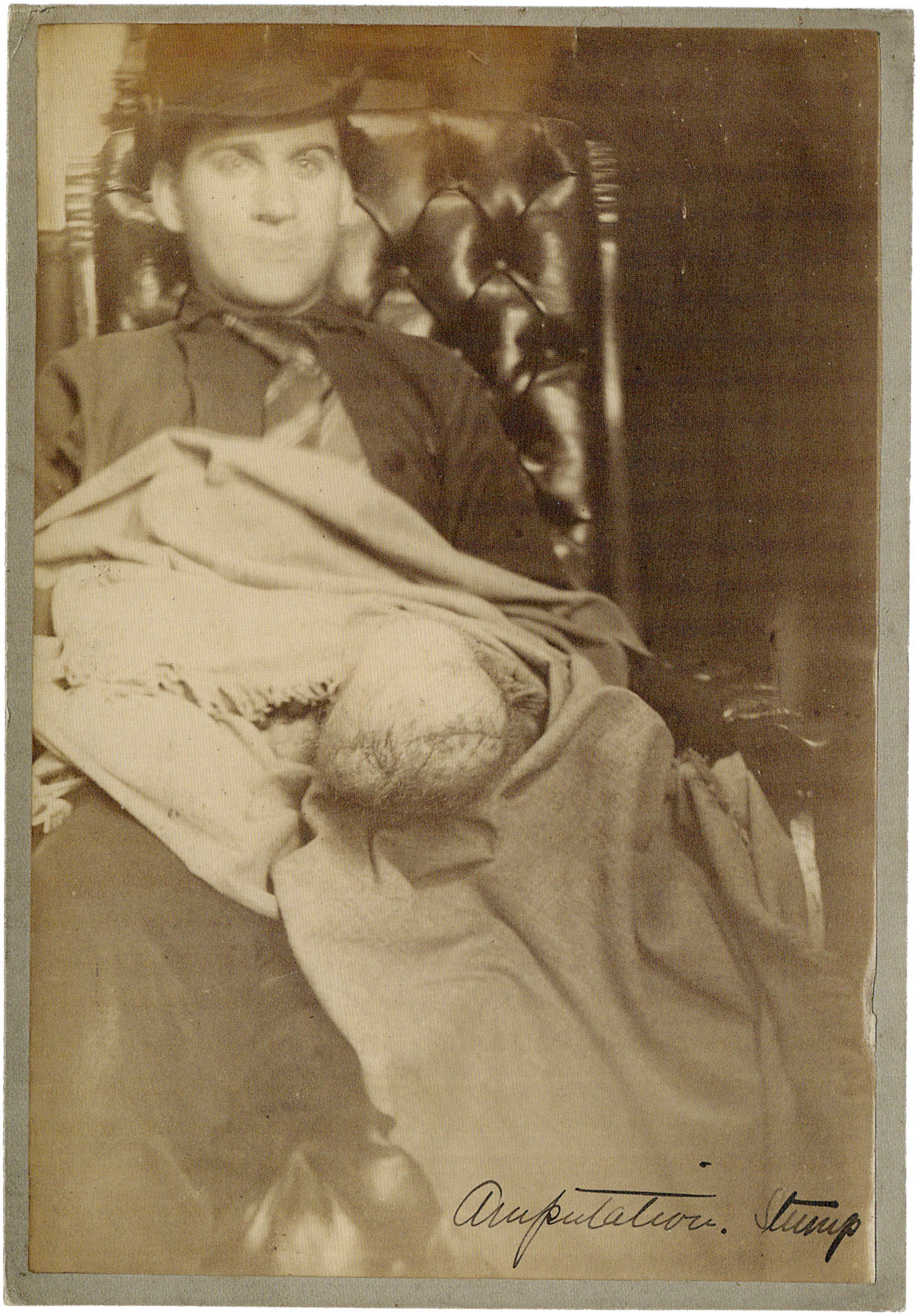

ABOVE: Amputation, stump. Photographed for Dr. DeForest Willard (1846–1910). Photographer and date unidentified.

OPPOSITE: Pirogoff amputation performed by Dr. Thomas George Morton (1835–1903). Photograph by A. Newman, Philadelphia, ca. 1867.

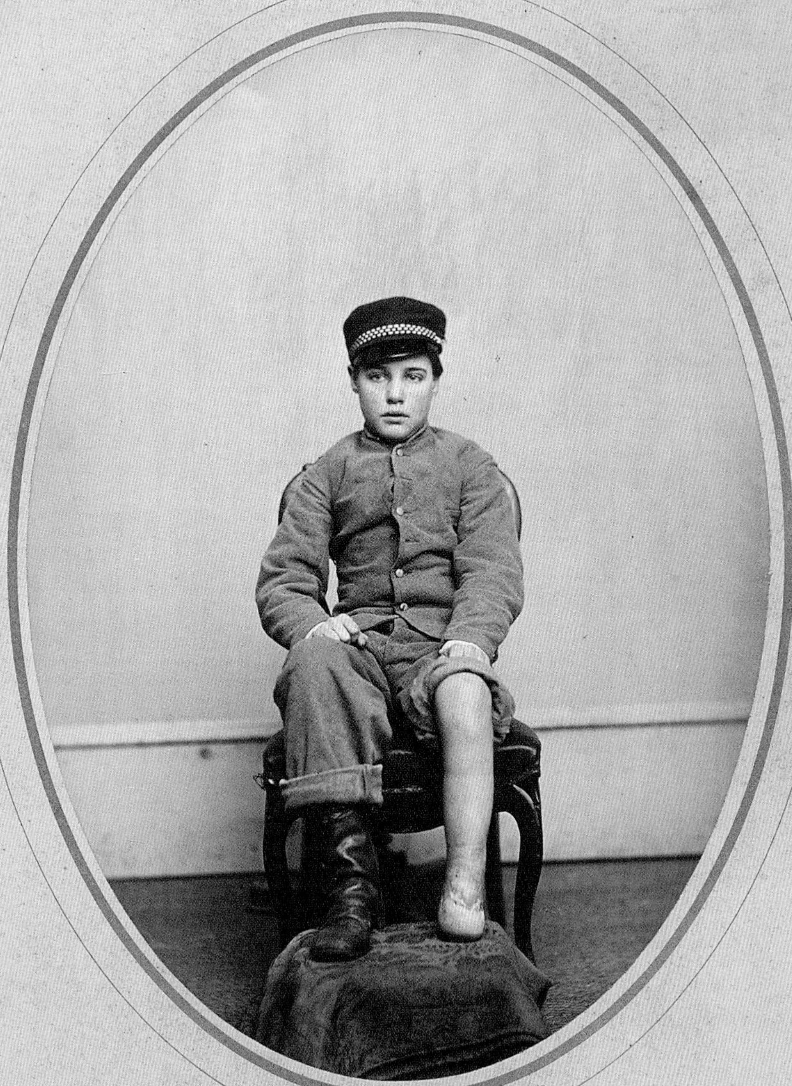

Photo. by A. NEWMAN, No. 127 S. 8th St. Philada.

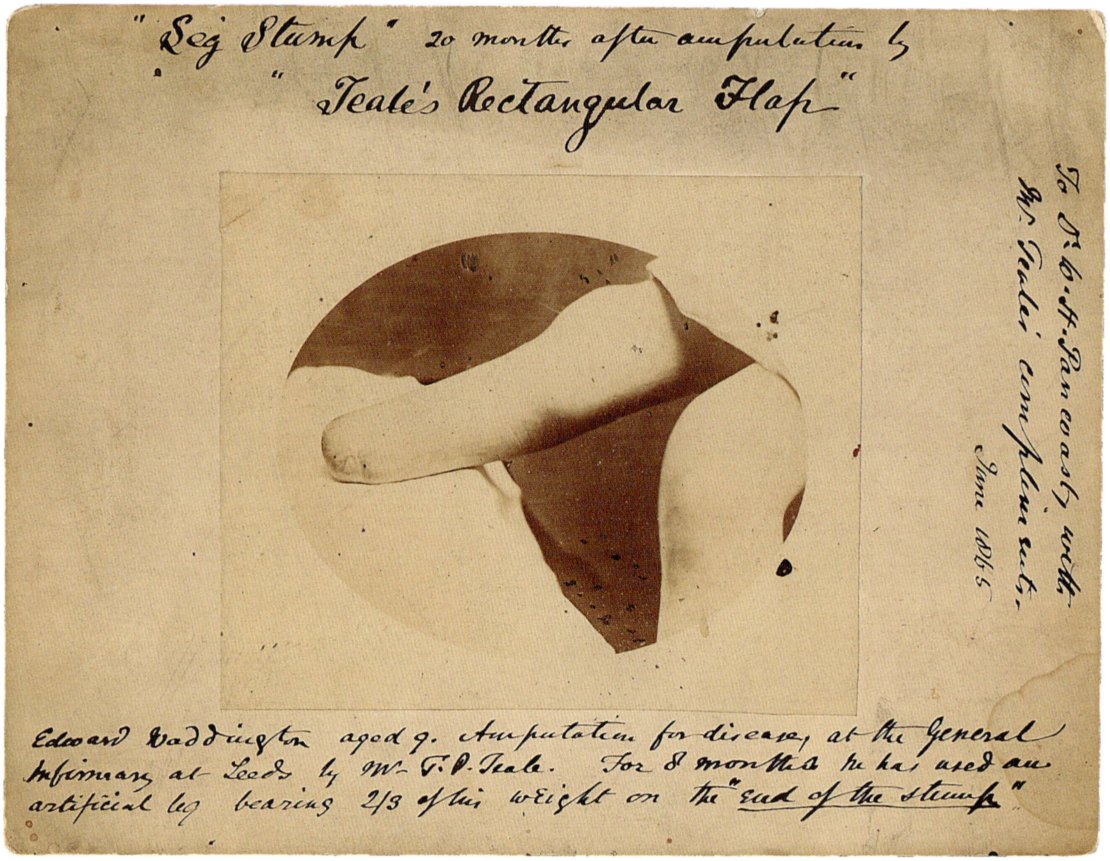

Leg stump, twenty months after amputation by Teale's rectangular flap. Teale's amputation preserves a long rectangular flap of muscle and skin on one side of the limb and a short rectangular flap on the other. Case of Edward Waddington, age nine, amputation for disease, at the General Infirmary at Leeds by Mr. Thomas Pridgin Teale (1801–1868). Notation on photograph records, "For eight months Waddington has used an artificial leg bearing two-thirds of his weight on the 'end of the stump.'" Photographer unknown. Photograph given by Mr. Teale to Dr. William H. Pancoast (1835–1897), June 1865. Donor: Dr. William H. Pancoast.

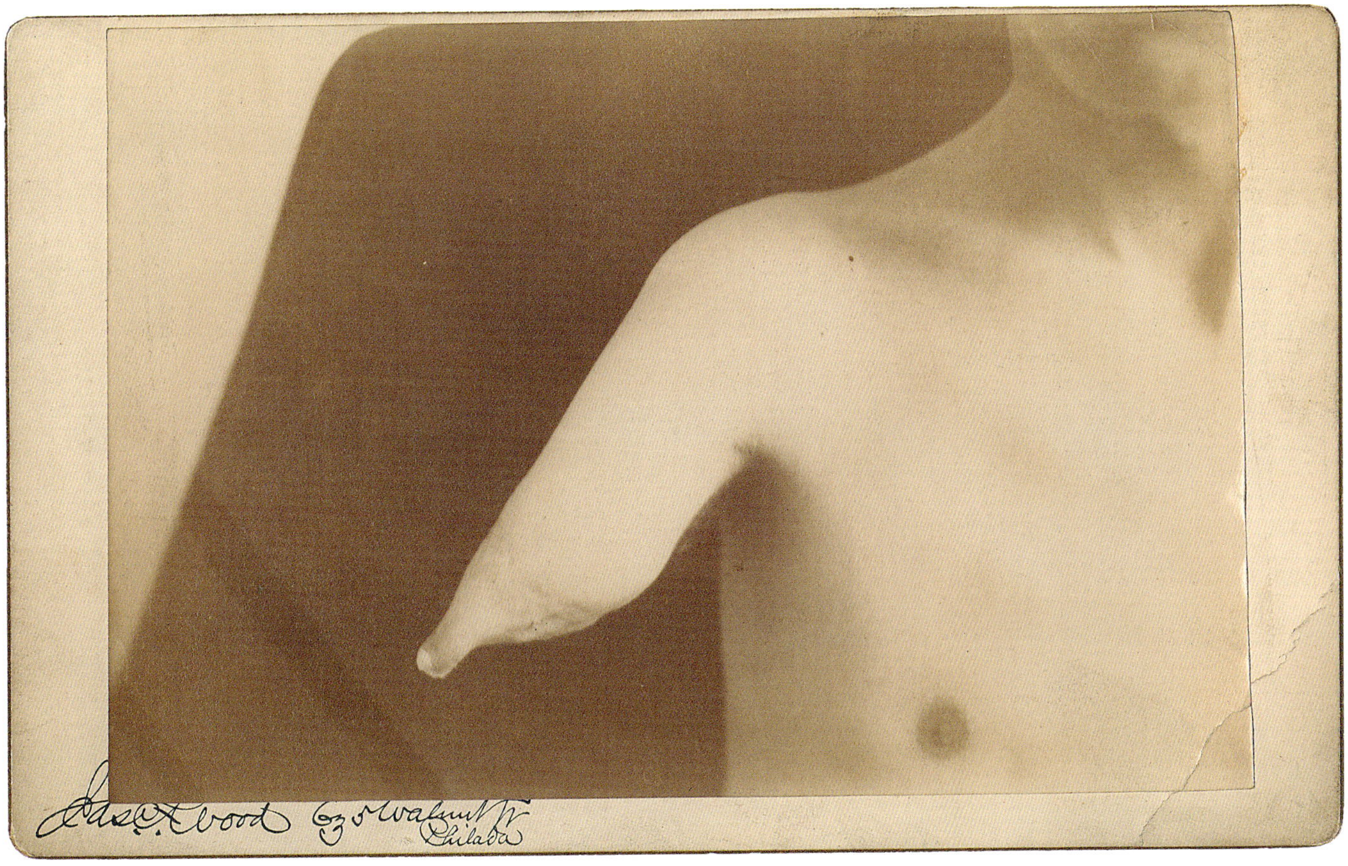

Conical stump from continued growth of bone after amputation in early life. Reamputated. University Hospital, Philadelphia, January 25, 1896. Photograph by James F. Wood, Philadelphia, ca. 1892–1900.

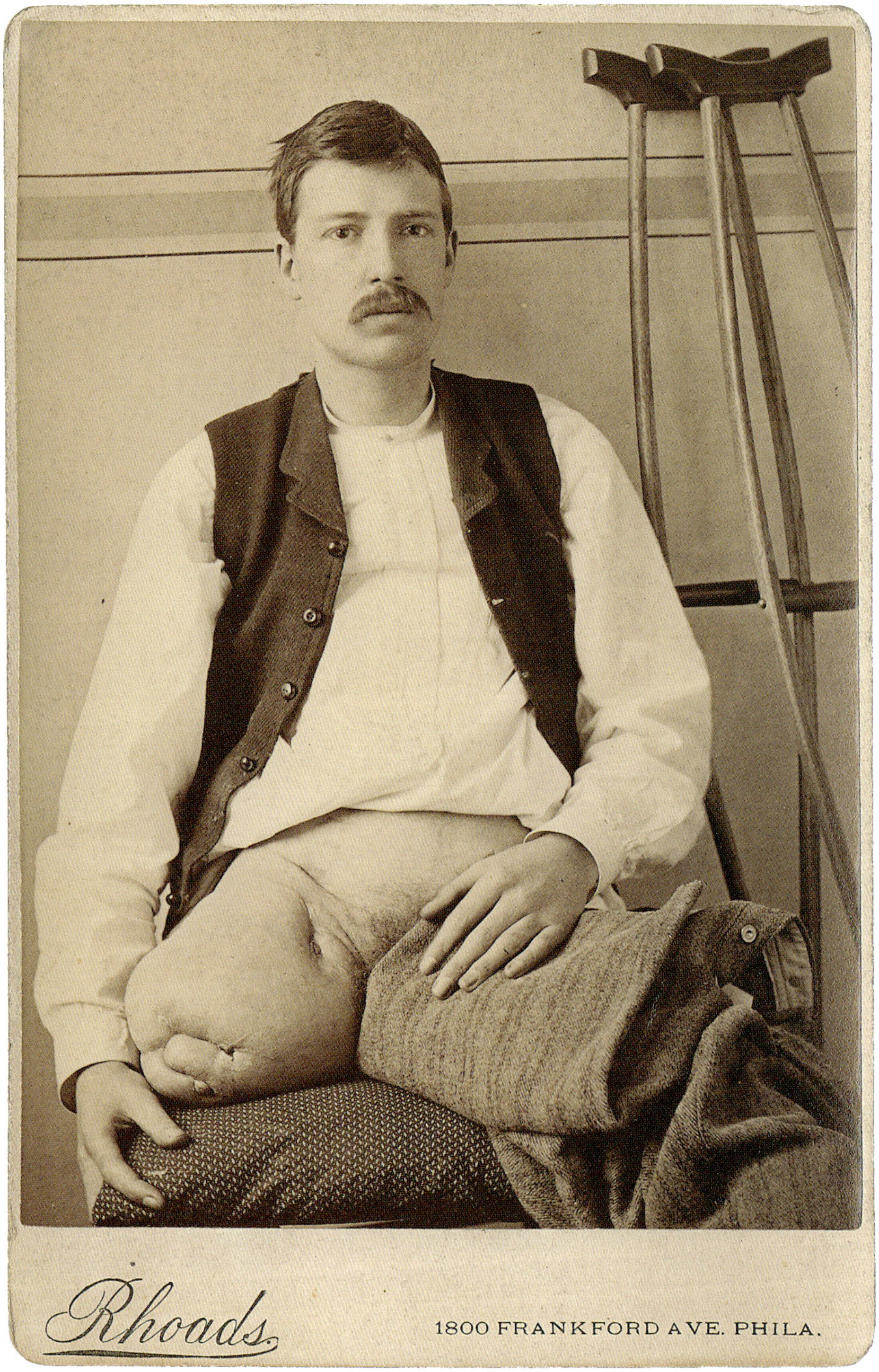

Leg amputation, Rudolph Kavanagh. Photograph by William H. Rhoads, Philadelphia, ca. 1866–98.

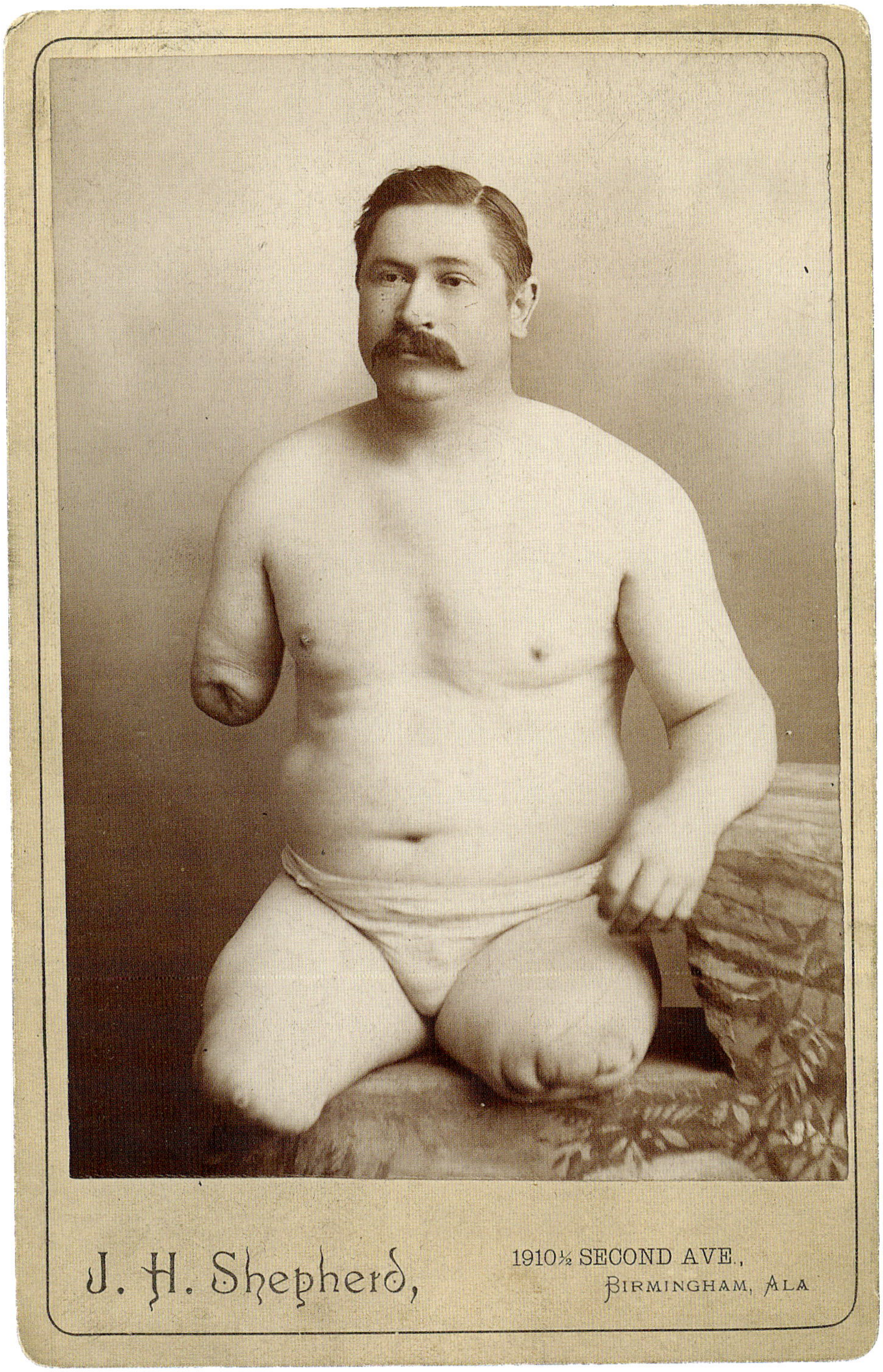

Dr. James Buckner Luckie's (1833–1908) second case of triple amputation, Birmingham, Alabama. Dr. Luckie performed the first and second successful triple amputations in the United States. Photograph by J. H. Shepherd, Birmingham, Alabama, undated.

Triple amputation. Photograph by J. H. Henning, Johnstown, Pennsylvania, 1880s.

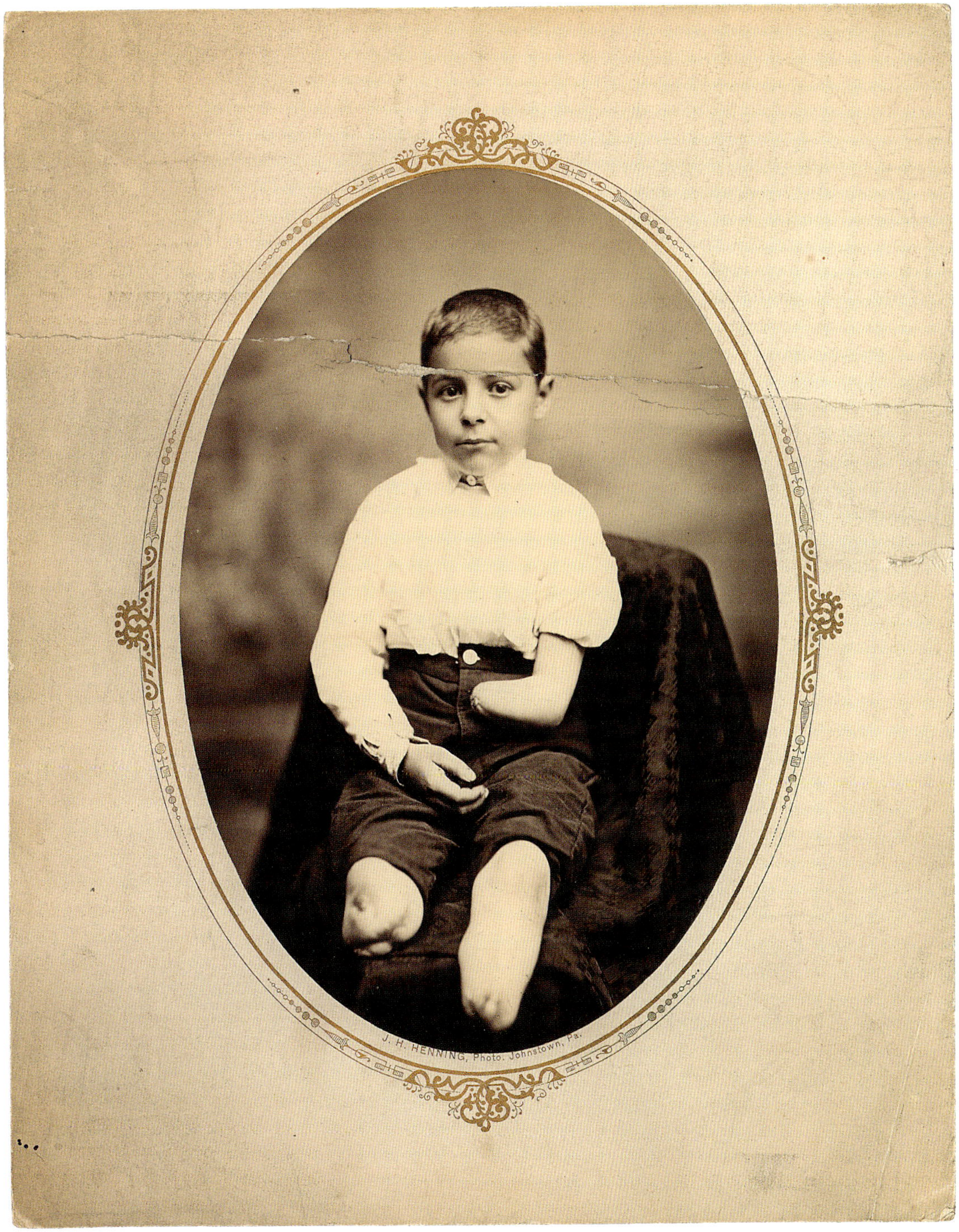
J. H. HENNING, Photo. Johnstown, Pa.

Hypertrophy, Malformation, and Excess Growth

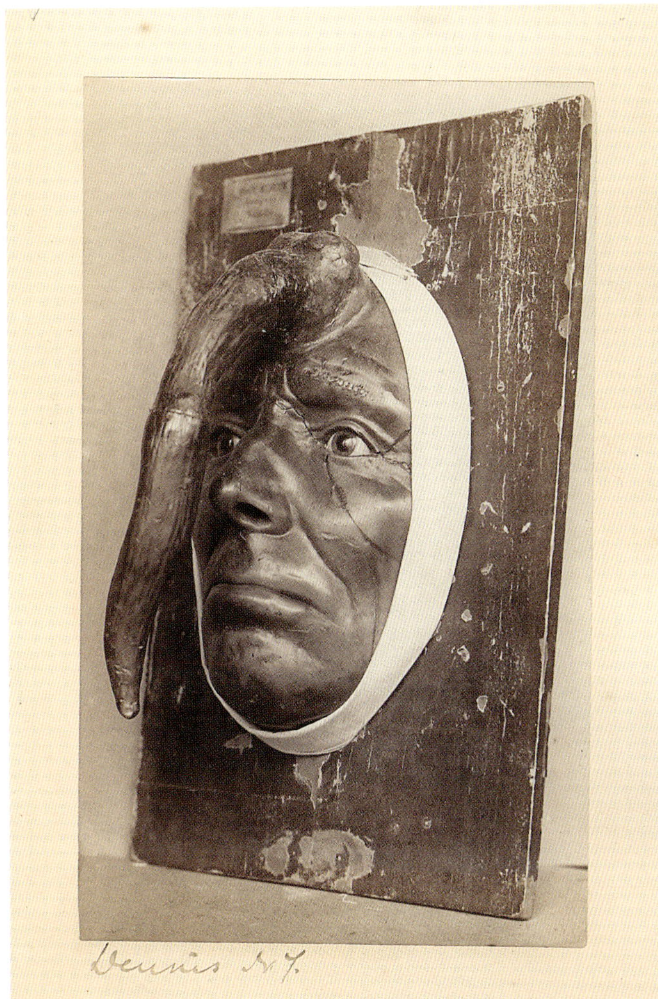

Wax model of Madame Dimanche, or Widow Sunday, who lived in Paris around the beginning of the nineteenth century. The horn on her forehead attained a length of 9.8 inches by her eighty-second year, having begun to form six years earlier. It was successfully removed by Dr. Joseph Souberbeille (1754–1846), a noted French surgeon. Models such as this one of Madame Dimanche are known to have been in a number of American medical and popular anatomic museums by the mid-nineteenth century. At present no model other than the one at the Mütter Museum (different from that pictured here and part of the original collection of Dr. Mütter) is known to exist. Photograph by James F. Wood, ca. 1892–1900, from the album of photographs by Wood presented to the Mütter Museum in 1898.

Inscription on back of photograph: "Photograph of a Filipino with a tail about five inches long. Taken by my grandson John Freeman in the spring or summer of 1925." Donor: Dr. William Williams Keen (1837–1932), a surgeon for the U.S. Army in 1862–64 during the Civil War, and in 1887 the first United States' surgeon to remove a brain tumor successfully.

The vestigial human tail is a very rare congenital abnormality often associated with other malformations. The vestigial tail contains adipose and connective tissue, blood vessels, and nerves covered by skin.

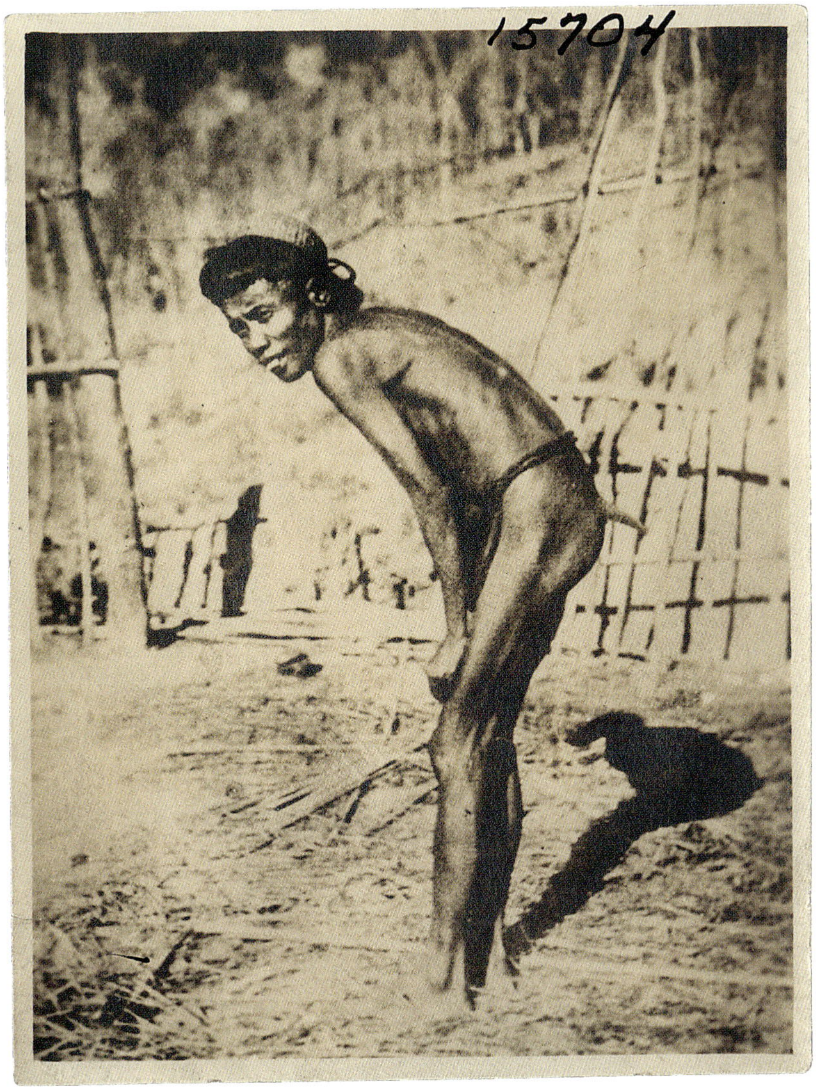
15704

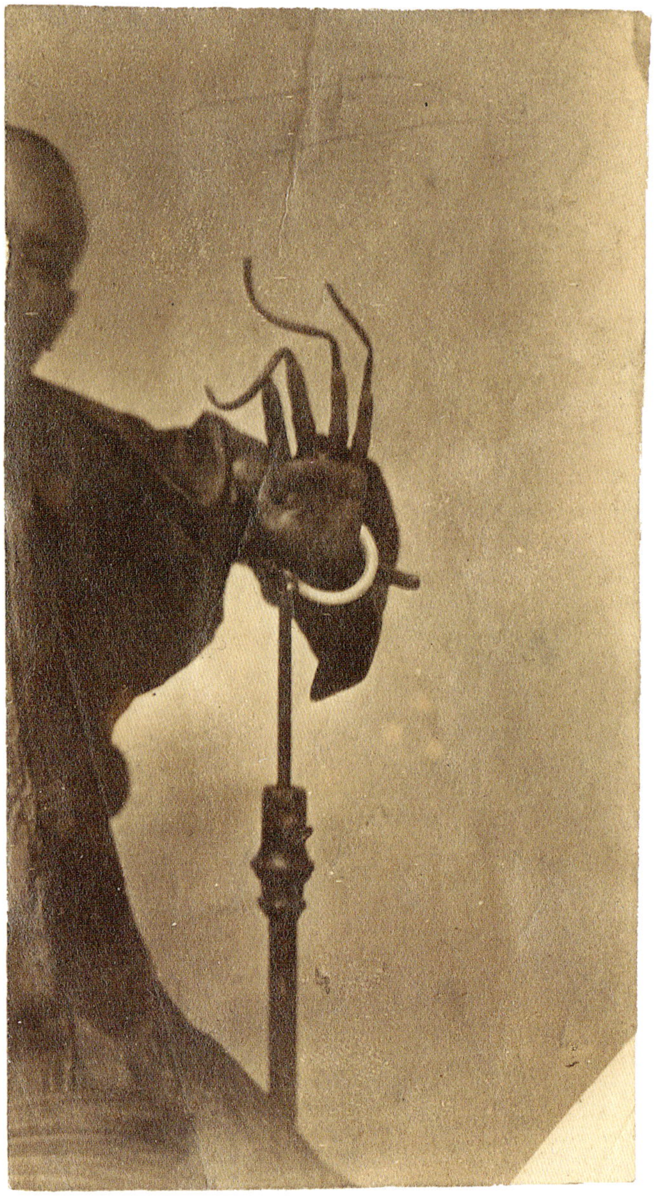

Photograph, second and third fingernails 6½ inches; fourth 5 inches. From an album by John Glasgow Kerr, M.D. (1824–1901), of photographs of his practice in Canton, China.

Fingernails were grown very long among some of the elite in China as a symbol of their high social standing.

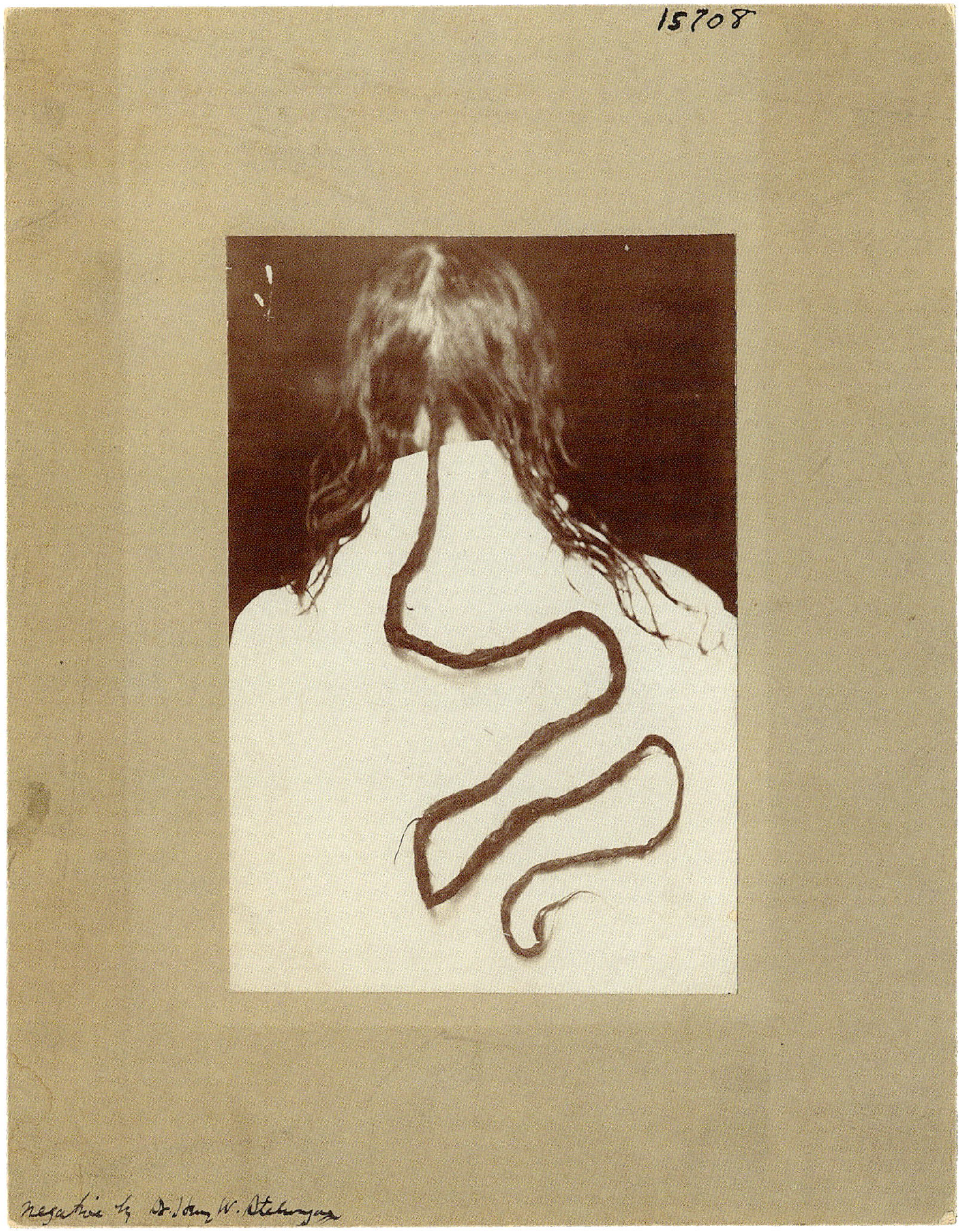

Case of plica (pilica neuropathica, or plica polonica) in an Irishwoman, aged forty, reported by Dr. Henry Weightman Stelwagon (1853–1919), clinical professor of dermatology at Jefferson Medical College, in *The American Journal of the Medical Sciences*, December 1892. Dr. Stelwagon reported that with the exception of a peculiar growth upon the patient's scalp, the hair was found to be normal and reached to the shoulders. From a dollar-sized area in the middle of the occipital region, however, the hair had begun to grow twelve years earlier into a felted lock, about the thickness of a thumb, and four feet one inch in length, extending to the patient's ankles. Careful investigation indicated the formation had been of spontaneous origin, and in this instance, as in all cases of plica, the patient and her friends and relatives looked upon it with more or less awe and superstition. Dr. Stelwagon's suggestion to cut the lock off to ascertain whether new-growing hair would exhibit the same tendency was met on all sides with fear and doubt and led to patient withdrawing herself from observation. Negative by Dr. Stelwagon, ca. 1892.

Inscription on back of photograph: “Louis Savidge: supernumerary auricle. Idiot, had incontinence of urine. June 20, 1891.” Extra folds of outer ear in region of antihelix. The outer ear forms during foetal development when many other vital organs are developing. Abnormal folds in the outer ear are sometimes associated with conditions such as Down syndrome. Photographer unidentified.

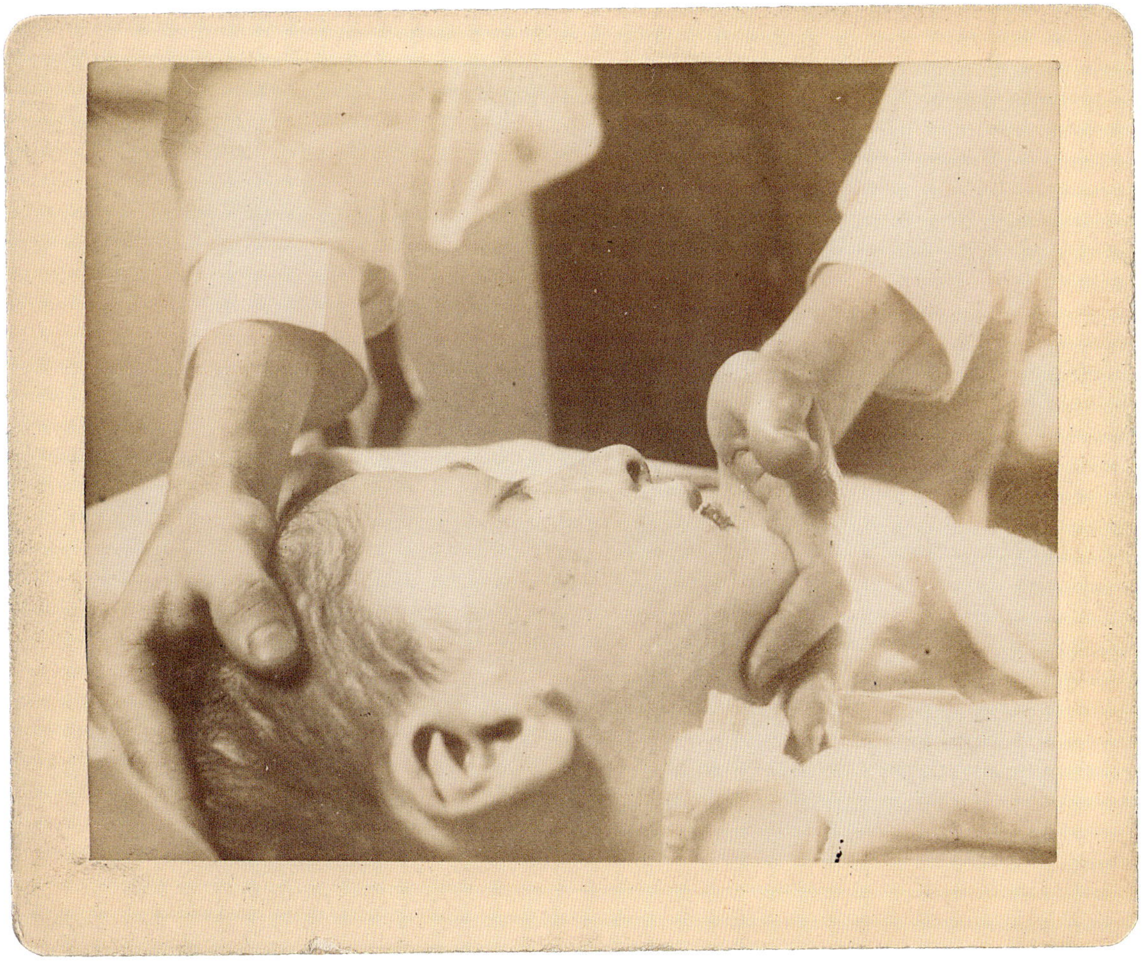

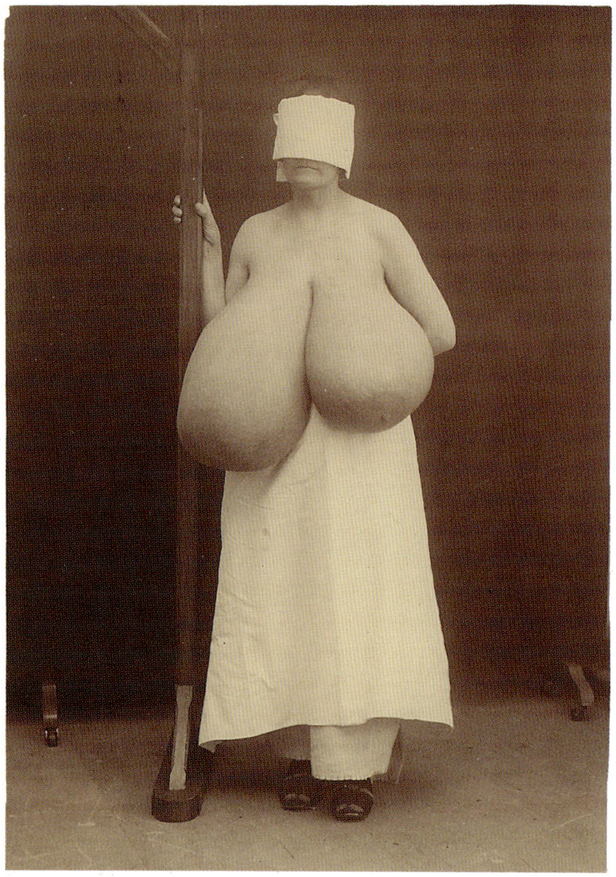

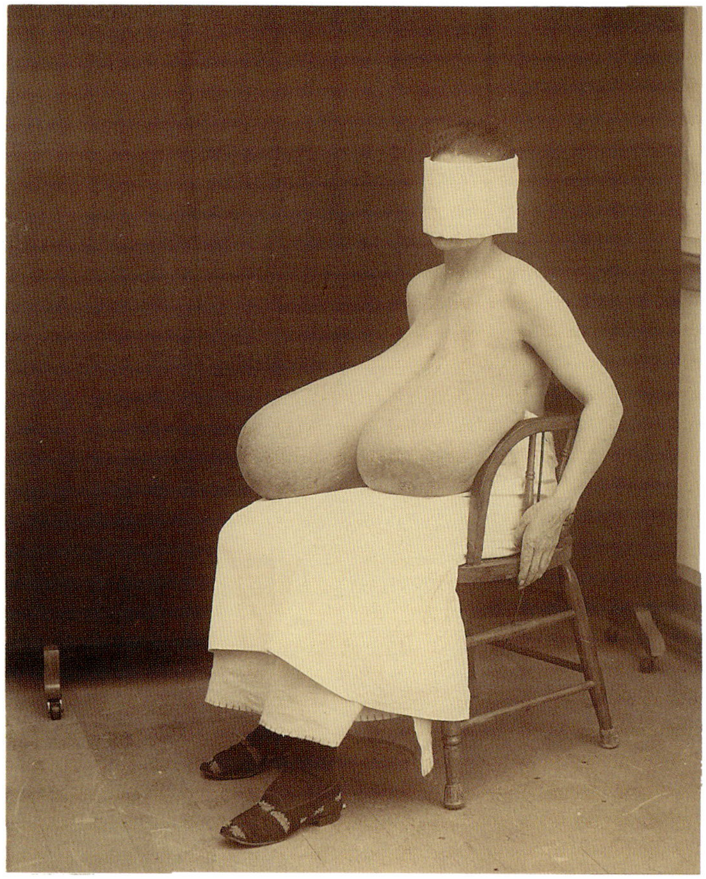

Bilateral hypertrophy of both breasts. Patient of Charles B. Porter, M.D. (1840–1909), Massachusetts General Hospital, ca. 1893. Photographs taken before a successful operation to remove the breasts. The patient was a married woman, age thirty-seven, with two children, the youngest ten years old, both nursed. Three years prior to time of photography, patient discovered a hard lump in outer part of right breast and, three months later, the same in the left breast. Since then both breasts continued to increase in size, but not symmetrically. No pain or soreness reported, but a constant dragging sensation in chest and at times difficulty in breathing. Locomotion and standing position for any length of time prevented by the weight of the breasts. Left breast removed first and the right after an interval of three weeks. Left weighed after removal seventeen pounds and the right forty-three pounds; combined weights sixty pounds. Excellent recovery after each operation. Discharged from the hospital, well, three weeks after second operation. Silver gelatin prints, photographer unidentified, ca. 1893.

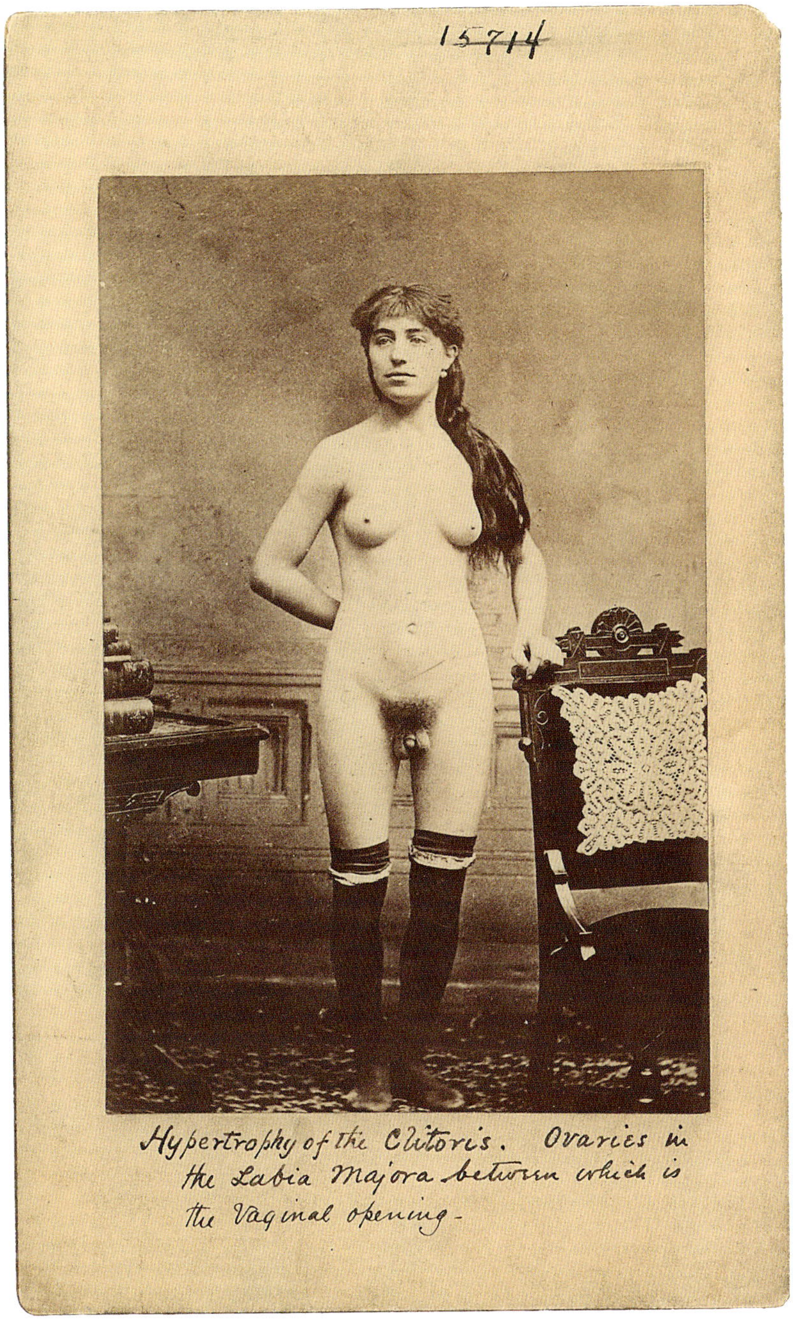

Congenital hypertrophy of the clitoris. Ovaries in the labia majora, between which is the vaginal opening. Photographer and date unidentified.

Precocious sexual development in four-year-old boy. Theodore Scrivener, born September 14, 1848, daguerreotyped September 16, 1852, in Washington, D.C. Scrivener is held in the photograph by Dr. Robert King Stone (1822–1872), professor of physiological anatomy in the National Medical College, and Abraham Lincoln's personal physician, present at Lincoln's deathbed. Stone wrote that Scrivener "was a man in genitals at one year—Daguerreotype bad as well as position but the boy is very restless. . . ." Samples of hair from Scrivener's head and pubes are included in "A collection of specimens of Hair representing Different Nationalities and Different Diseases," mounted and described by Peter Arrell Browne, L.L.D. (1782–1860), presented to the Mütter Museum by Dr. S. Weir Mitchell (1829–1914). A report on the case of Scrivener by Dr. Stone appeared in *The American Journal of the Medical Sciences*, October 1852. Photographer unidentified.

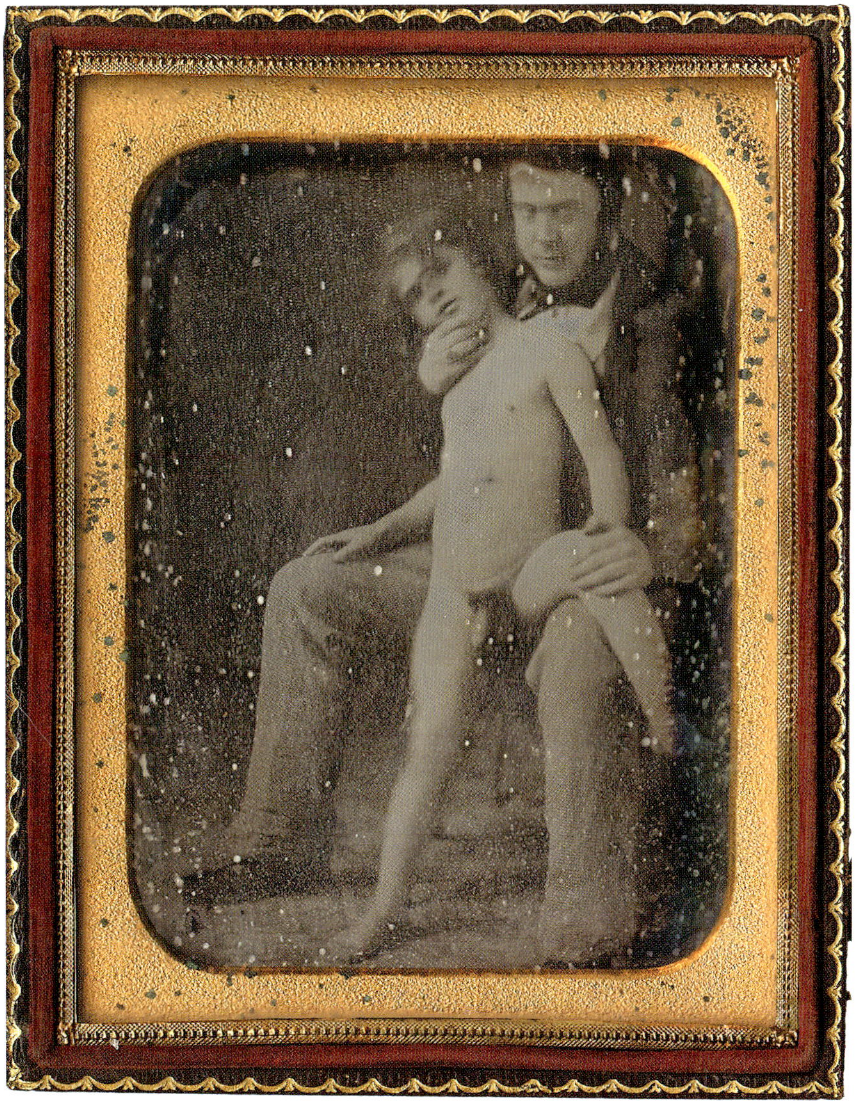

Mr. Chauncey Morlan (1869–1912), also known as The Indiana Fat Boy, age twenty-five, weight 602 pounds, and Mrs. Morlan (1873–1904), also known as Anna Bell, The Fat Wonder, age twenty-two, weight 526 pounds. Married in 1892, Mr. and Mrs. Morlan toured in Europe with the Barnum & Bailey Circus. Photograph by Frank Wendt, Boonton, New Jersey, ca. 1894.

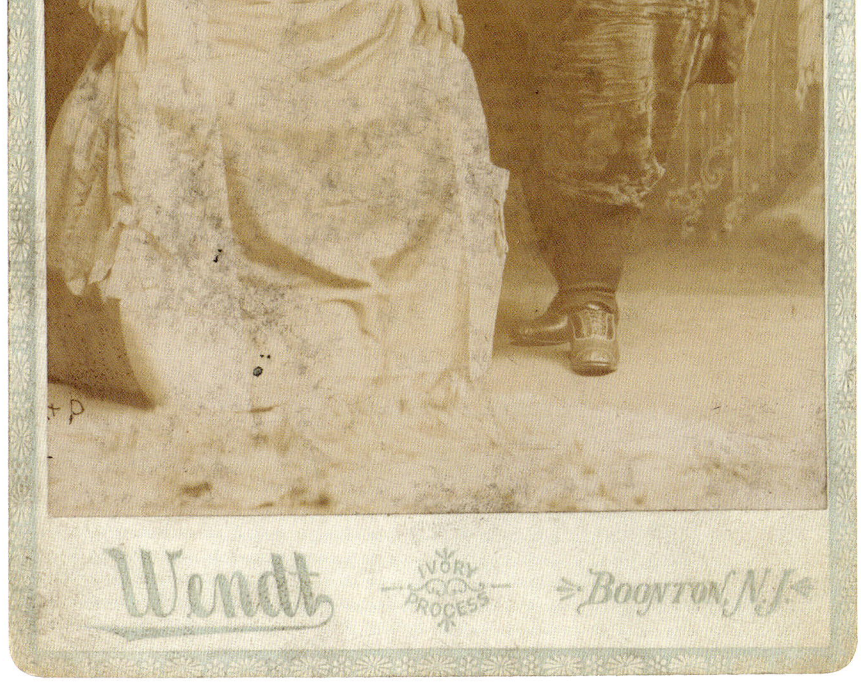
15713.
Wendt
IVORY PROCESS
BOONTON, N.J.

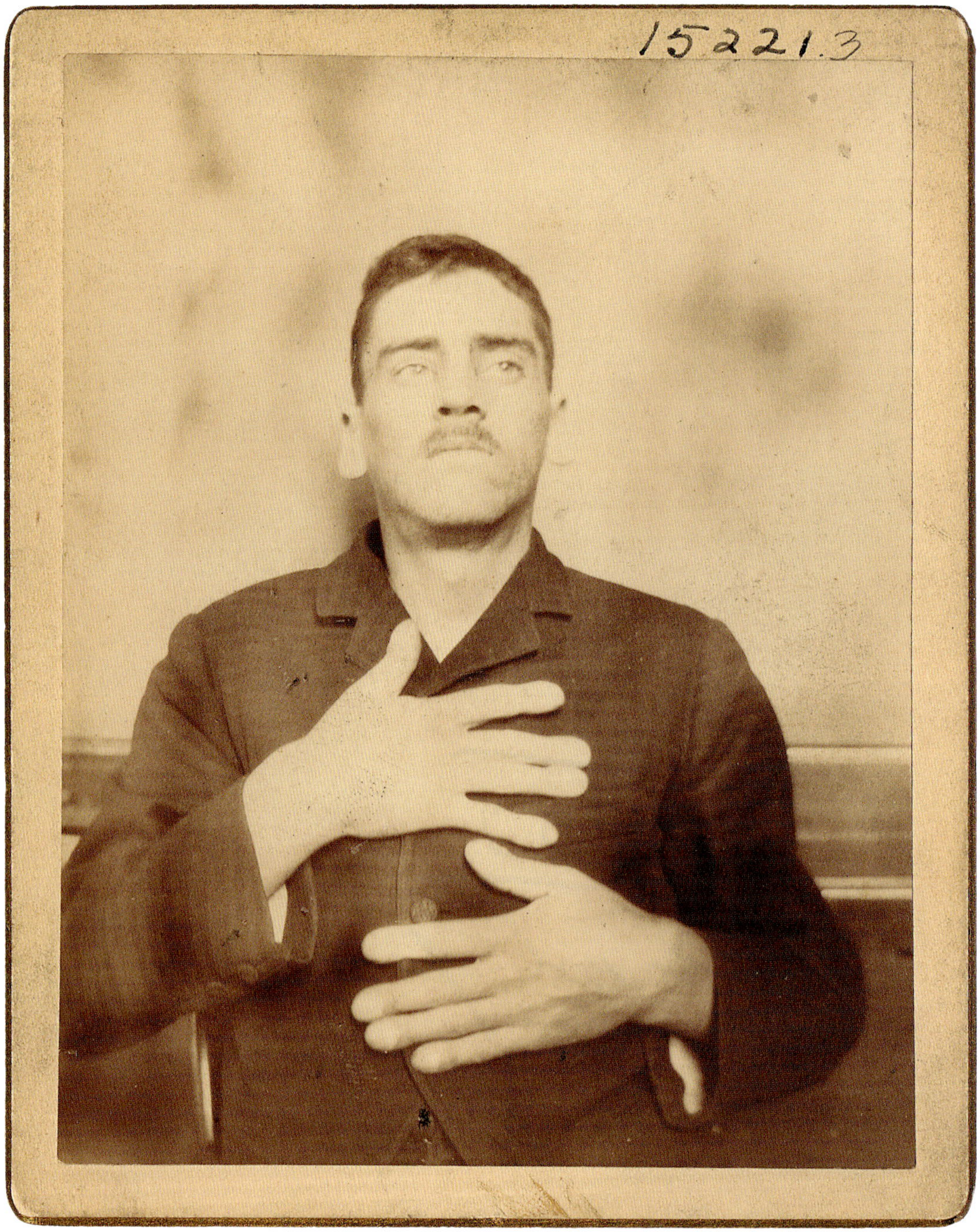

Acromegaly, a hormonal disorder resulting from excess growth hormone (GH) production in the pituitary gland. Acromegaly most commonly occurs in middle-aged adults, with abnormal growth of hands and feet and prominence of mandible among the most common signs. Photographer and date unidentified.

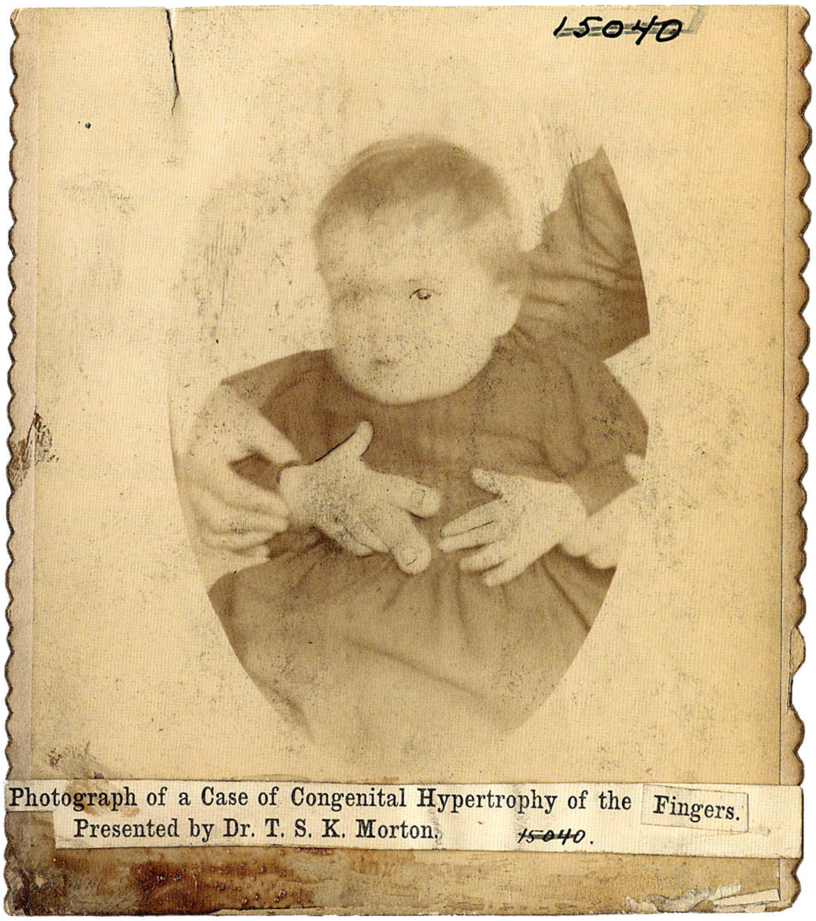
15040
Photograph of a Case of Congenital Hypertrophy of the Fingers.
Presented by Dr. T. S. K. Morton. 15040.

Congenital hypertrophy of the fingers. Donor: Dr. Thomas Story Kirkbride Morton (1865–1930). Photographer and date unidentified.

Mütter Museum giant, photographed June 24, 1941, by Dr. Charles D. Humberd (1897–1960) of Barnard, Missouri, June 24, 1941, from an album of photographs and newspaper clippings of giants and acromegalic cases compiled 1942 by Dr. Joseph McFarland (1868–1945), curator of the Mütter Museum.

The skeleton of the Mütter Museum giant is that of a male, estimated to be aged between twenty-two and twenty-four, and approximately 7' 6" tall. The curvature of the spine (kyphoscoliosis) has decreased the potential height. The skeleton was acquired in 1877 from Professor A. E. Foote, a purveyor of anatomic preparations to museums and medical schools, at a cost of $50. It had been on display at the Academy of Natural Sciences in Philadelphia, and Professor Joseph Leidy (1823–1891) suggested its purchase. Nothing was known of its history except that it came from Kentucky; the terms of the sale specified that no questions were to be asked that might lead to its identification. It is the second tallest human skeleton on display in the world, the tallest being that of Charles Byrne in the Royal College of Surgeons of England, which is 7' 7".

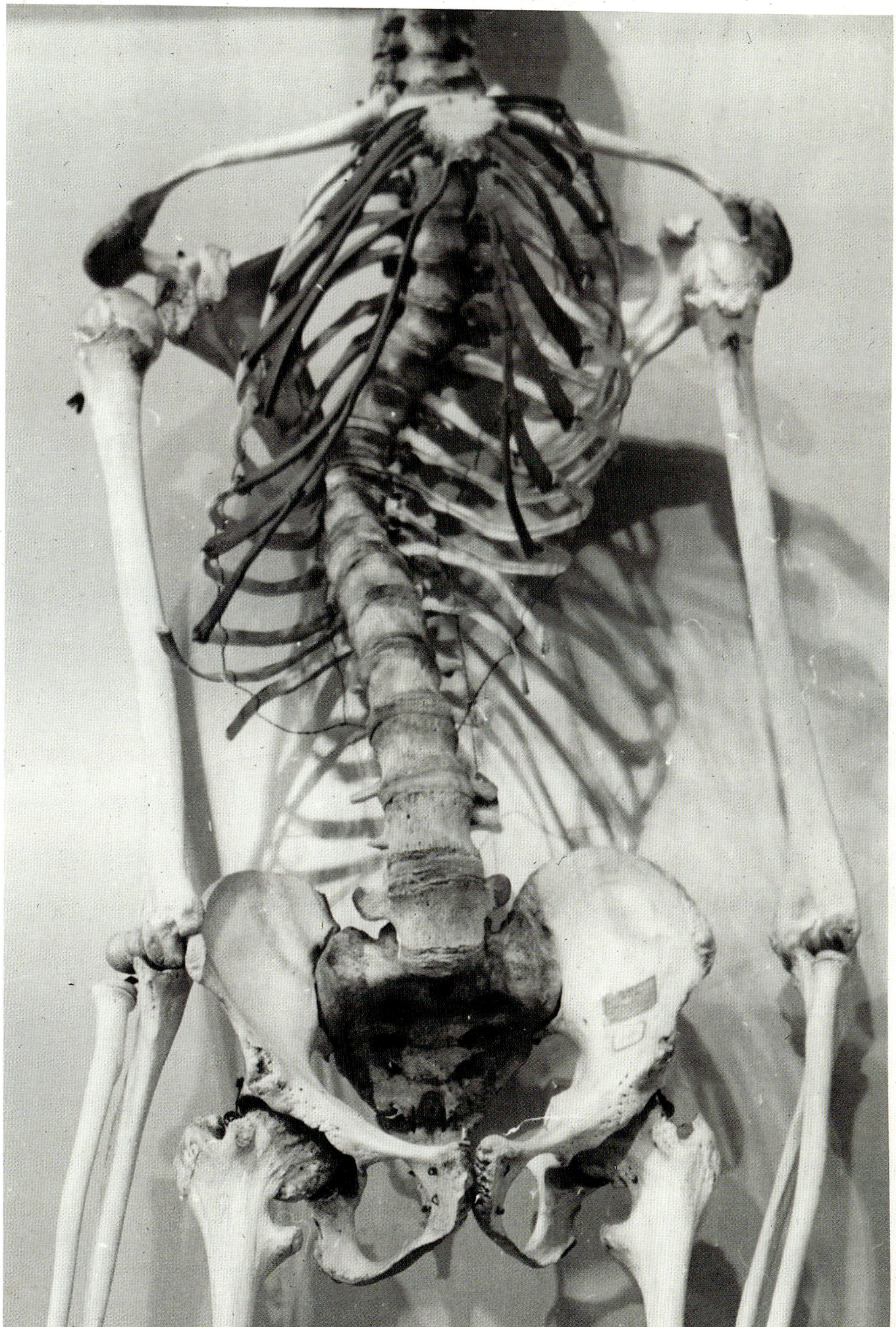

Mütter Museum Giant June 24, 1941

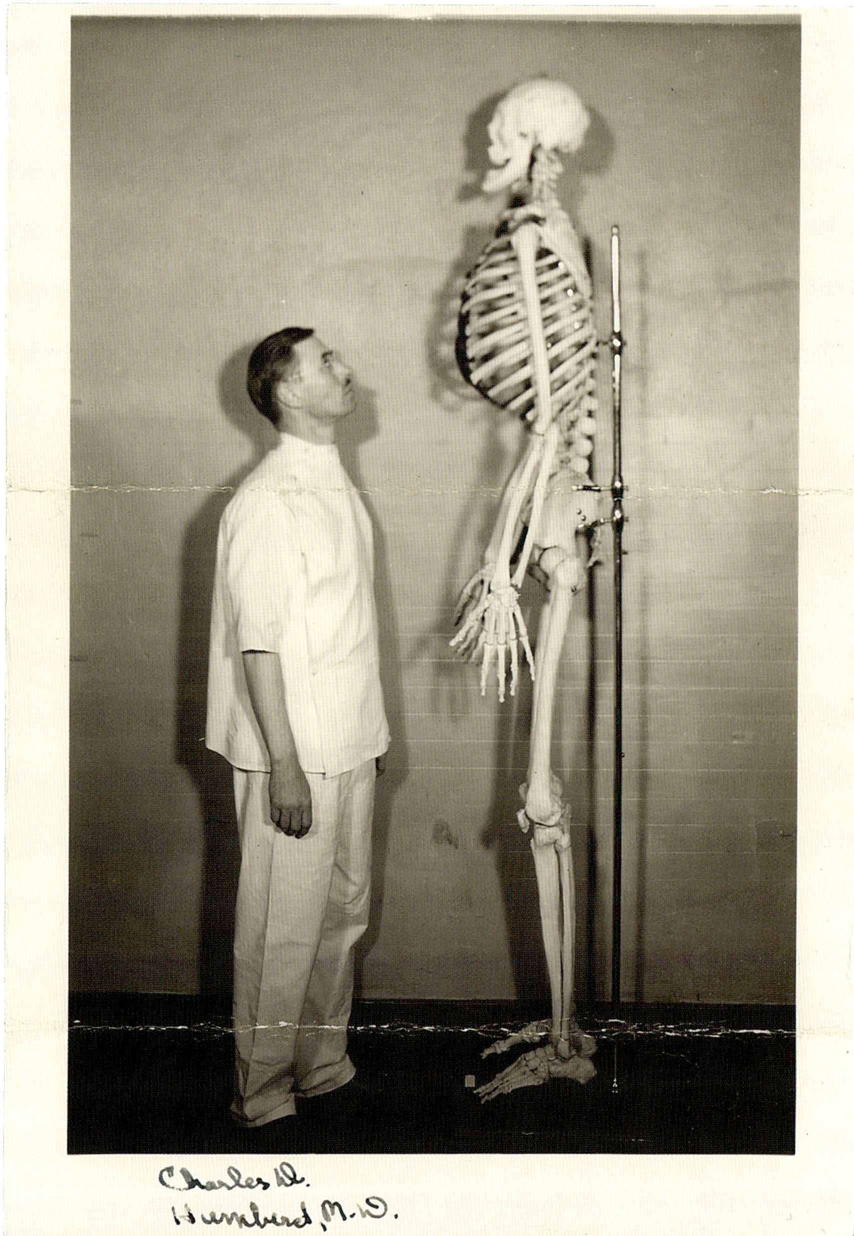

ABOVE: Skeleton of John Aasen (1890–1938), former circus giant and Hollywood movie actor. Aasen was cast as "Colosso" by Hal Roach in the 1923 film *Why Worry?* starring Harold Lloyd. The film was one of the biggest box-office attractions of 1923. Skeleton in the possession of Dr. Charles D. Humberd (1897–1960) (photographed with Aasen's skeleton) at the time the photograph was made is described as 214 cm (7' ¼") in height. From an album of photographs and newspaper clippings of giants and acromegalic cases compiled 1942 by Dr. Joseph McFarland (1868–1945), curator of the Mütter Museum.

OPPOSITE: Stanley Rosinski, Tommy Lowe, Dr. Charles D. Humberd, and Henry M. Mullins (1915–?), photographed December 30, 1939, from an album of photographs and newspaper clippings of giants and acromegalic cases compiled 1942 by Dr. Joseph McFarland. Henry M. Mullins measured 7' 6¾" and weighed 280 pounds. Humberd reported of Mullins, who had been on the stage and in movies (*The Sideshow Mystery*, 1932), "It is indeed amazing to watch so vast a personage doing a whirlwind acrobatic act.... He dances, fast and furiously, and engages in a comedy knock-about 'business' that would be found strenuous by any trained 'Physical culturist.'... He is alert, intelligent, well read, affable and friendly."

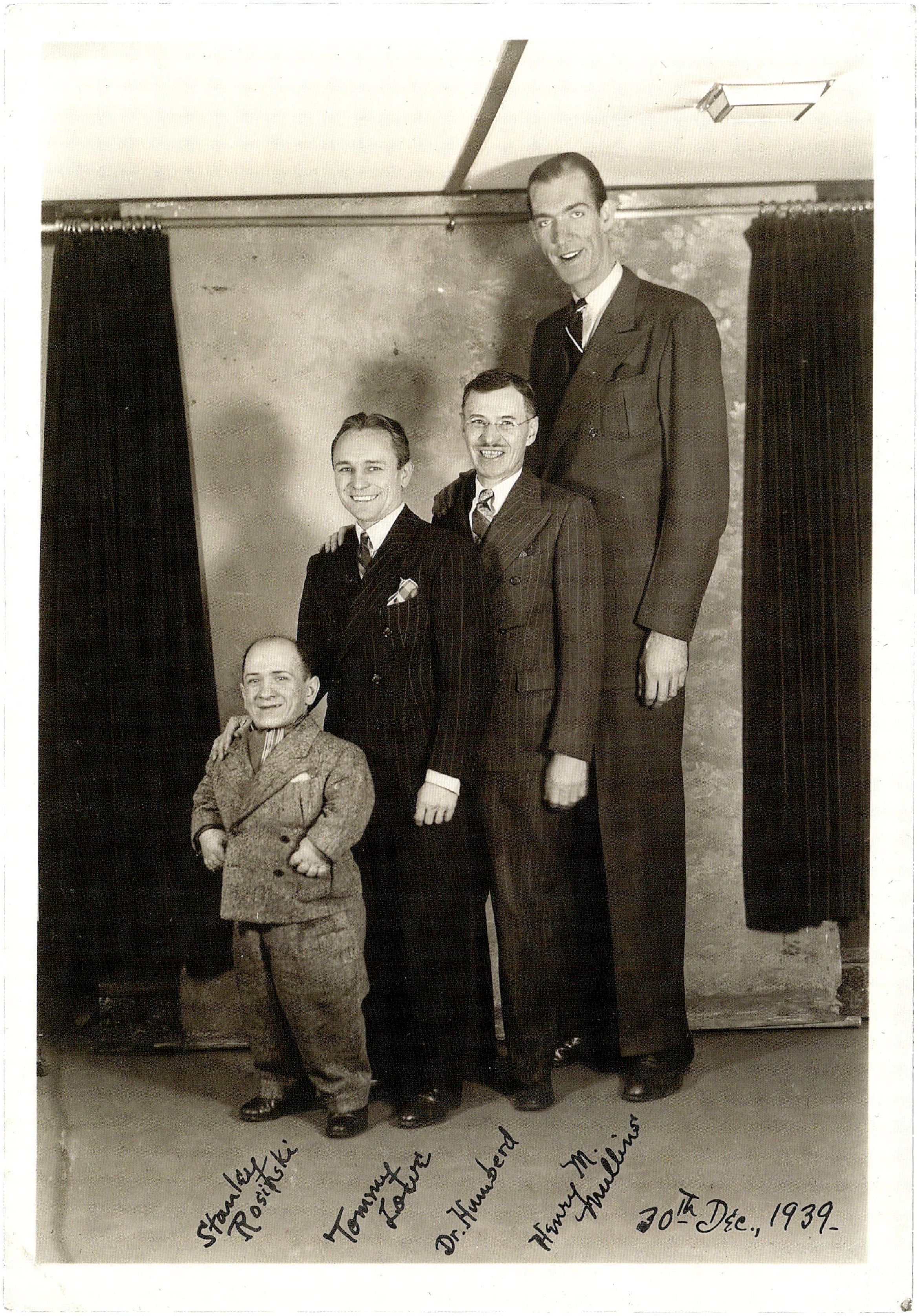
Stanley
Dr. Humberd
Henry M. Mullins
30th Dec., 1939

Congenital Deformity, Deficiency, and Disorder

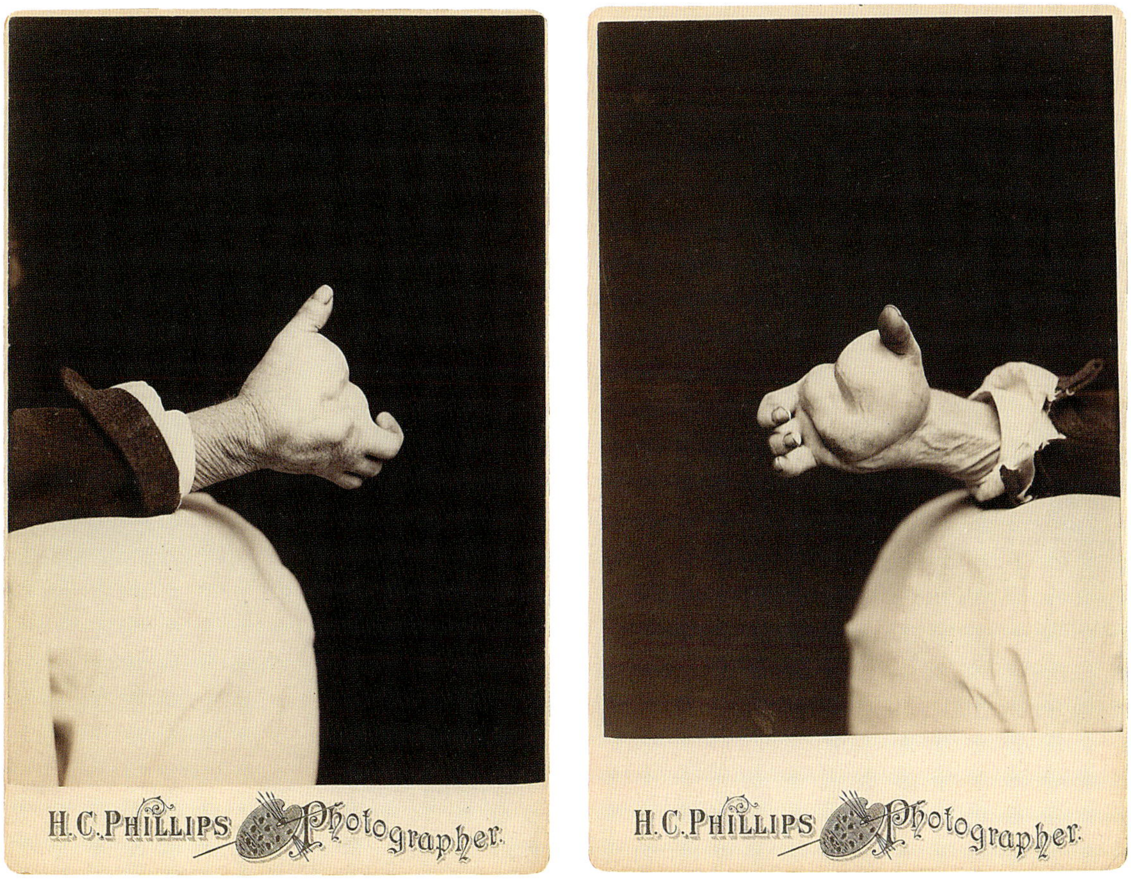

Congenital deformity of the hand. Albumen print, photographed by Henry C. Phillips, Philadelphia, ca. 1869 or 1882–90.

Varicose veins of the right hand, forearm, arm, shoulder, and upper part of the right side of the chest. Inscription on photograph: "John Aldrich, aged sixty-one, soldier during the late war, has been affected with varicose enlargement of the veins of the upper extremity, shoulder, and chest for many years. The enlargement and varicosity are enormous and no doubt of congenital origin. The lower extremities are free from vein disease. The left upper extremity is affected in a very slight degree. The man in other respects is healthy and suffers no special inconvenience from the enlargement." Photographer unidentified, clinical case September 1877.

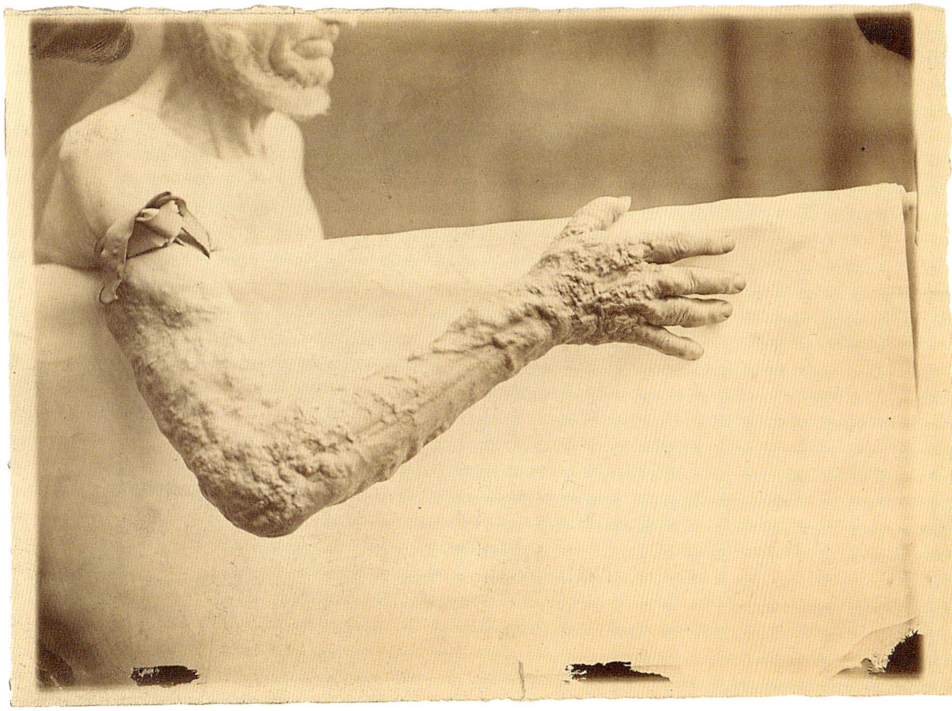

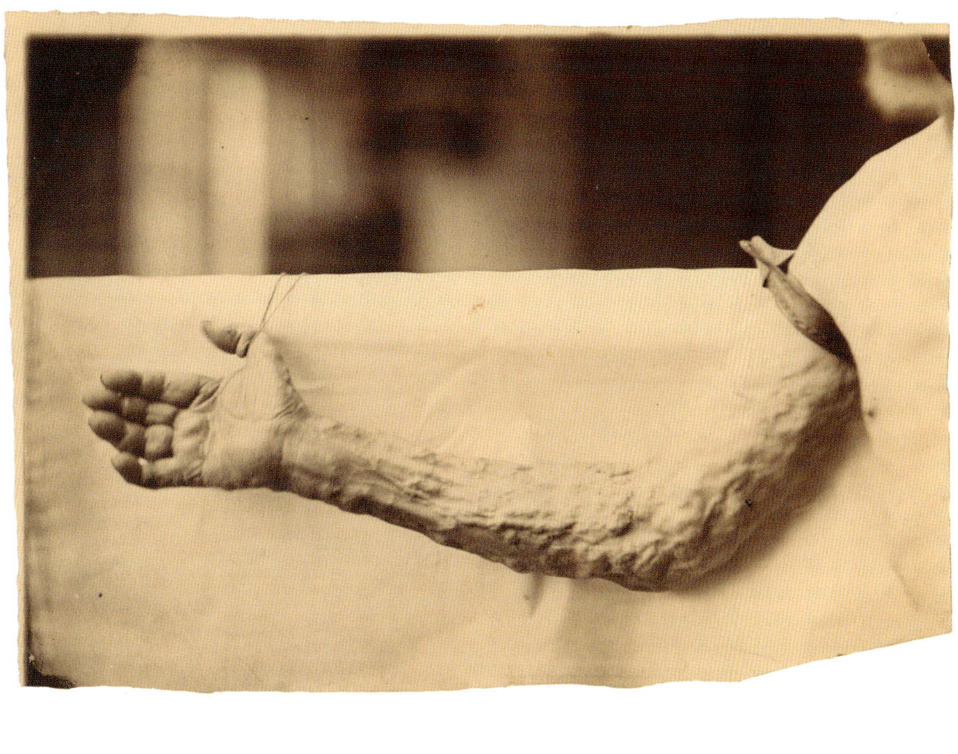

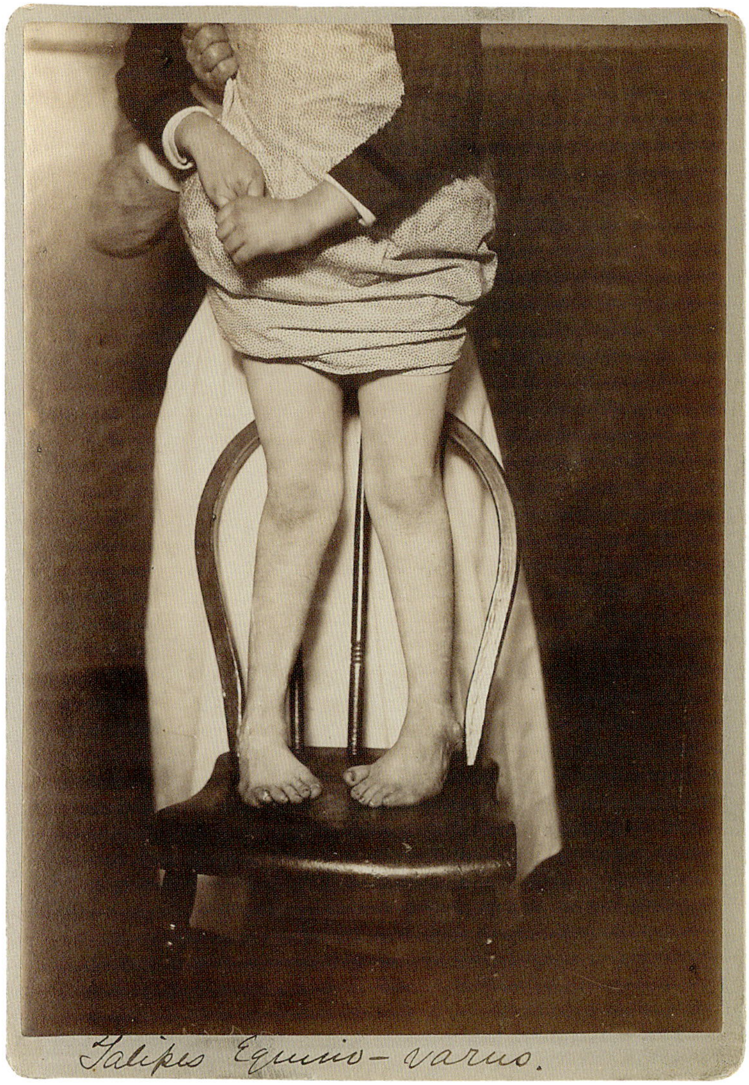

Talipes equino varus, corrected by multiple tenotomies. Patient of DeForest Willard, M.D. (1846–1919). Dr. Willard pioneered in the specialty of orthopedic surgery, delivering the first course of lectures in the subject at the University of Pennsylvania, 1887. Albumen print, photographed by John R. Laughlin, Philadelphia, ca. 1869–91.

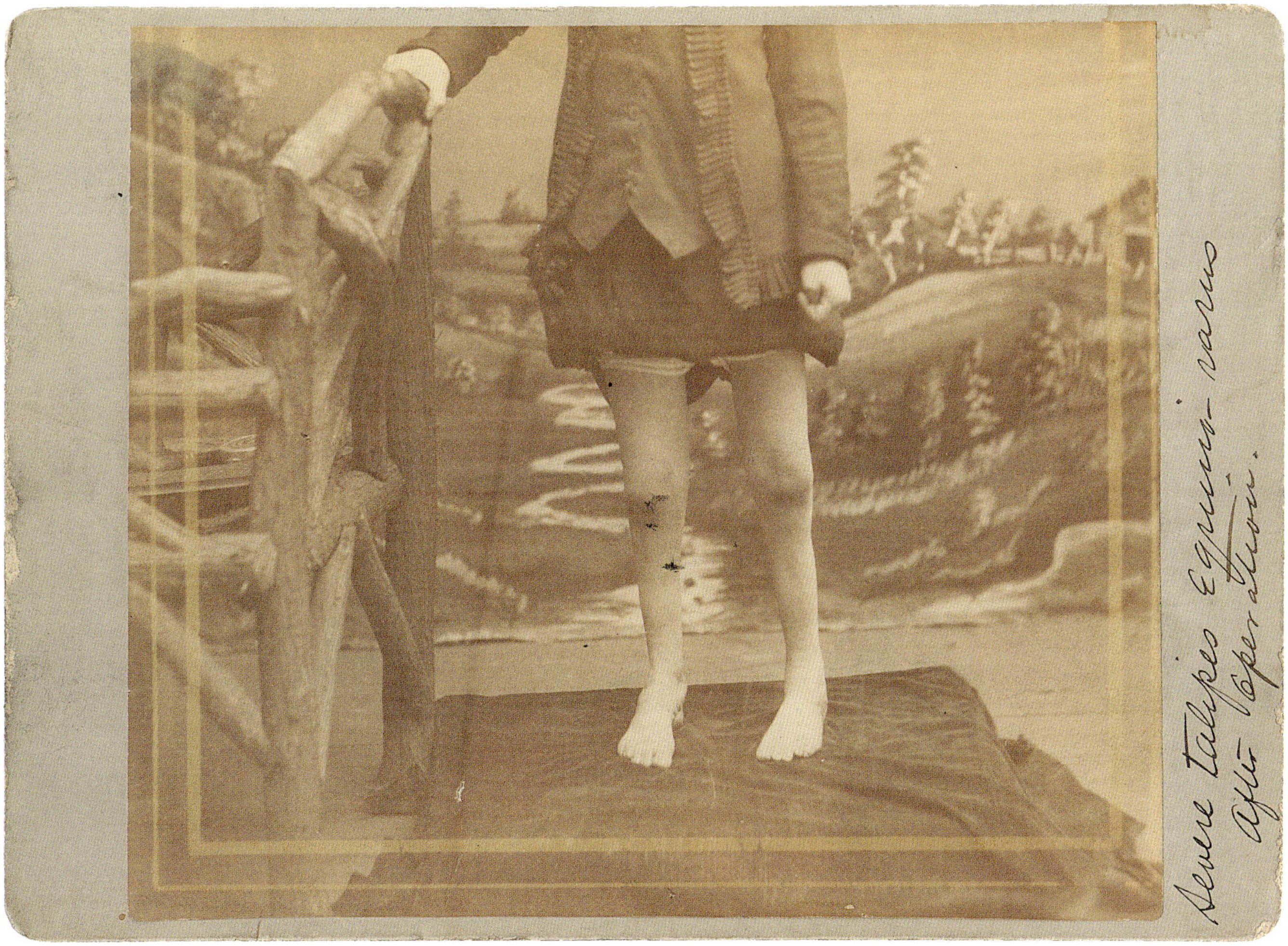

Severe talipes equino varus, after multiple tenotomies operation. Patient of Dr. DeForest Willard. Photograher and date unidentified.

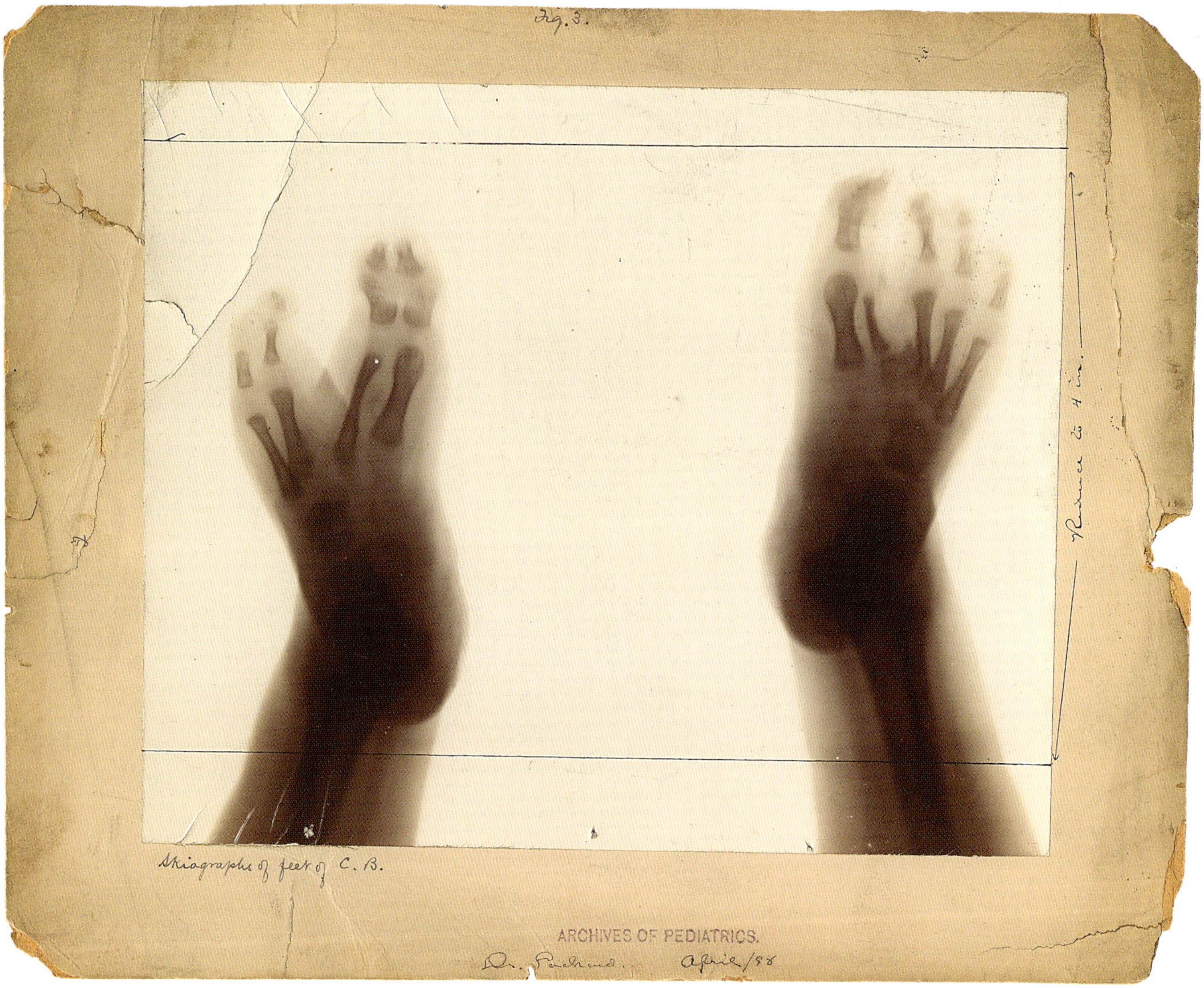

ABOVE: Skiagraph of feet of C. B., a four-year-old mentally deficient boy of premature birth, one of only three surviving of fourteen born to the mother. Reported by Frederick A. Packard, M.D. (1864–1902), in *Archives of Pediatrics*, April 1898. Dr. Packard noted that although the explanation of such defective formations was one of great difficulty, he attributed them to a defect of germ or sperm, foetal vascular disease, or destructive pressure by the umbilical cord or adventitious intrauterine bands and rejected the maternal impression theory in dispute at the time. Radiograph by J. C. Starbuck, M.D.

OPPOSITE: Congenital deformity of feet. Albumen print, photographed by Henry C. Phillips, Philadelphia, ca. 1869 or 1882–90.

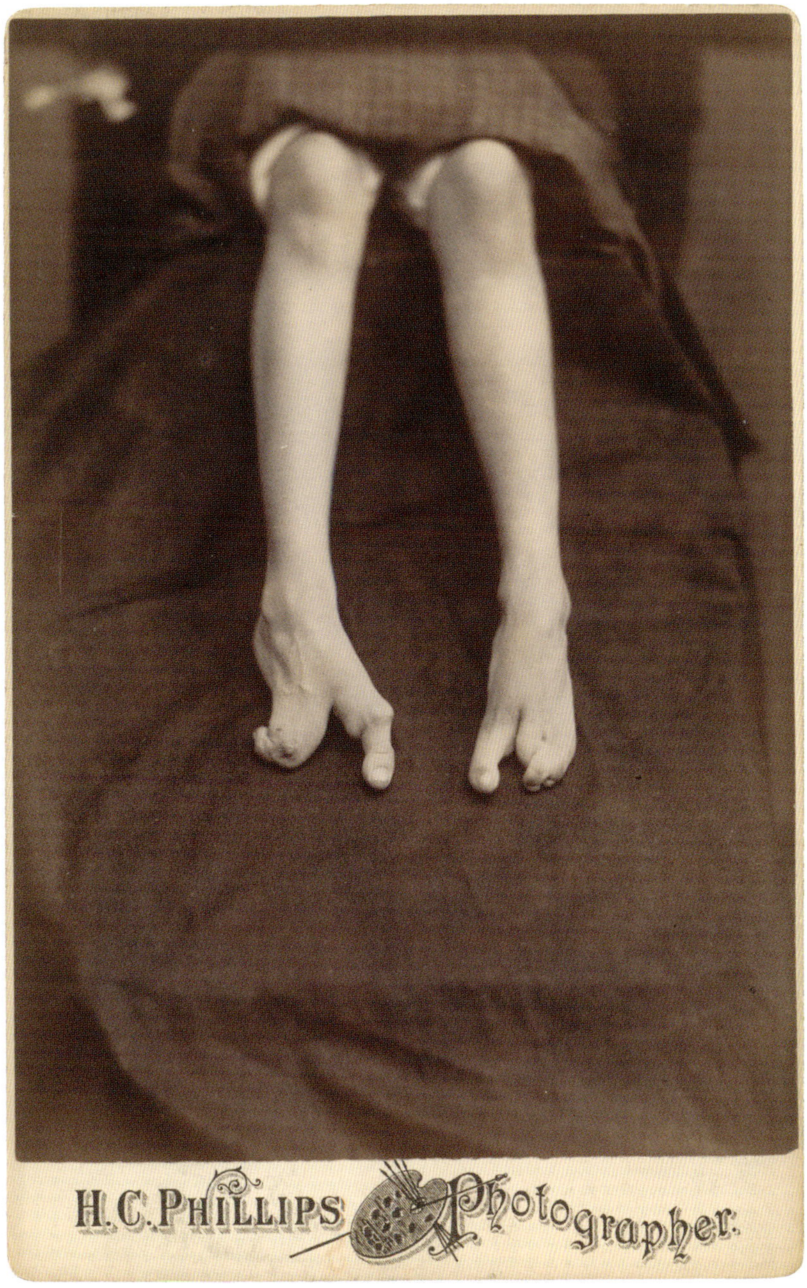
H. C. PHILLIPS Photographer.

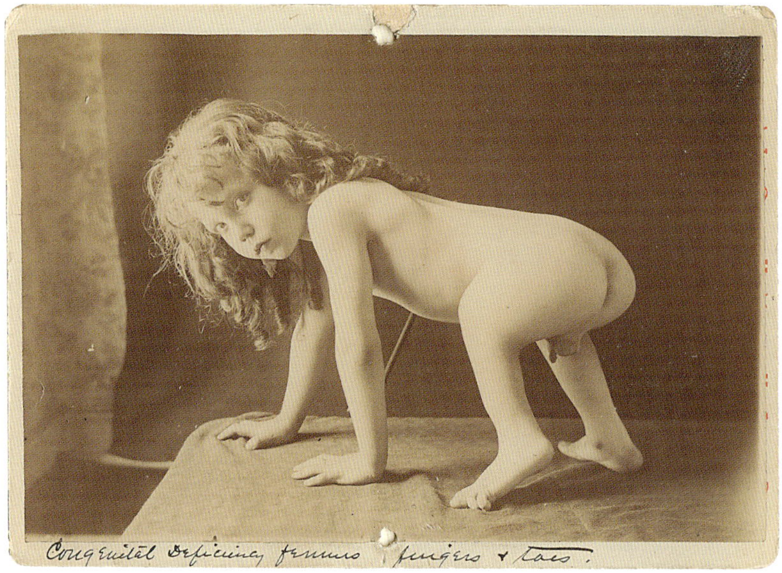

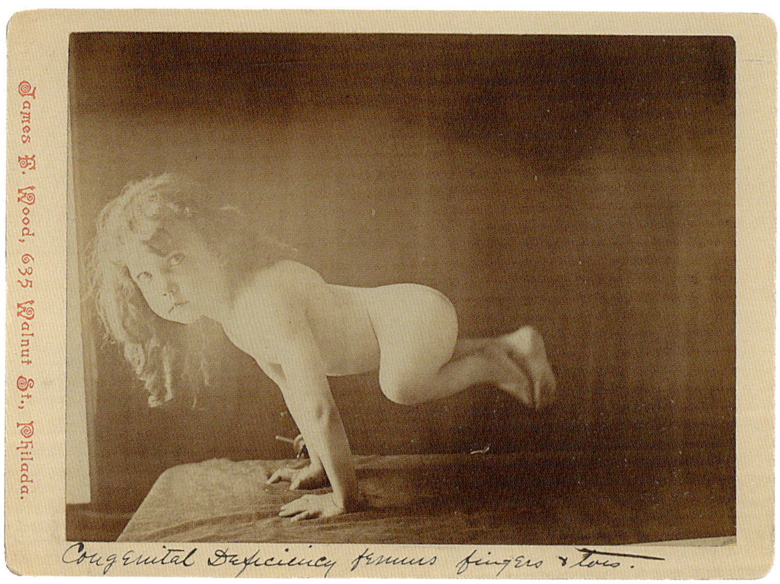

ABOVE AND OPPOSITE: Case of congenital deficiency of the femurs, fingers, and toes. Patient of Dr. DeForest Willard (1846–1910). Photograph by James F. Wood, Philadelphia, ca. 1892–1900.

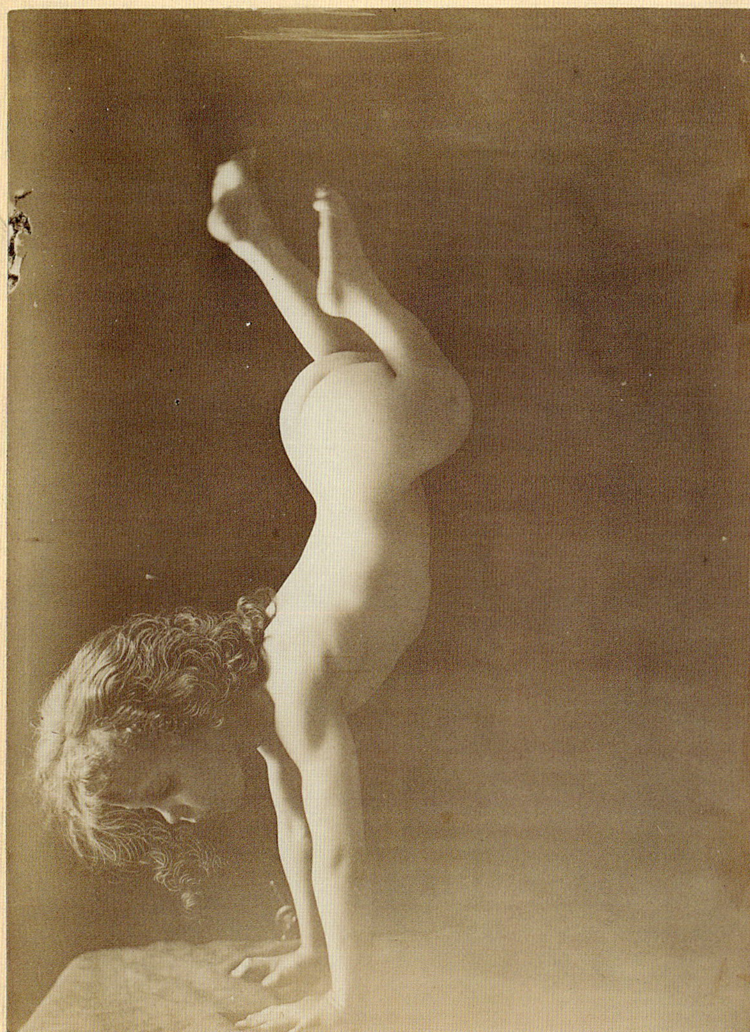

Congenital Deficiency femurs fingers & toes.

James F. Wood, 635 Walnut St., Philada.

Congenital deficiency of the bones of the hand, fingers absent. Skiagraphs by Edward Pennock, optician, Philadelphia. Lower photograph accompanied article by Dr. DeForest Willard (1846–1910) in *Transactions of American Surgical Association*, vol. 14, 1896. Donor: DeForest Willard, M.D.

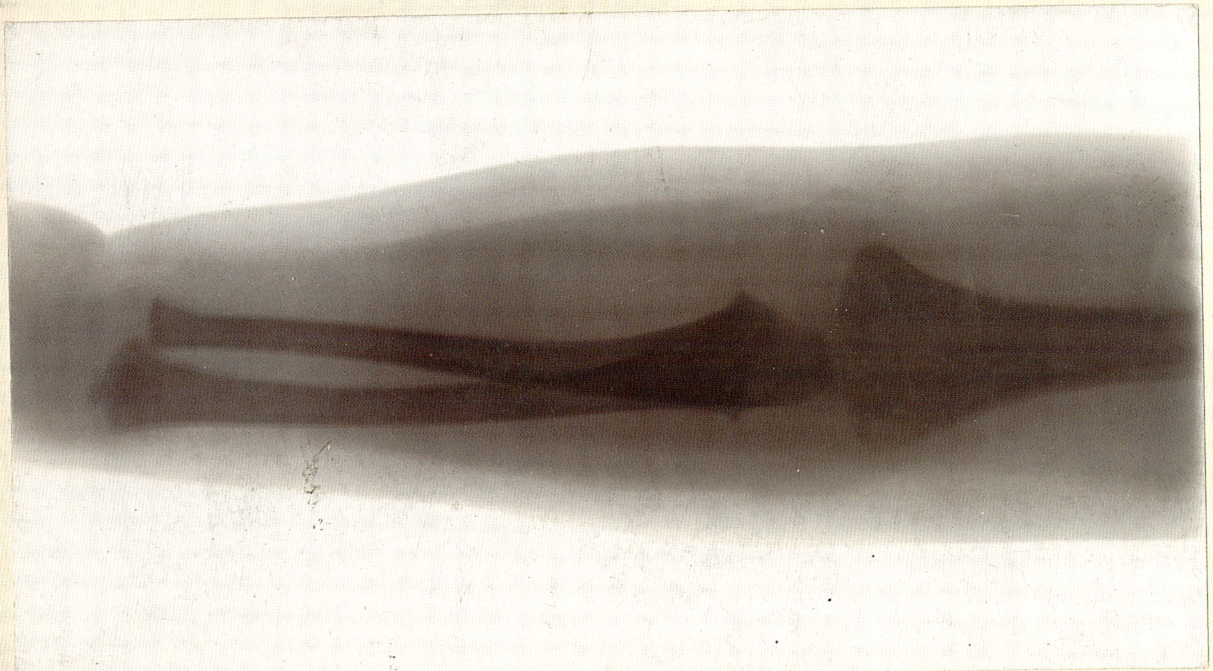

Cong. Deficiency bones of hand. Fingers absent.

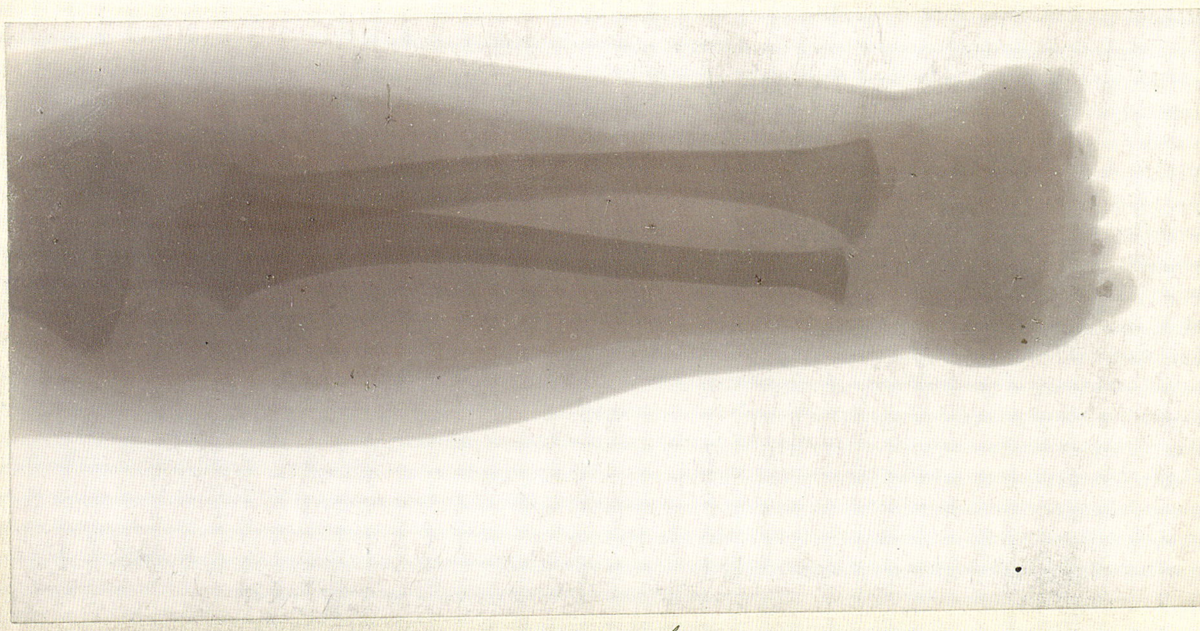

Cong. Deficiency bones of hand. Fingers absent.

Presented by Dr. Willard.

Epispadias, a congential defect in which the urethra opens upon the upper surface of the penis (note origin of urinary stream). This condition may also be associated with bladder malformation (fissure). Herold Alfont, age approximately twelve, July 25, 1905. Inscription on photograph reports boy retains urine for two hours. Silver gelatin print, photographer unidentified.

27.C.

No 3.

Epispadia with fissure of neck of bladder.
Fissure of pelvis.
Boy retains urine for two hours.

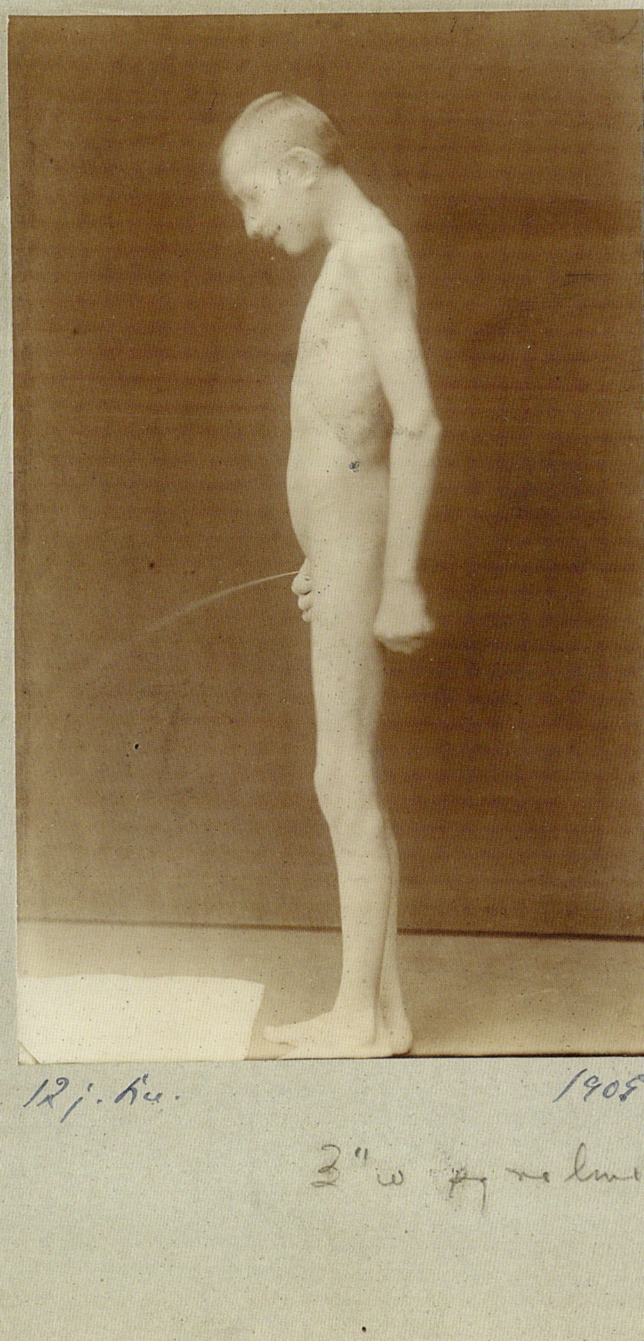

5

12 j. Ku.

1905

3" w [illegible]

Dipygus tripus (parasitic twin), case of Blanche Dumas [mislabeled on photographs as "Dumont"], born 1860. Photo left by A. Liebert, right by Pierre Petit, Paris. Inscription on photograph notes: "Pelvis so broad a pelvimeter cannot span it." An illustration of Dumas was published in Part IV (page 168) of the collection of pictures of congenital abnormalities that form the basis of the four-volume atlas *Human Monstrosities*, by Barton Cooke Hirst (1861–1935) and George Arthur Piersol (1856–1924), published 1891–93. Blanche Dumas also appears in *Anomalies and Curiosities of Medicine* (1896) by George Milbury Gould (1848–1922) and Walter Lytle Pyle (1871–1921).

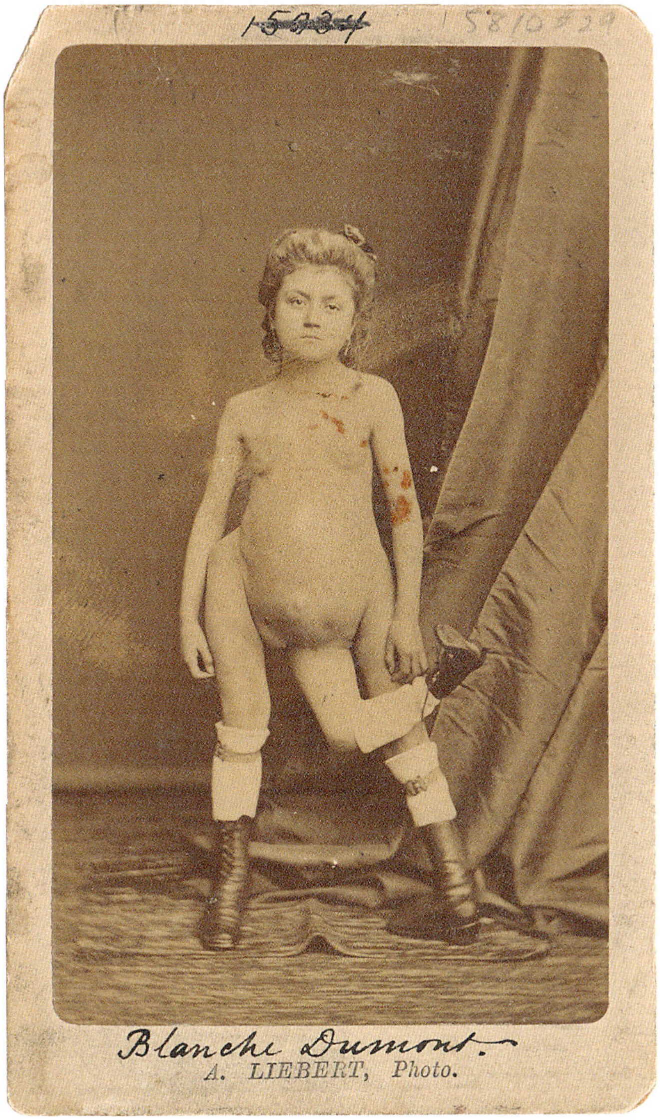
~~15034~~ 15810#29
Blanche Dumont.
A. LIEBERT, Photo.

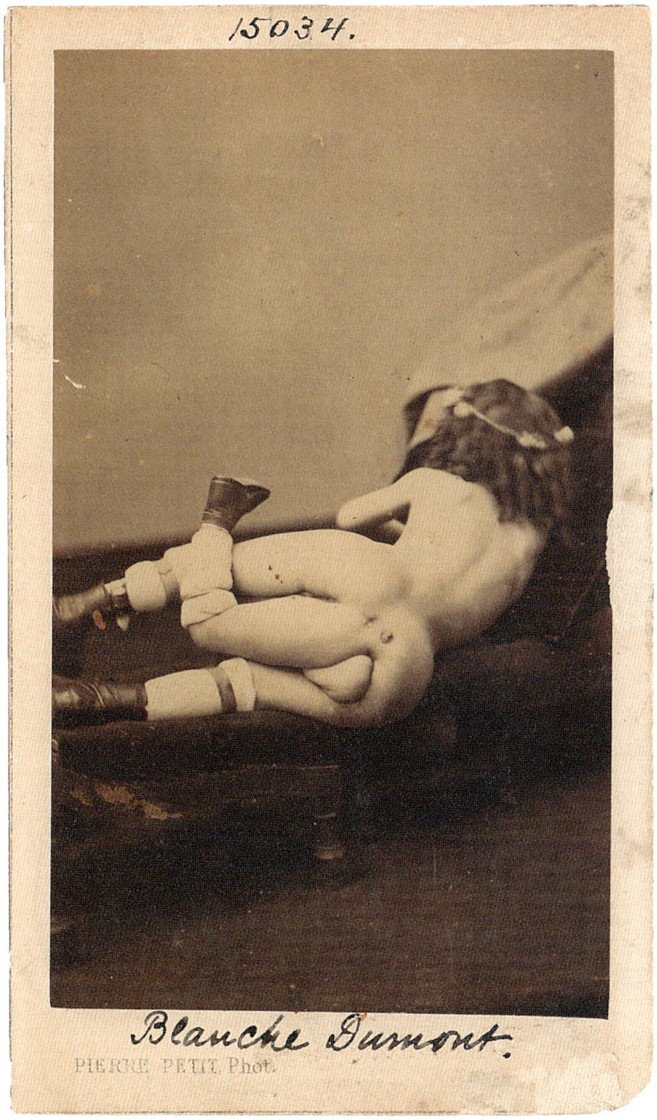
15034.
Blanche Dumont.
PIERRE PETIT, Phot.

Case of amelus (congenital absence of one or more limbs), Albert Pilgrim, age about one year at time of photograph; inscription on back of photograph reports Pilgrim was about four years old as of September 29, 1885. Photograph by H. Frank Beidel, Shippensburg, Pennsylvania, ca. 1882.

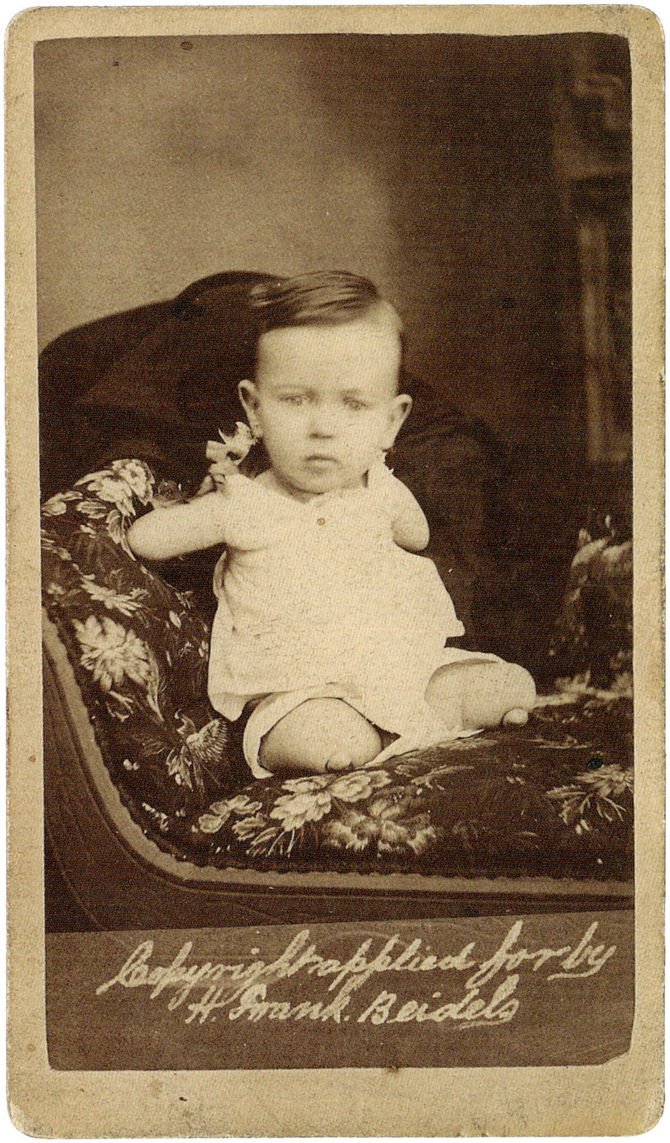
Copyright applied for by
H. Frank. Beidels

Paralysis

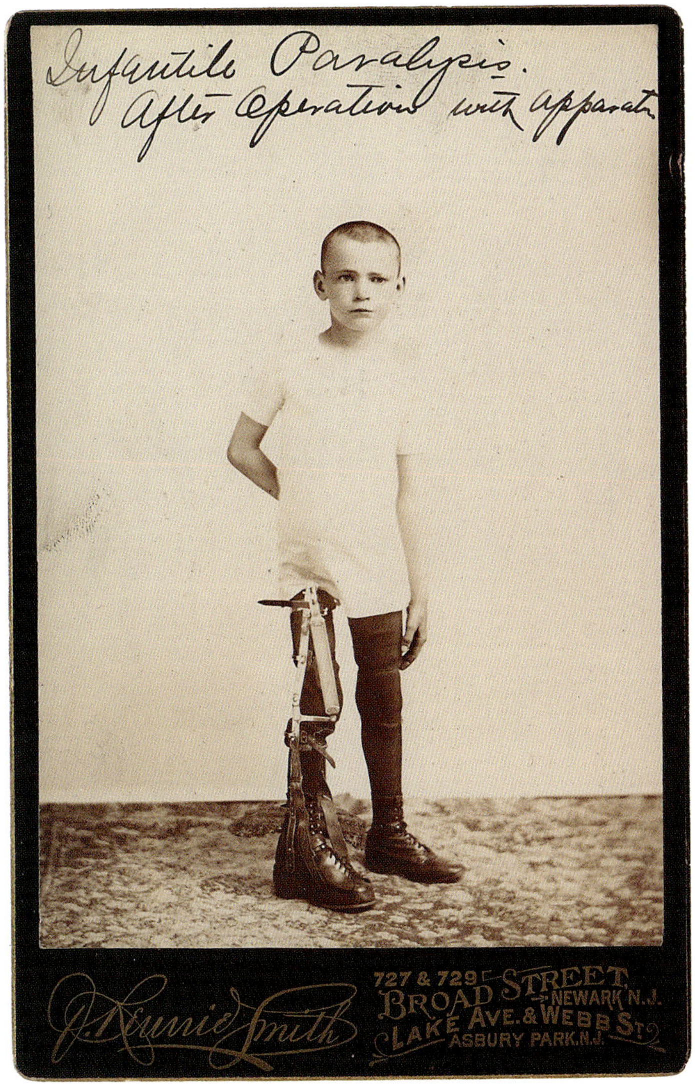

Infantile paralysis (polio) after operation, with apparatus (leg brace). Photograph by J. Rennie Smith, Newark and Asbury Park, New Jersey, ca. 1880s. Donor: Dr. DeForest Willard (1846–1910).

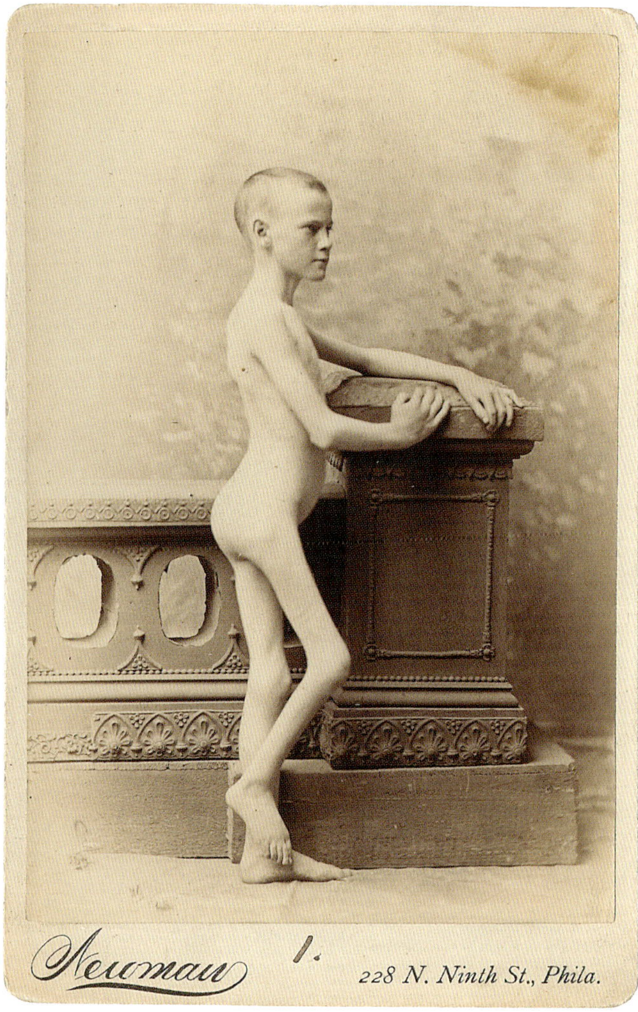

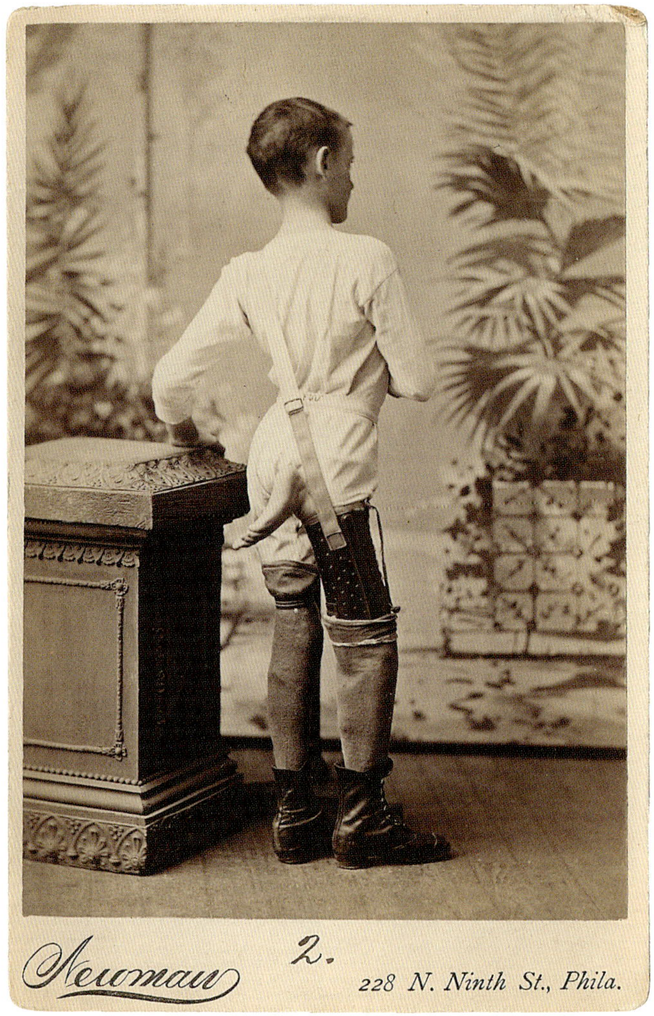

ABOVE AND OPPOSITE: Case of paralytic deformity (polio) before and after treatment with artificial limb manufactured by D. W. Kolbe & Son, Philadelphia. Patient of Dr. Thomas George Morton (1835–1903), a founder of and surgeon at the Orthopedic Hospital and Infirmary for Nervous Diseases, Philadelphia. Albumen prints, photographs by A. Newman, Philadelphia, ca. 1879–88.

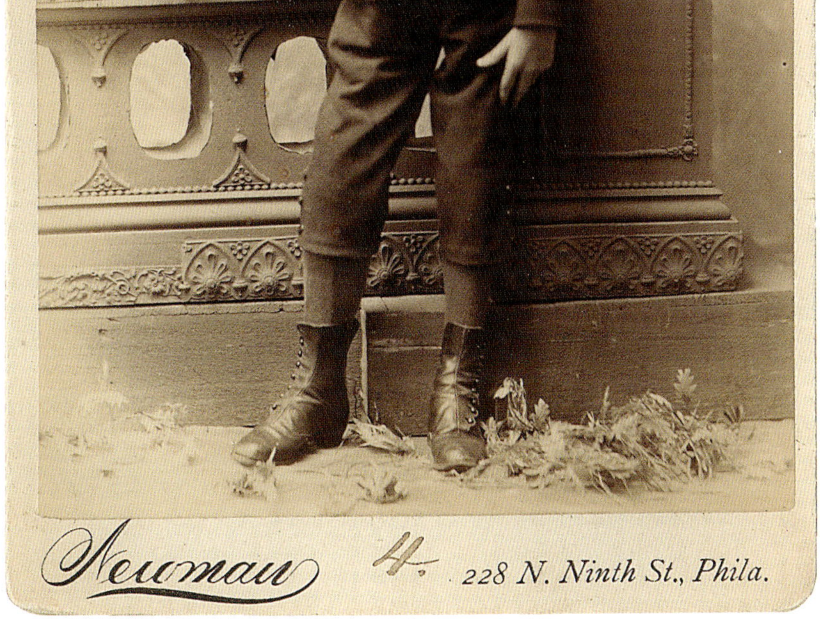
Newman
228 N. Ninth St., Phila.

Wheeled crutch for infantile paralysis (polio). Photographer and date unidentified. Donor: Dr. DeForest Willard (1846–1910).

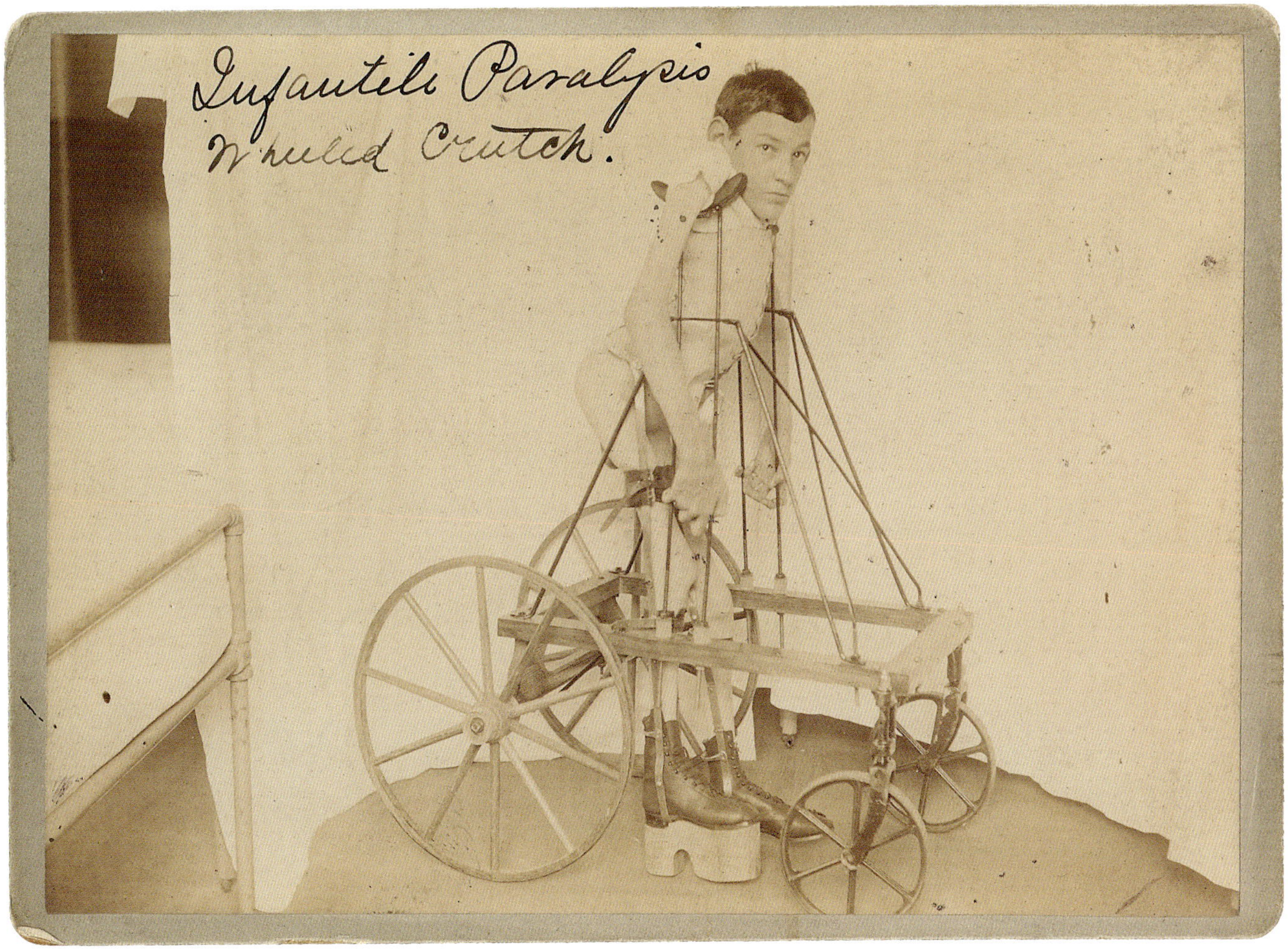
Infantile Paralysis
Wheeled Crutch.

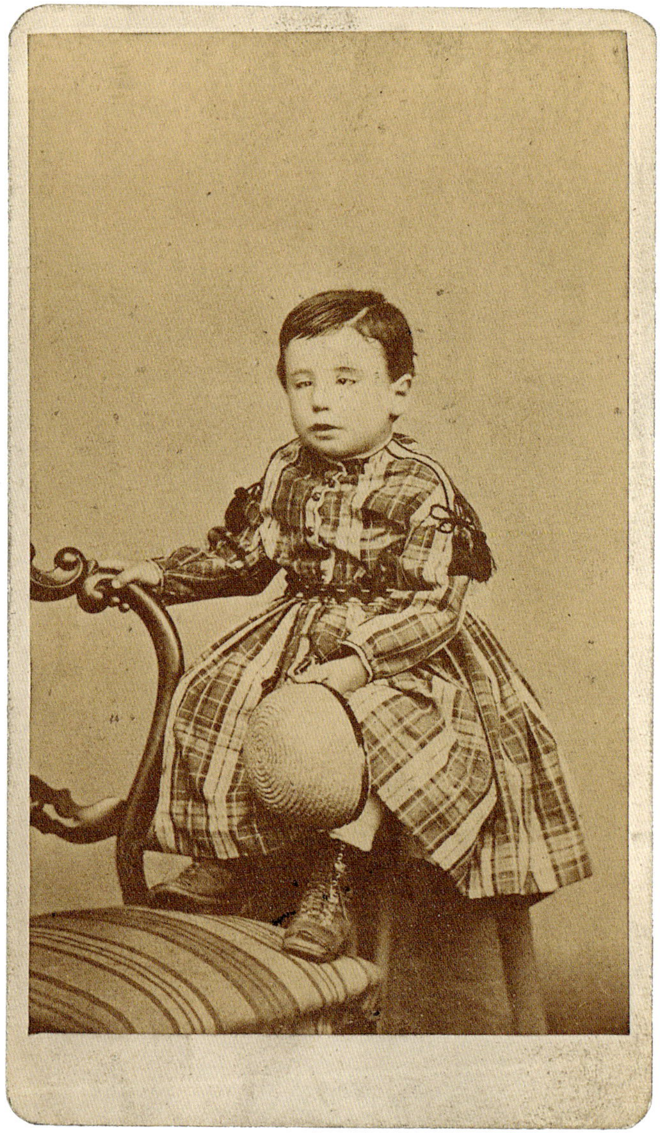

ABOVE AND OPPOSITE: Case of congenital complete bilateral paralysis of the abducent (sixth) and seventh facial nerves. Paralysis of the abducent nerve causes inward turning of the eye leading to double vision. Photographed above as a boy by Samuel Broadbent and Henry C. Phillips, Philadelphia, ca. 1870–80, and opposite as a man, photographer and date unidentified. Donor: Dr. George C. Harlan (1835–1909).

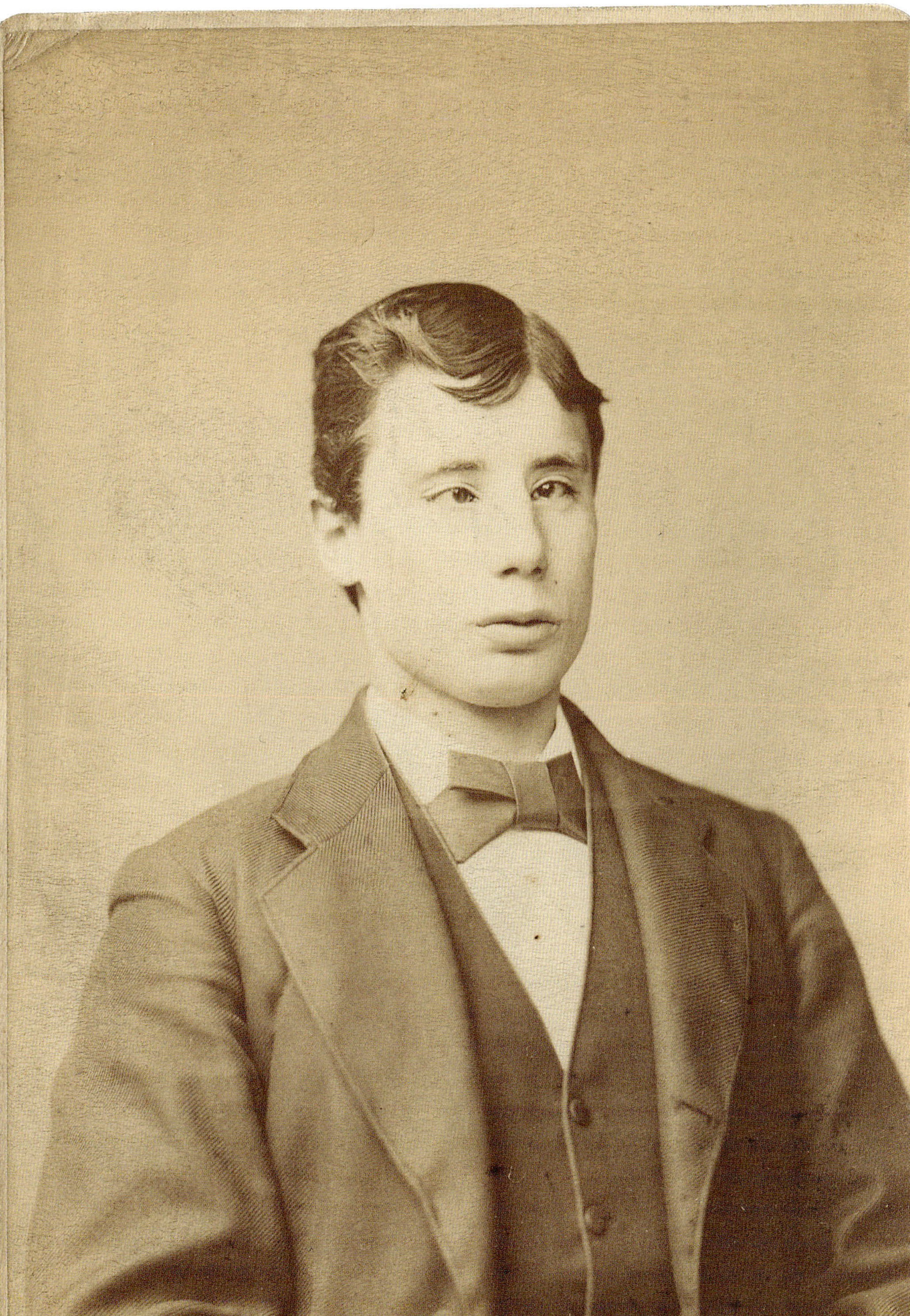

Photographs of a case of complete bilateral paralysis of the sixth and seventh nerves. Dr. Harlan.

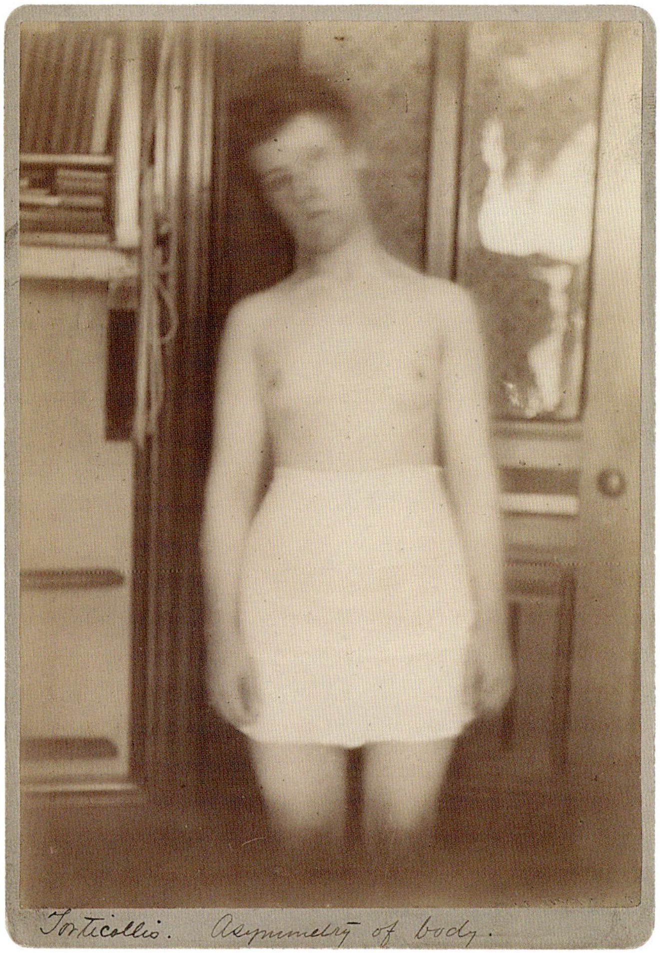

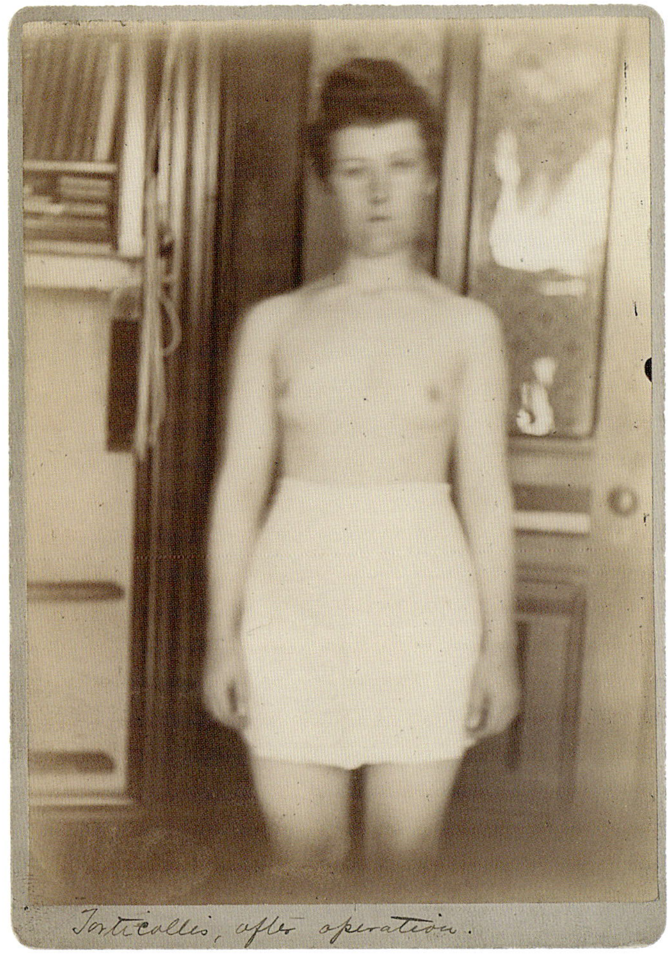

ABOVE: Lateral curavature from torticollis (also known as wryneck), asymmetry of body, caused by spasm of the sternocleidomastoid muscle. Photographed before and after operation. Photographer and date unidentified. Donor: Dr. DeForest Willard (1846–1910).

OPPOSITE: Torticollis. Photographed by Harry Phillips, Atlantic City, New Jersey, ca. 1878–97.

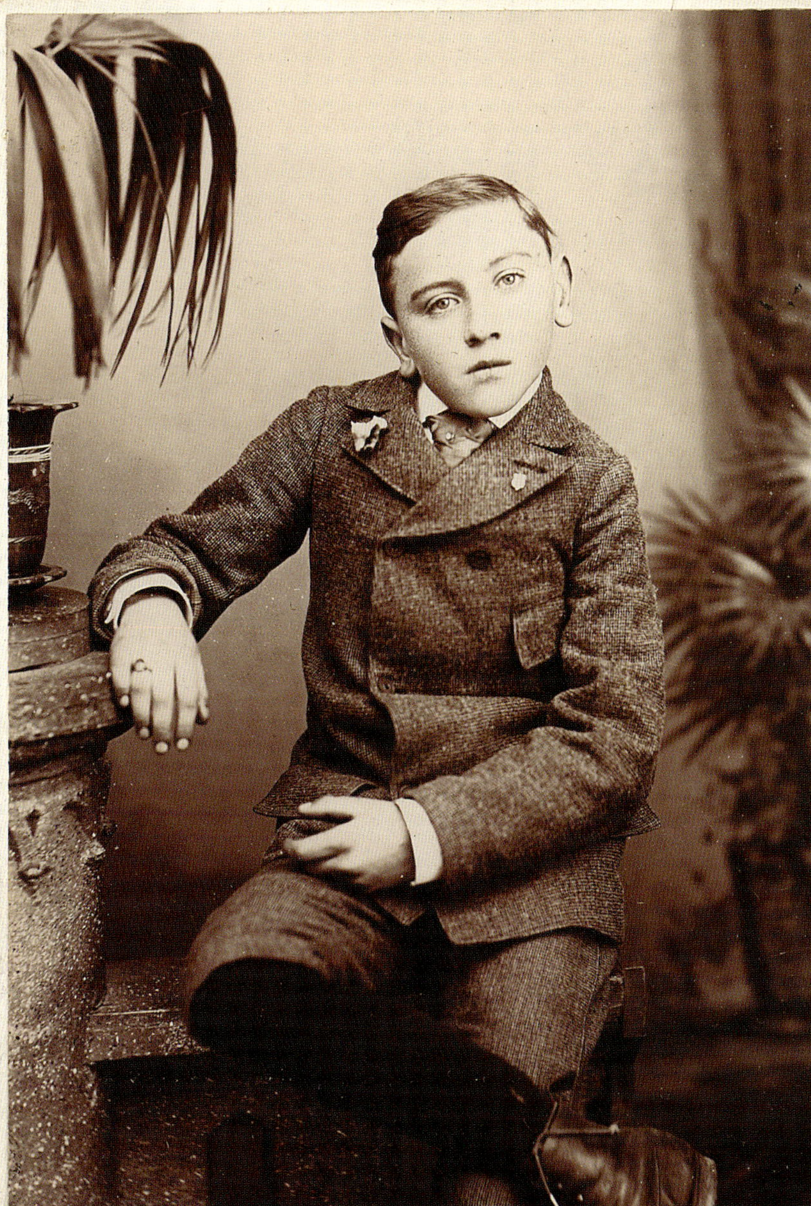

Harry Phillips PHOTO Bet. Kentucky & Illinois Aves ATLANTIC CITY, N. J.

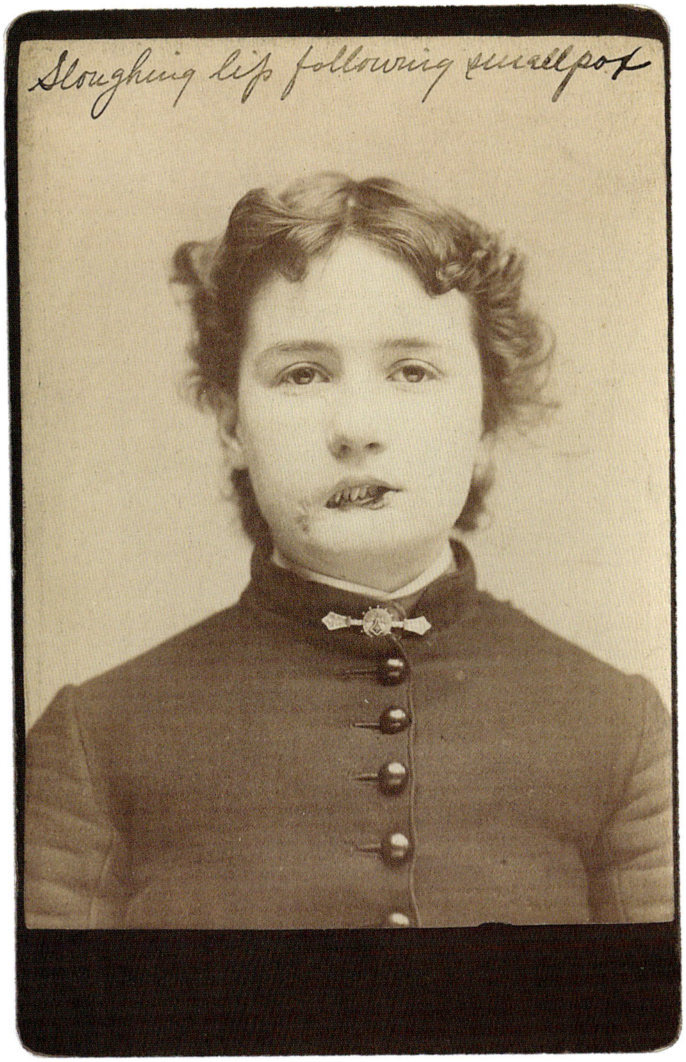

Sloughing lip following smallpox. The smallpox virus commonly caused extensive facial scarring in survivors. Photographer and date unidentified. Donor: Dr. DeForest Willard (1846–1910).

Hodgkin's disease, James K., age twenty. Patient admitted to Montreal General Hospital June 30, 1880, and examined by William Osler, M.D. (1849–1919), who noted enlarged lymph nodes on the left side of the neck, in both axillæ, and with marked bulging of the upper two-thirds of the sternum. Patient died August 20. Autopsy performed by Dr. Osler. Albumen print, photograph by Field, Montreal, 1880. Published in *Canada Medical and Surgical Journal*, February 1881. Donor: William Osler, M.D.

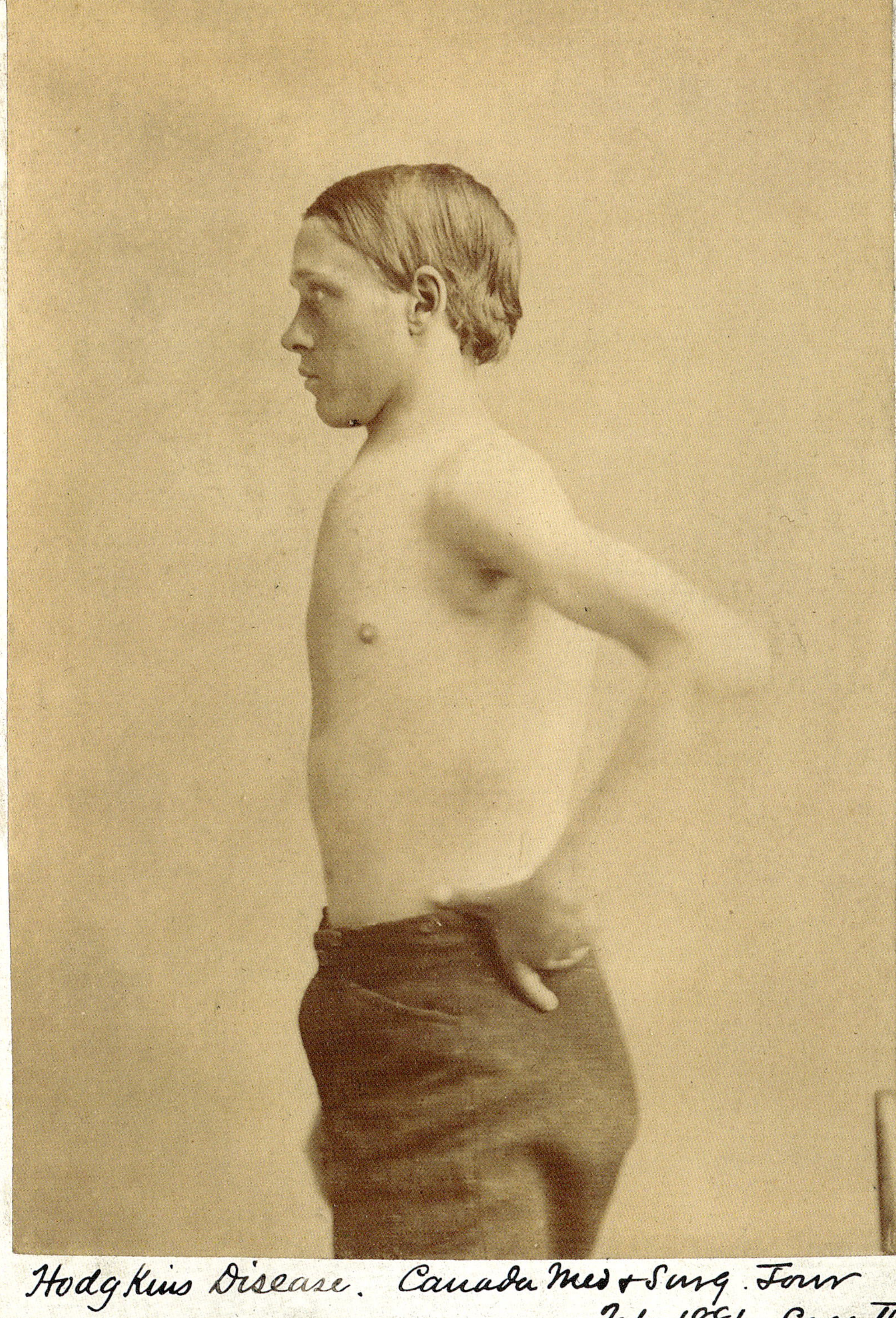

Hodgkins Disease. Canada Med & Surg. Jour
Feb. 1881 Case II.

Field Presented by Dr. Osler. Montreal.

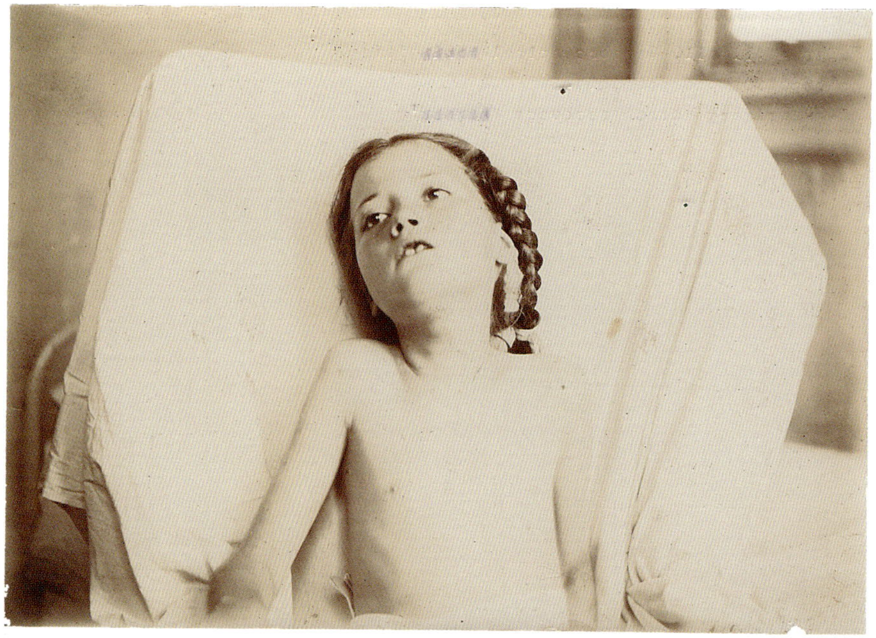

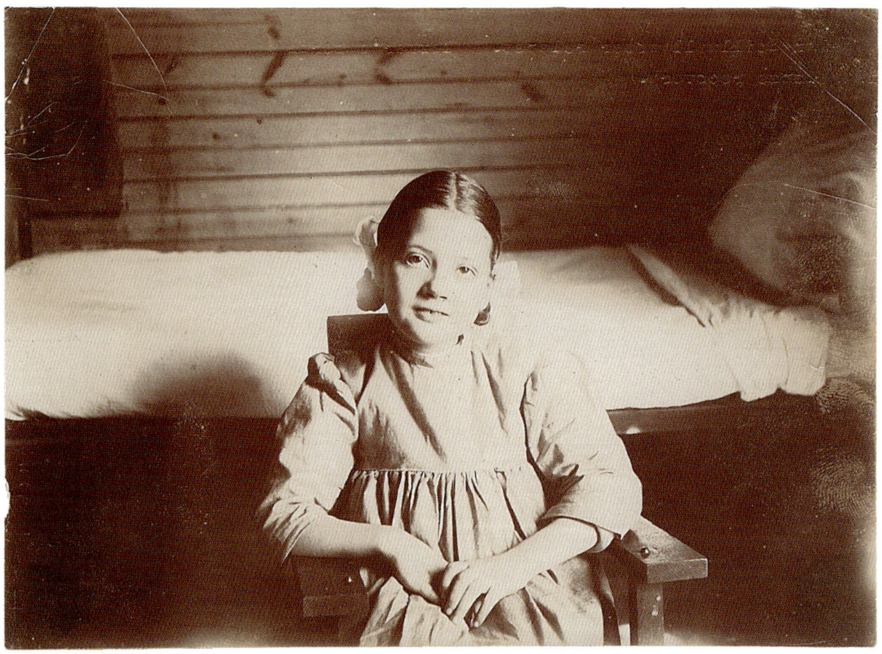

ABOVE AND OPPOSITE: Two cases of epidemic cerebrospinal meningitis. From an album prepared by B. Franklin Royer, M.D. (1870–1961), for an annual meeting of the American Medical Association in Atlantic City, New Jersey, ca. 1908. Photographer unidentified. Donor: B. Franklin Royer, M.D.

ABOVE: Case of H.S., age nine, photographed (top) on third day of primary attack. Onset December 18, 1907: nausea, vomiting, high fever, delirium unconsciousness; next day petechiæ on skin of trunk, neck, and on bulbar and conjunctivæ, deafness, retraction of head and neck, positive Kernig's sign. Rapid recovery under Flexner's serum. Discharged December 31, 1907. Relapse January 5, 1908; rapid recovery under Flexner's serum, discharged January 31, 1908. Municipal Hospital, Philadelphia. Bottom photograph taken forty days after primary attack, twenty-two days after relapse. Simon Flexner, M.D. (1863–1946), studied the disease during a severe epidemic in 1905 and 1906 in New York City and by 1907 developed a serum that reduced the mortality rate by 50 percent.

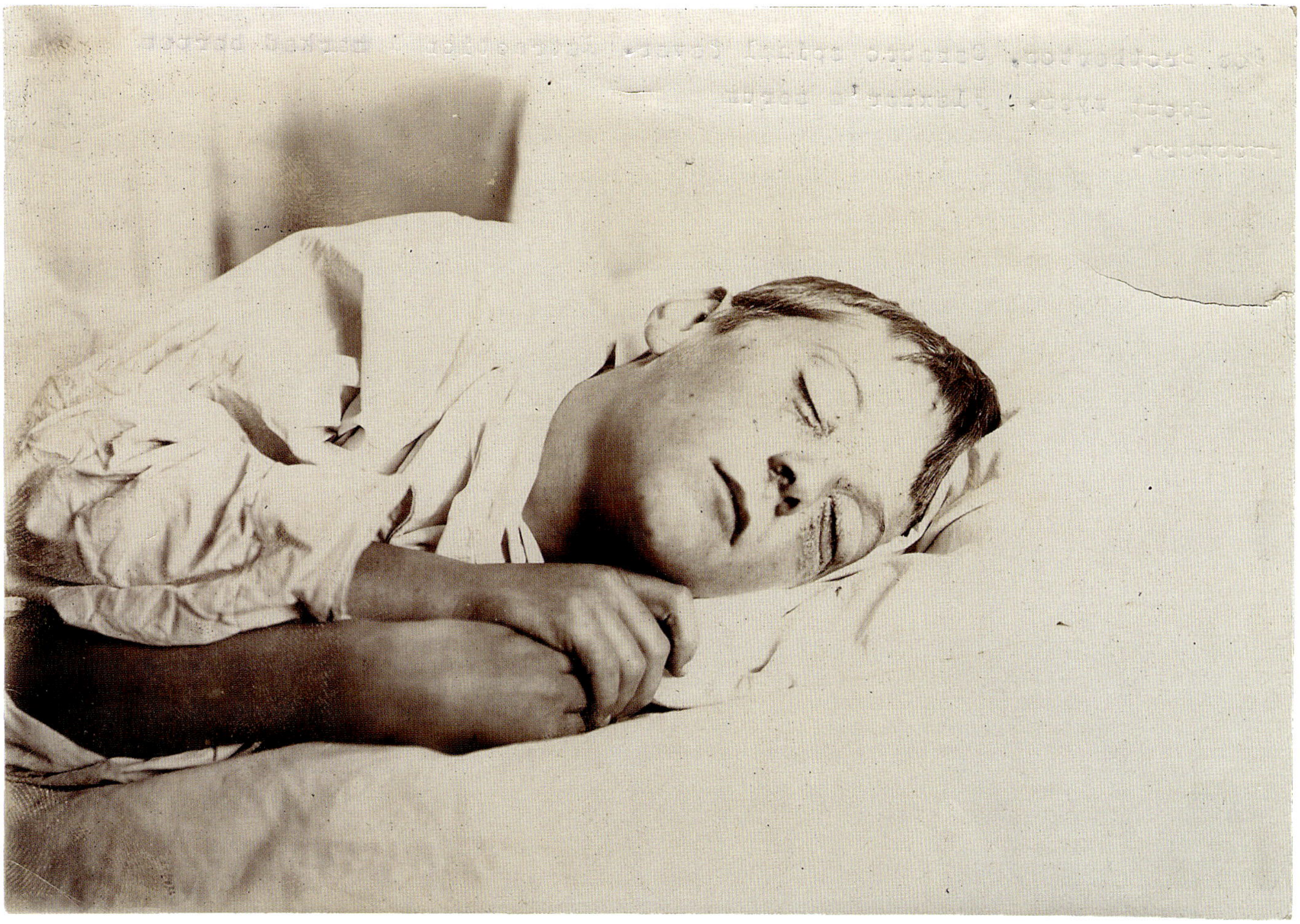

Case of J.B., age thirteen. Onset August 21, 1908: severe headache afternoon, fever at night, vomiting and stiff back next day. On admission August 23, 1908, retraction of neck, arching of spine, marked herpes about both eyes and nostrils, anesthesia both corneas, spinal fluid cloudy, meningococci. Recovery under Flexner's serum, discharged September 5, 1908, in good condition. Photograph taken fourth day of disease.

Case of double nephrotomy. Patient of Louis McLane Tiffany, M.D. (1844–1916), Baltimore, March 14, 1890. Letter from Dr. Tiffany to John Ashhurst, Jr., M.D. (1839–1900), of Philadelphia accompanying the photograph states: "The patient whose photograph is enclosed had an abscess in each kidney, they were opened, drained, and recovery followed. I cannot know whether the next edition of your *Principles & Practice* needs a nephrotomy illustration but it will give me pleasure if you will add the photo to your own collection." Dr. Ashhurst used the photograph in his sixth edition of *The Principles and Practice of Surgery*, 1893. Dr. Tiffany made important contributions to surgery of the kidney and maxilla; he reported the first successful nephrolithotomy in America. Photograph opaqued for reproduction; photographer unidentified.

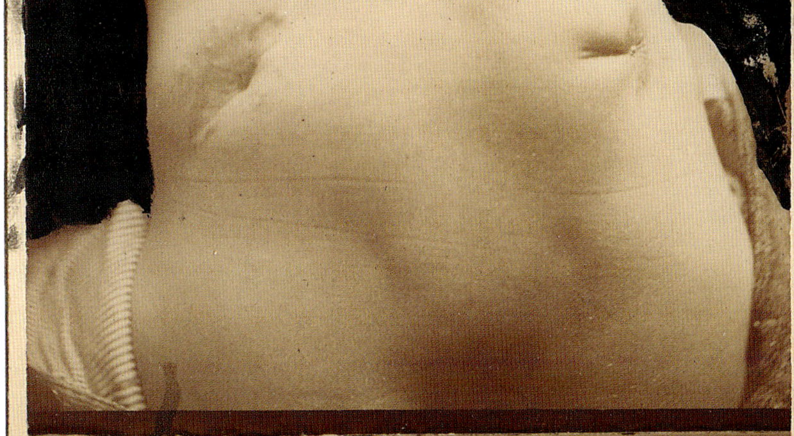

Dr. L. McLane Tiffany's case of double nephrotomy — March 15. 1890.

Enlarged heart. Jennie Savage, Children's Hospital. Albumen print, photographer unidentified, ca. December 15, 1899.

Medicine

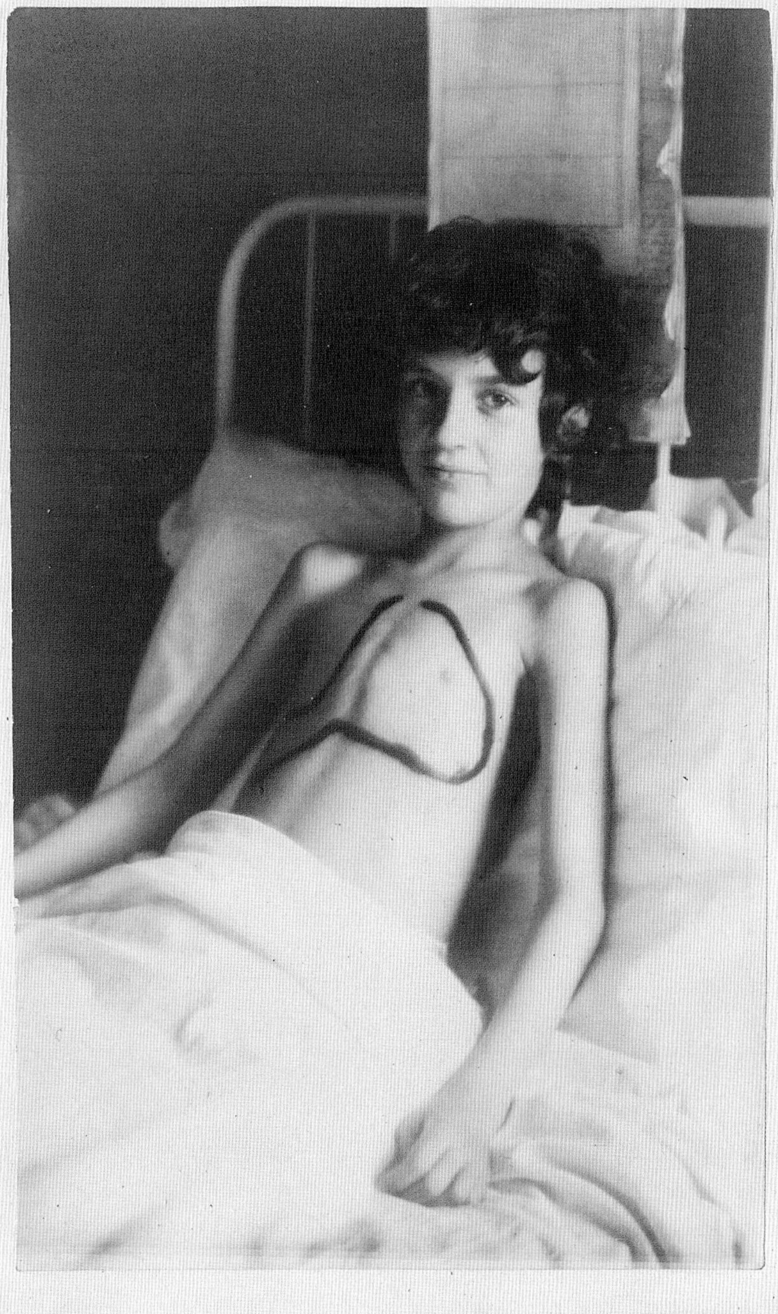

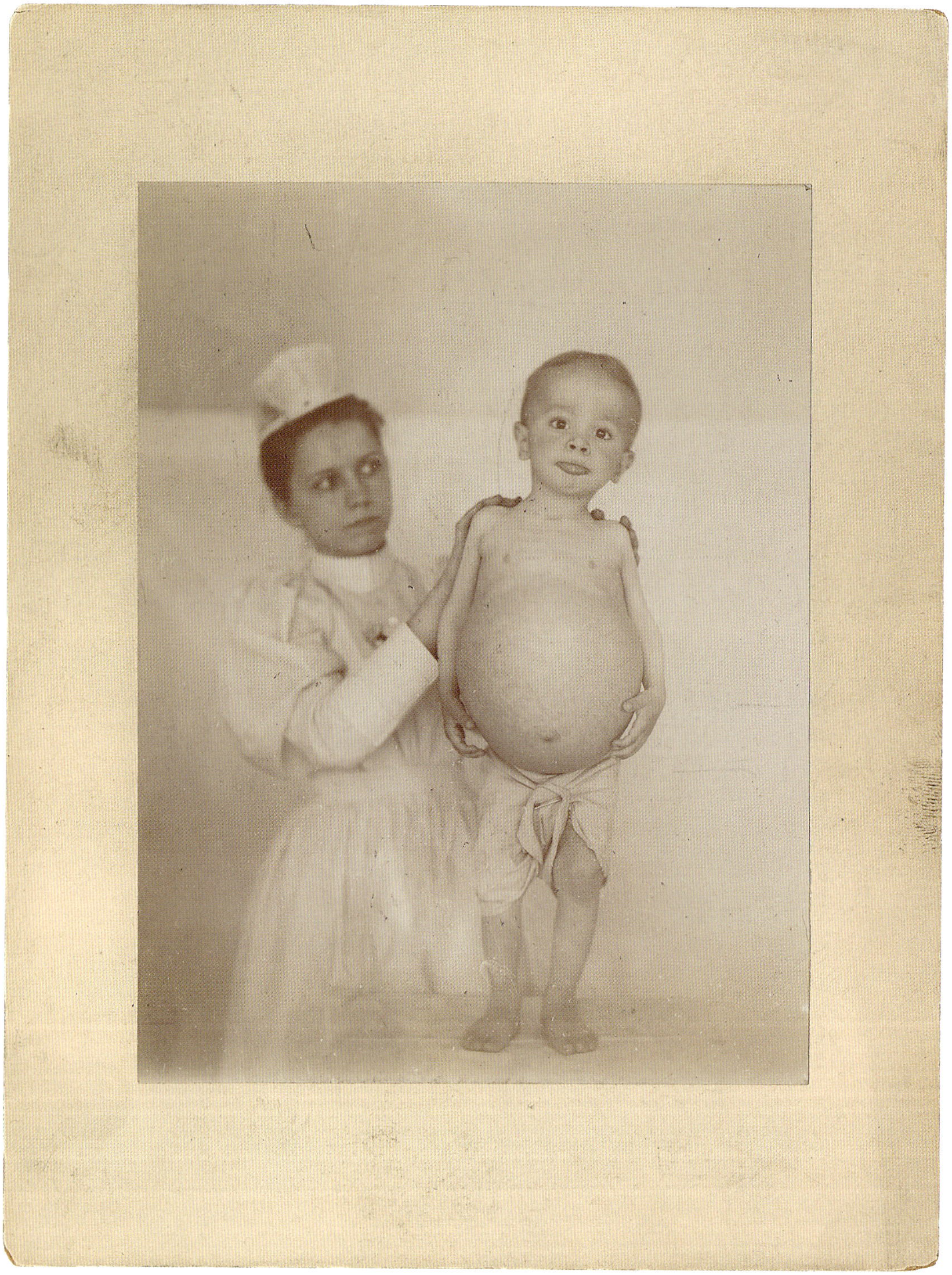

Chronic intestinal obstruction and paralytic tympany. University Hospital, Philadelphia, patient of Dr. J. P. Crozer Griffith (1856–1941). Caecatomy performed June 11, 1897, by Dr. John Ashhurst, Jr. (1839–1900). Photograph by Edward Pennock, optician, Philadelphia, ca. 1897.

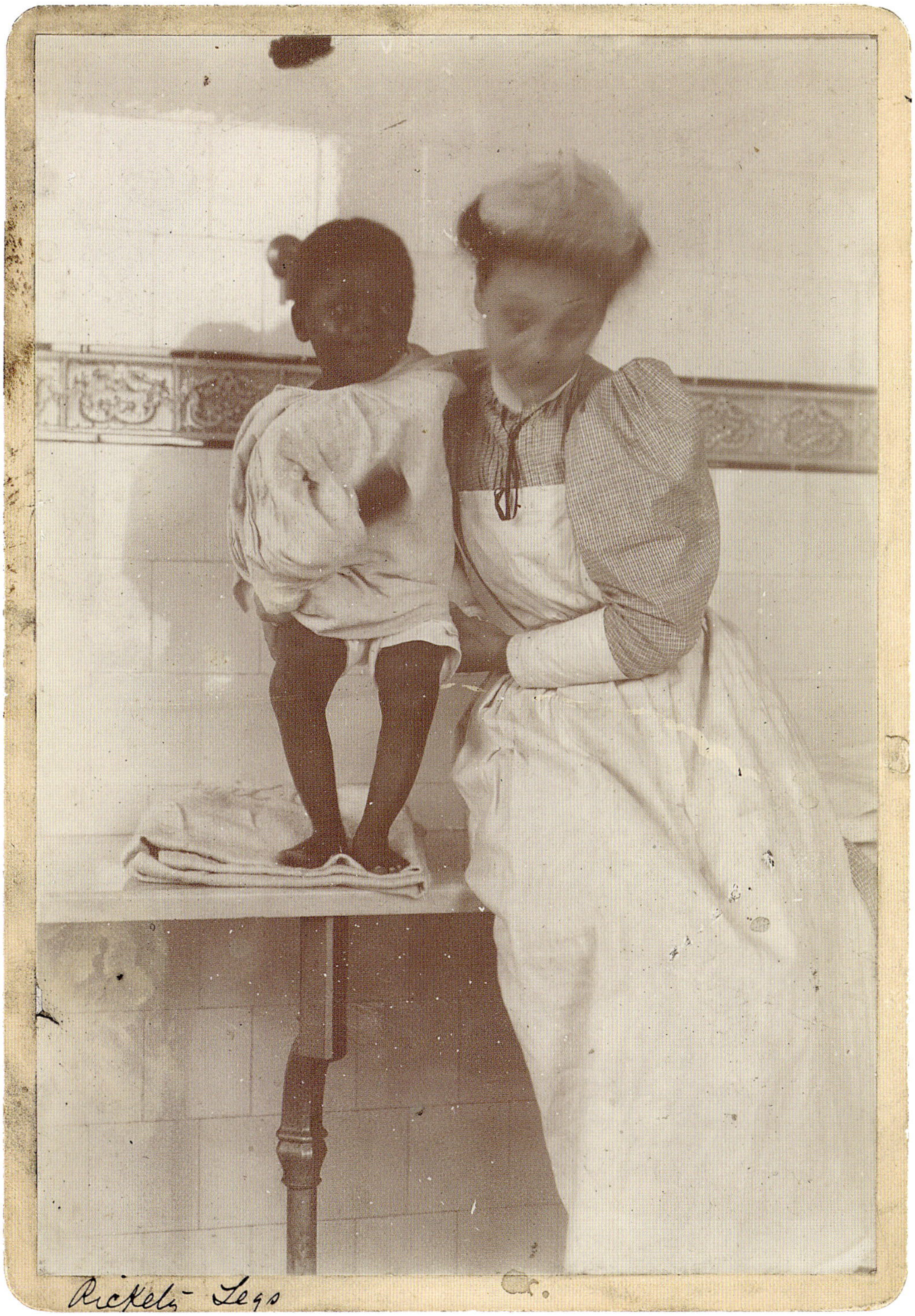

Weak legs from rickets resulting from vitamin D deficiency. Child delivered by cesarean section. Photographer unidentified, 1899. Donor: DeForest Willard (1846–1910).

Osteitis deformans (Paget's disease of bone), a bone disease disrupting the normal process of bone remodeling, causing an overly rapid remodeling producing softer, weaker bone and resulting in bowing of the long bones and deformation of the flat bones. Sir James Paget (1814–1899), alongside Rudolf Virchow, M.D. (1821–1902), was one of the founders of modern pathology. Photograph by William L. Suddards & George H. Fennemore, Philadelphia, ca. 1870–79.

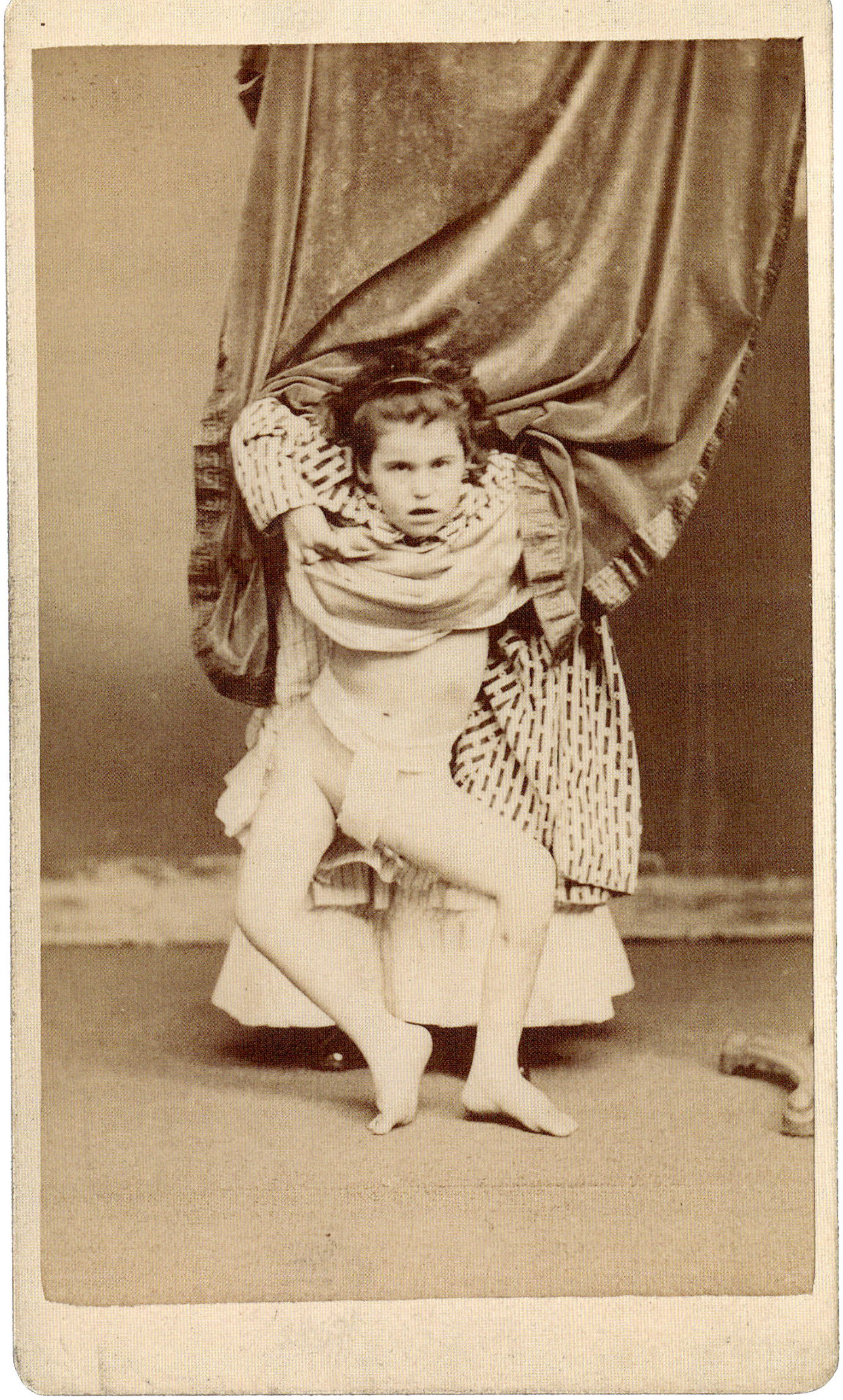

Osteitis deformans (Paget's disease of bone). Patient of Col. Arthur Harper Grimshaw, M.D. (1824–91), of Wilmington, Delaware, regimental commander for the Union in the American Civil War. Albumen print. Probably photographed by Eadweard Muybridge (1830–1904) at the University of Pennsylvania, ca. 1885. Donor: Richard Hickman Harte, M.D. (1855–1925).

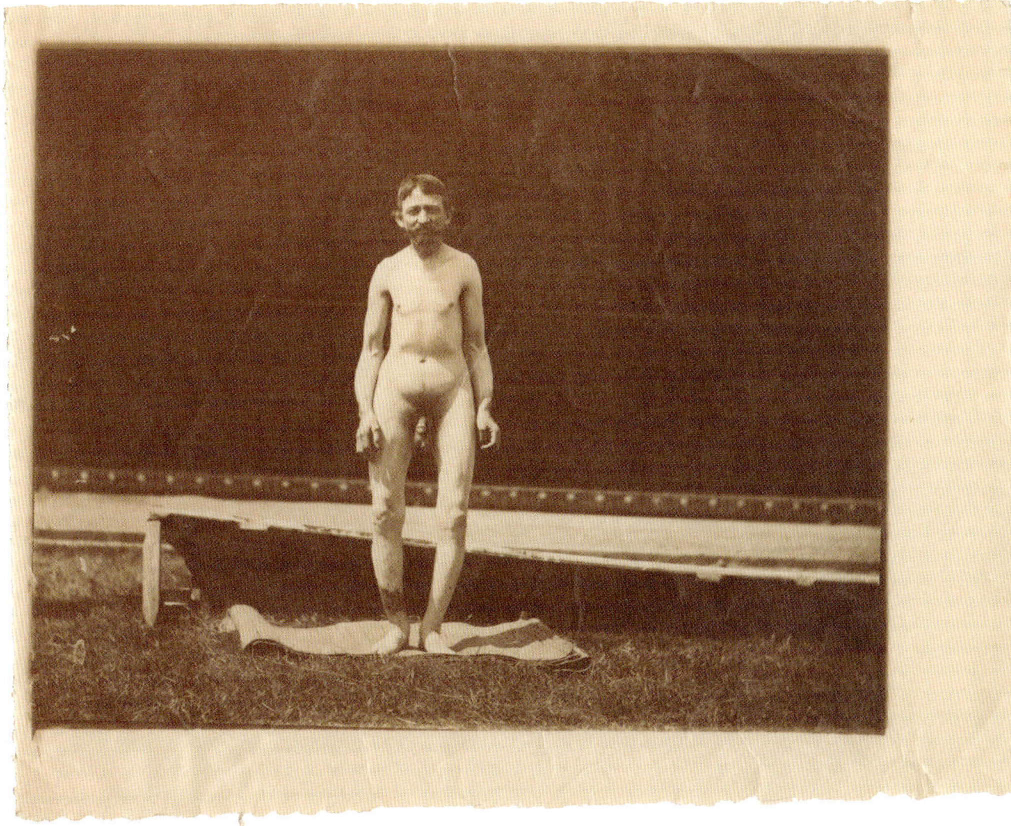

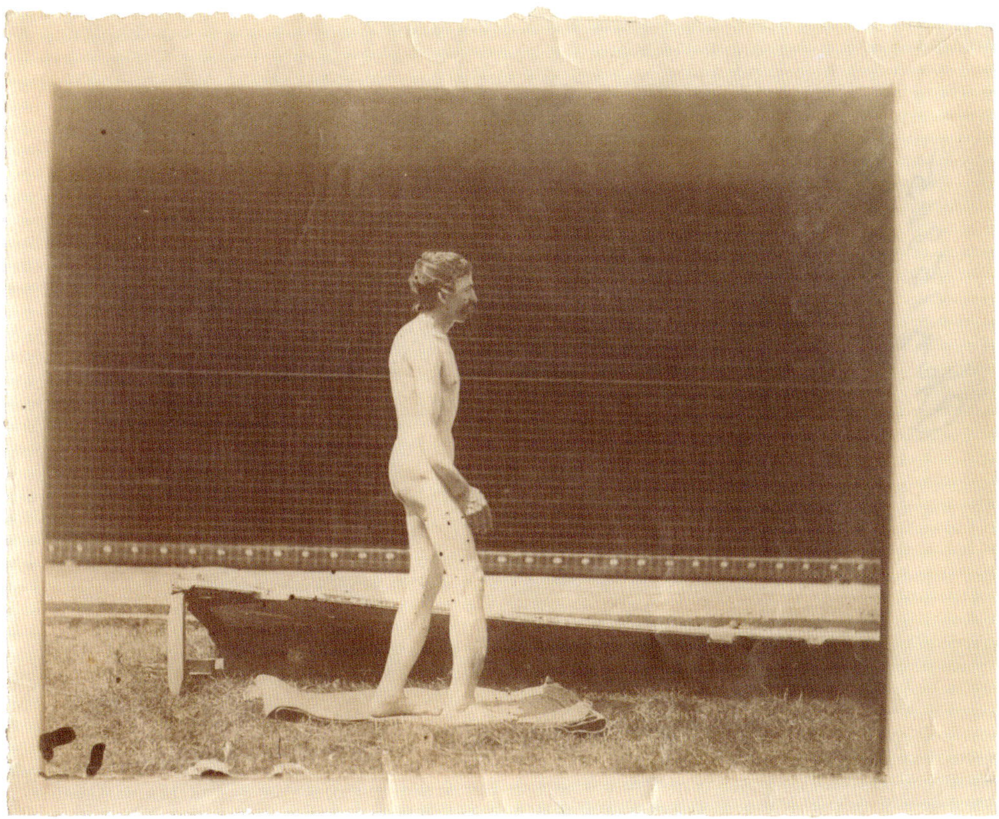

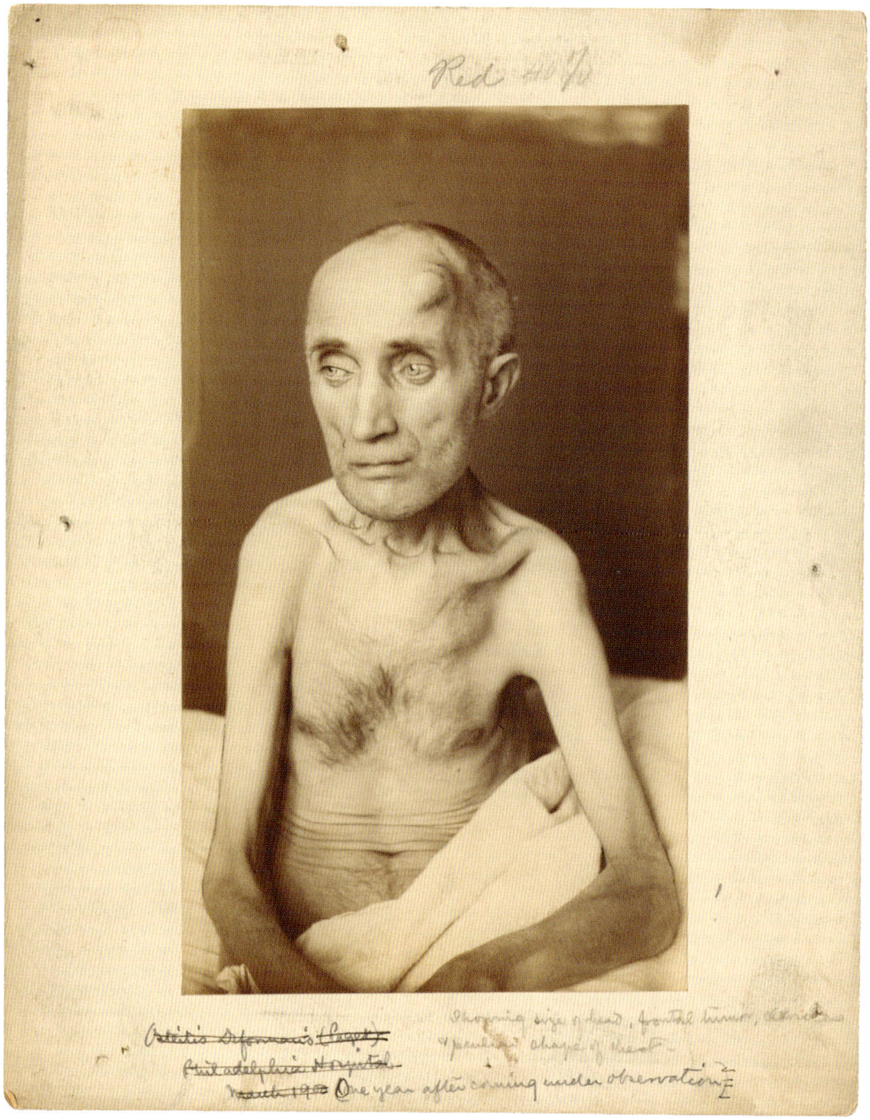

ABOVE AND OPPOSITE: Osteitis deformans (Paget's disease of bone). Anthony Roth, sixty-two, admitted to men's ward of the Philadelphia Hospital April 1899. Photographs taken in March 1900, one year after patient came under observation, showing (above) size of head, frontal tumor, clavicles, and peculiar shape of chest, and (opposite) separation of the knees when ankles are in contact. The patient died shortly afterward. Background in photograph opposite opaqued for reproduction. Reported by Frederick A. Packard, M.D. (1864–1902), J. Dutton Steele, M.D. (1868–1908), and Thomas Story Kirkbride, Jr., M.D. (1869–1900), in *The American Journal of the Medical Sciences*, November 1901. Photographer unidentified.

< 6"7

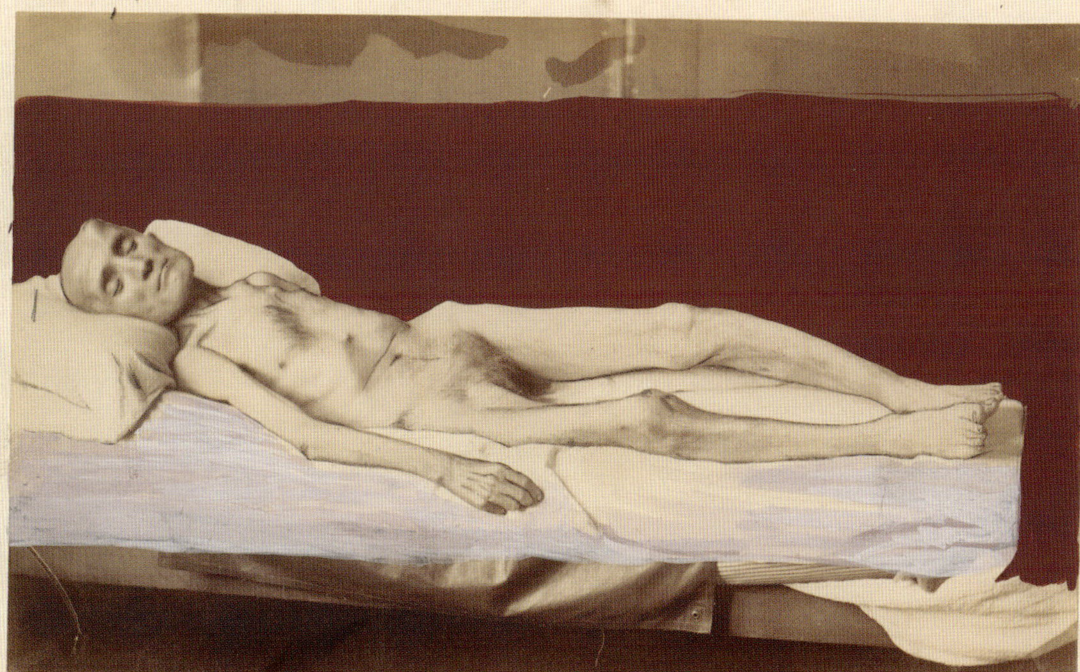

Showing especially seperation of the knees when ankles were in contact.

~~Osteitis Deformans (Paget)~~
~~Philadelphia Hospital~~
~~March 1900~~ One year after coming under observation

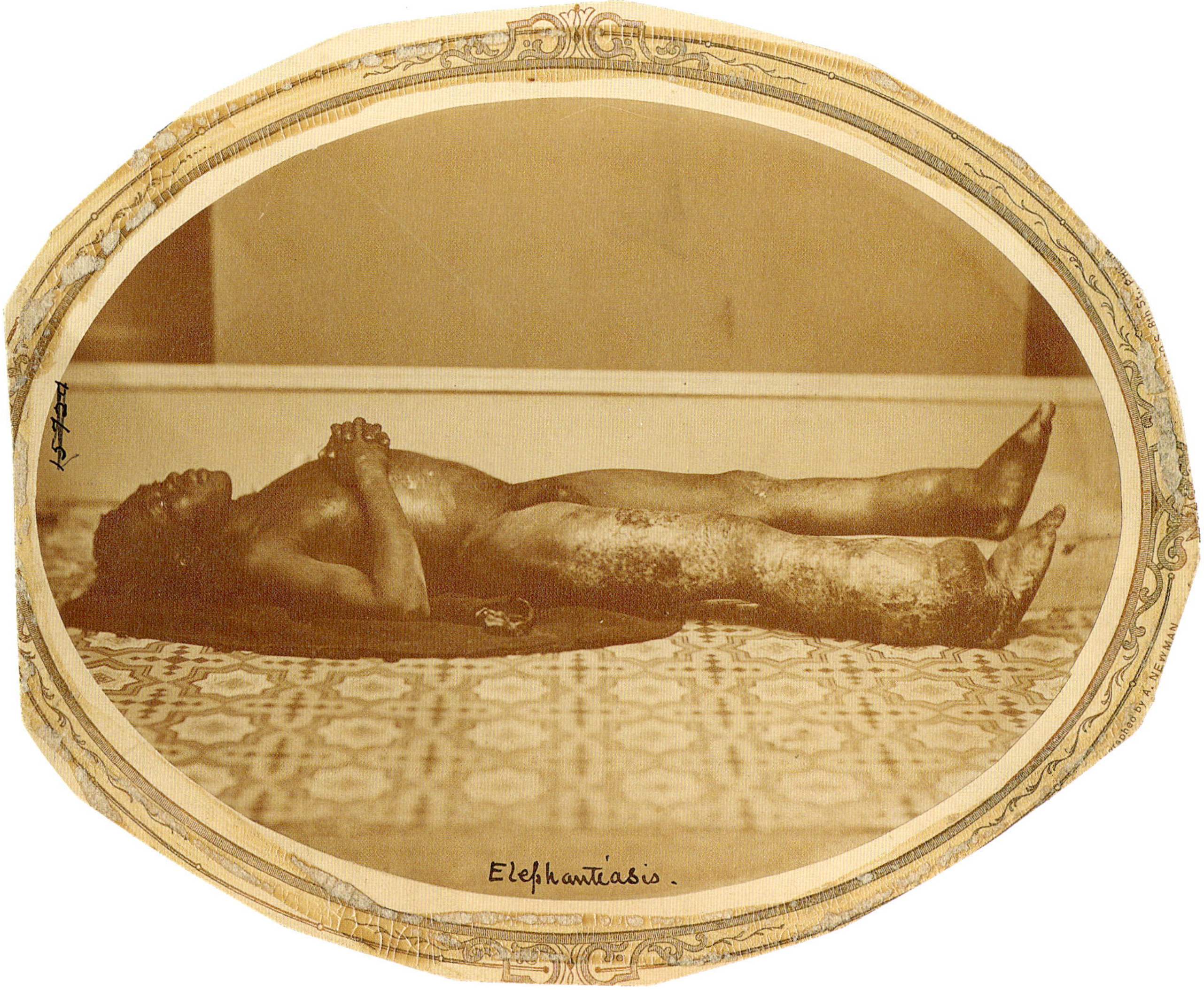

ABOVE AND OPPOSITE: Elephantiasis, or lymphatic filariasis, a disease caused by an infestation of mosquito-borne filarial worms that block lymphatic channels and cause an accumulation of fluid in the tissues resulting in chronic severe swelling and enlargement. Photograph above by A. Newman, Philadelphia, ca. 1867–78; photograph opposite unidentified.

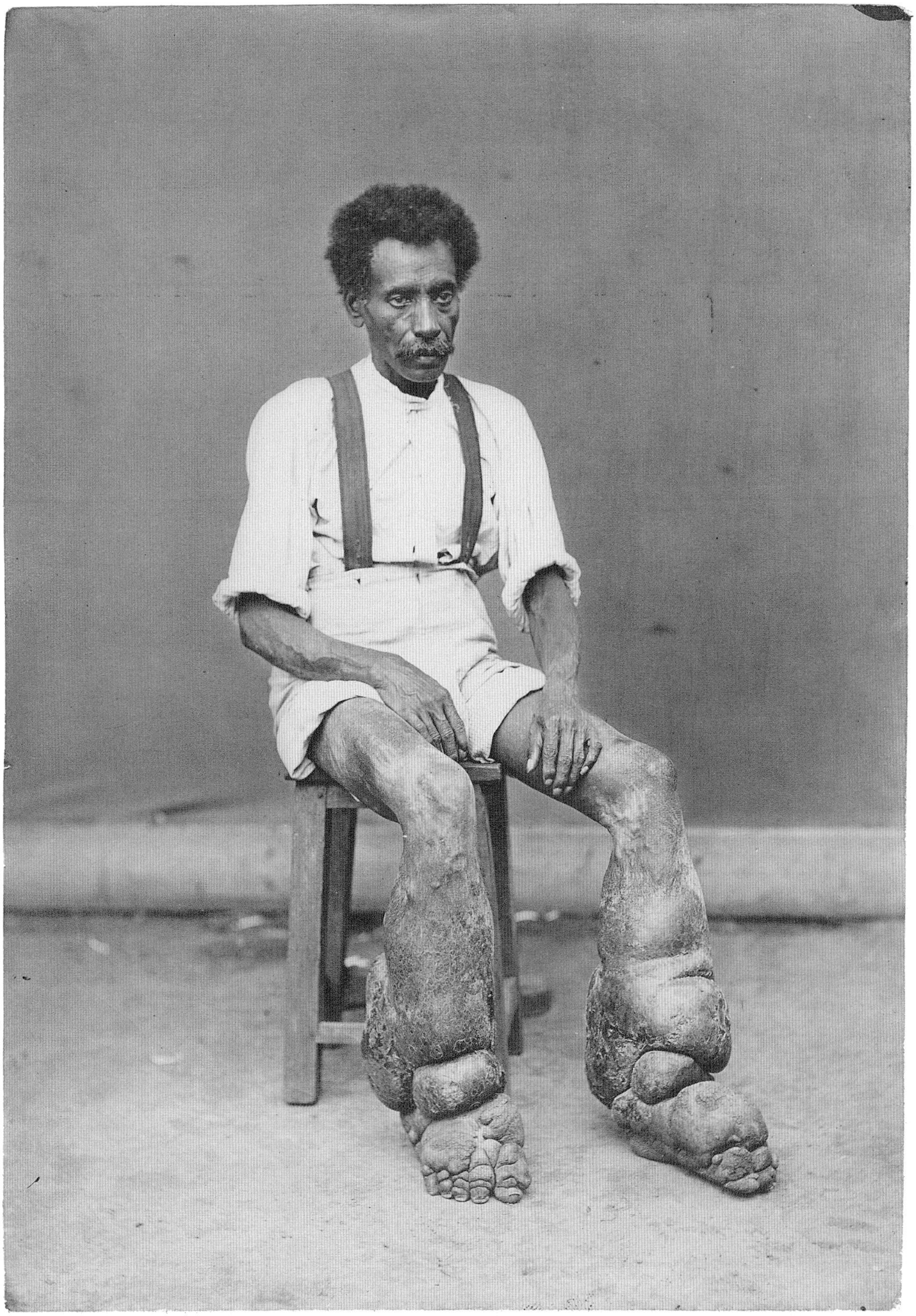

Tuberculosis of joints. Richard Pendlebery. A highly variable infectious disease caused by mycobacteria, tuberculosis can affect the lungs (pulmonary tuberculosis), the central nervous system, the lymphatic, circulatory, and genitourinary systems, the bones, joints, and skin (extrapulmonary tuberculosis). Photographs by William H. Rhoads, Philadelphia, ca. 1866–98.

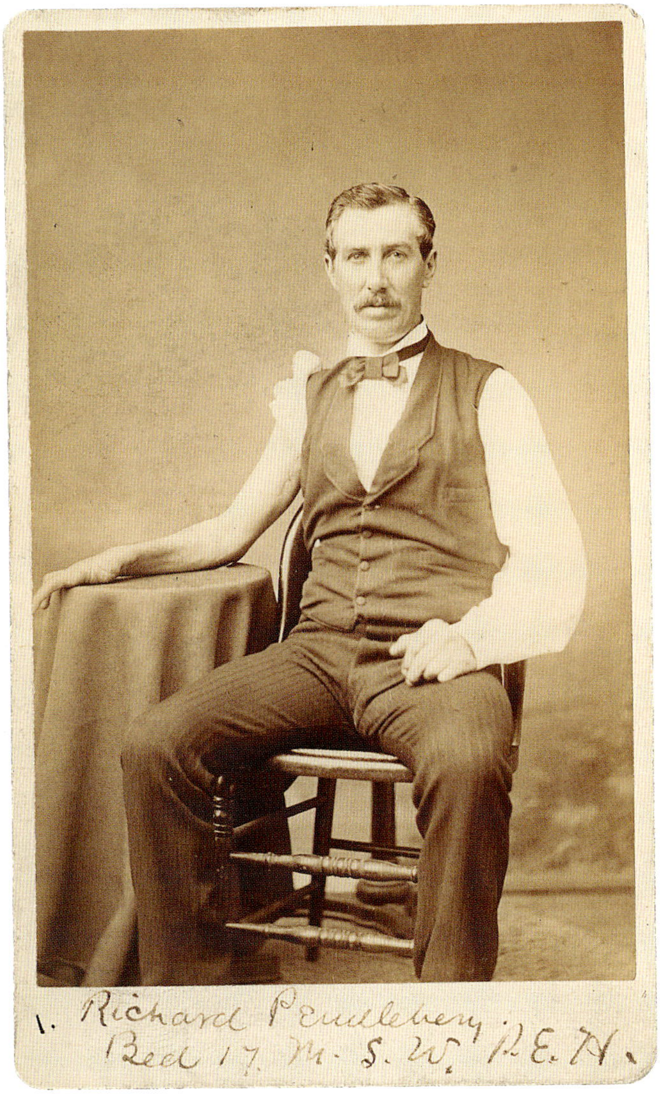
1. Richard Pendlebery
Bed 17. M. S. W. P.E.H.

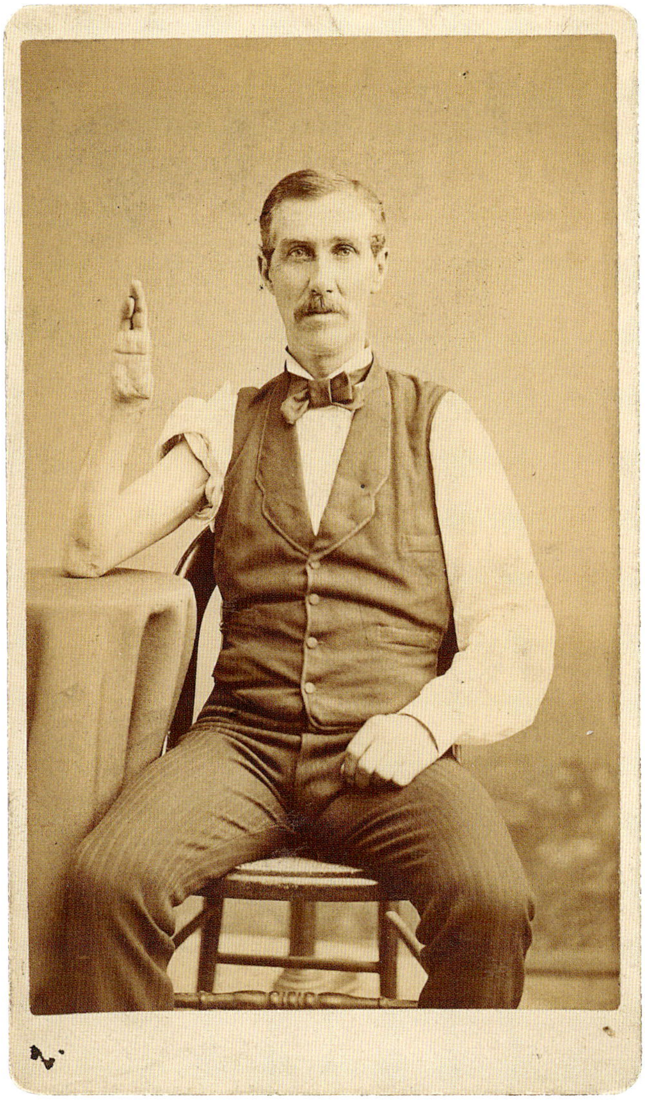

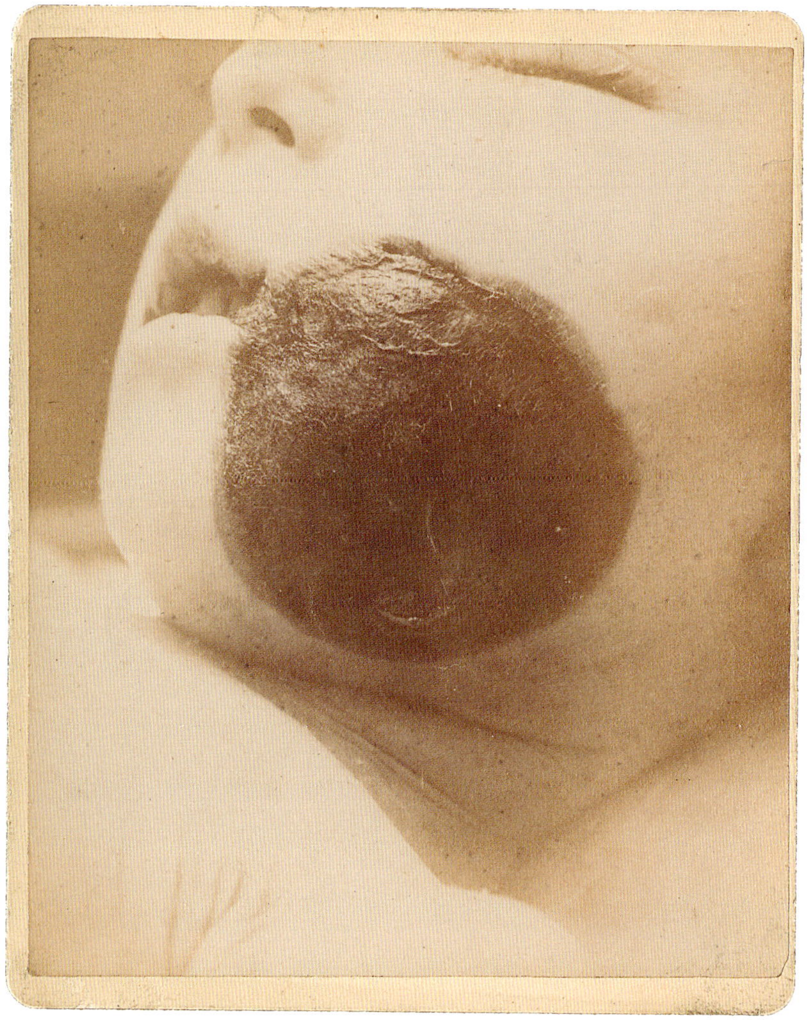

ABOVE: Cancrum oris (gangrene). Becky Goldman, girl about three, June 6, 1891, postmortem. Antecedent measles and broncho pneumonia. Photographer unidentified.

OPPOSITE: Necrosis of the skull, probably syphilitic. W. B. Metcalfe, University Hospital. Photograph by H. J. Harman, Pennsylvania, December 1879. Donor: John Ashhurst, M.D. (1839–1900).

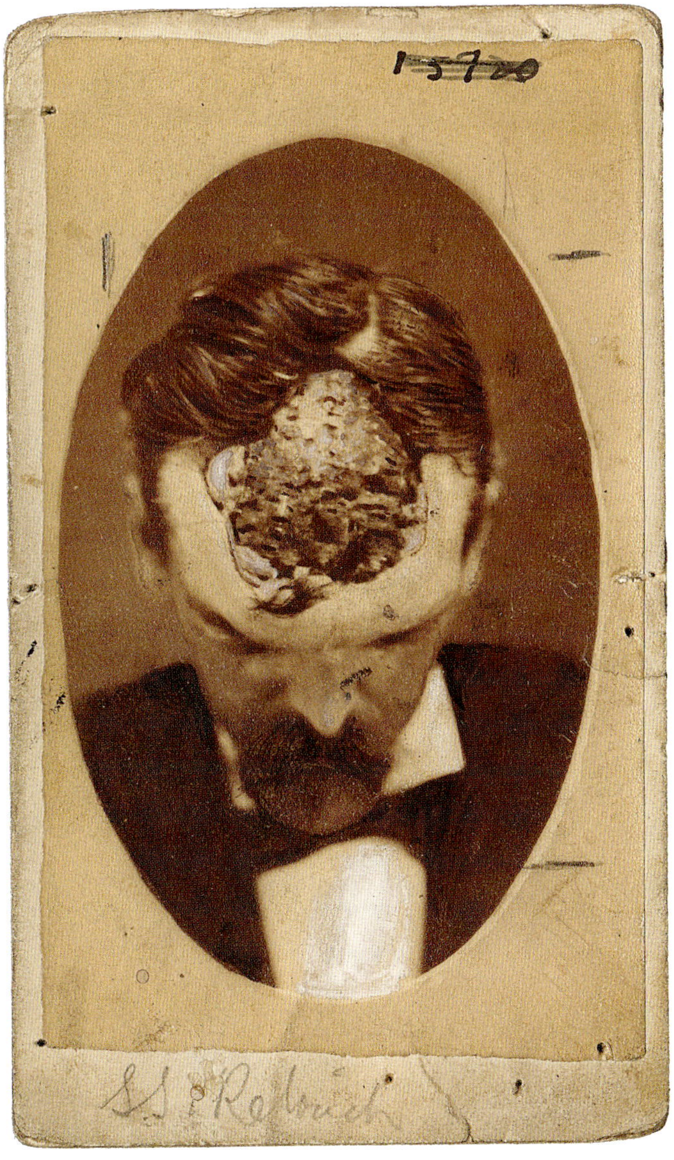

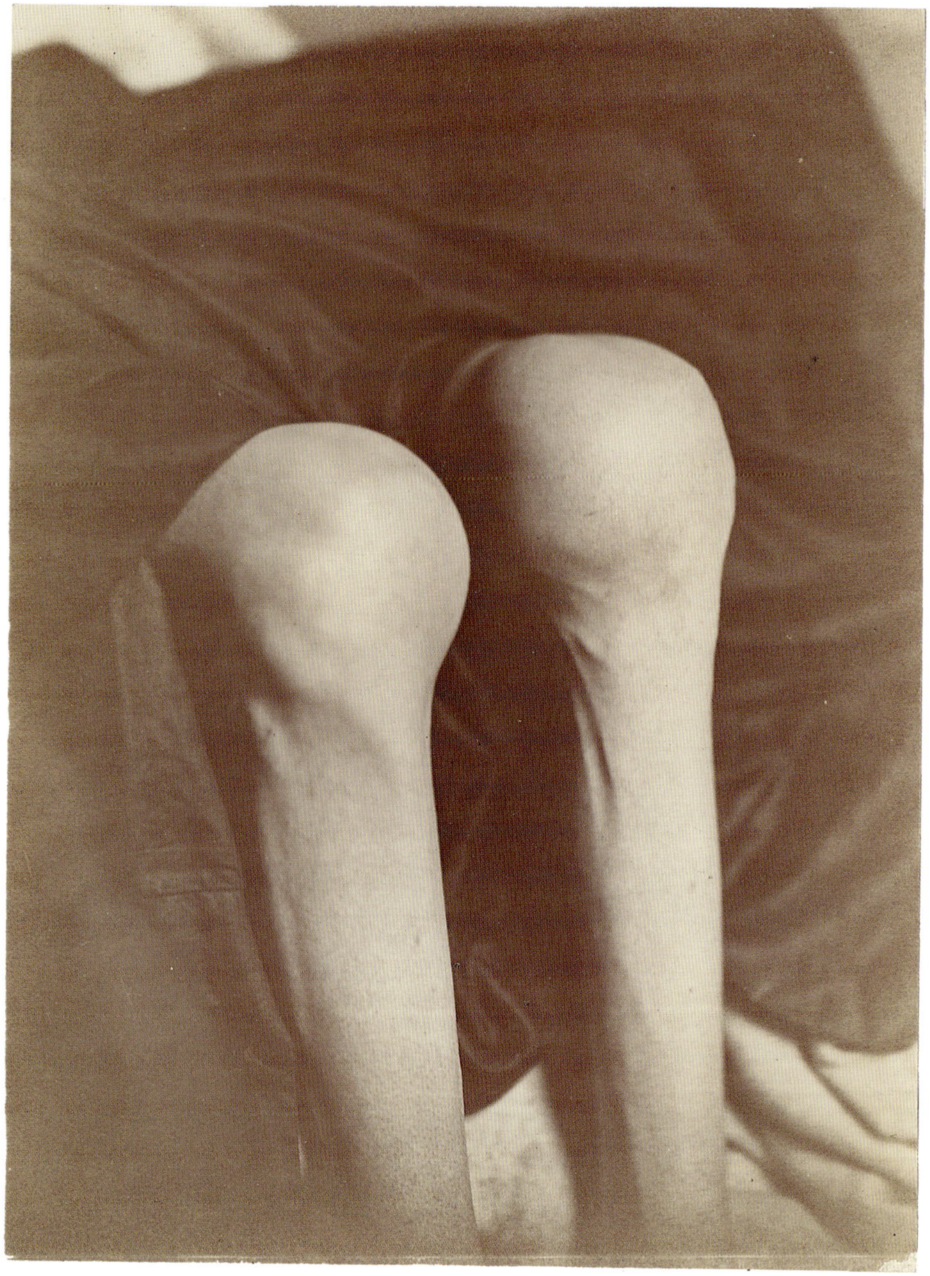

ABOVE AND OPPOSITE: Rheumatic polyarthritis of knees (above) and smaller joints (opposite). George Granger, age thirty-eight, admitted to Pennsylvania Hospital September 21, 1900. Photographer unidentified, ca. 1900.

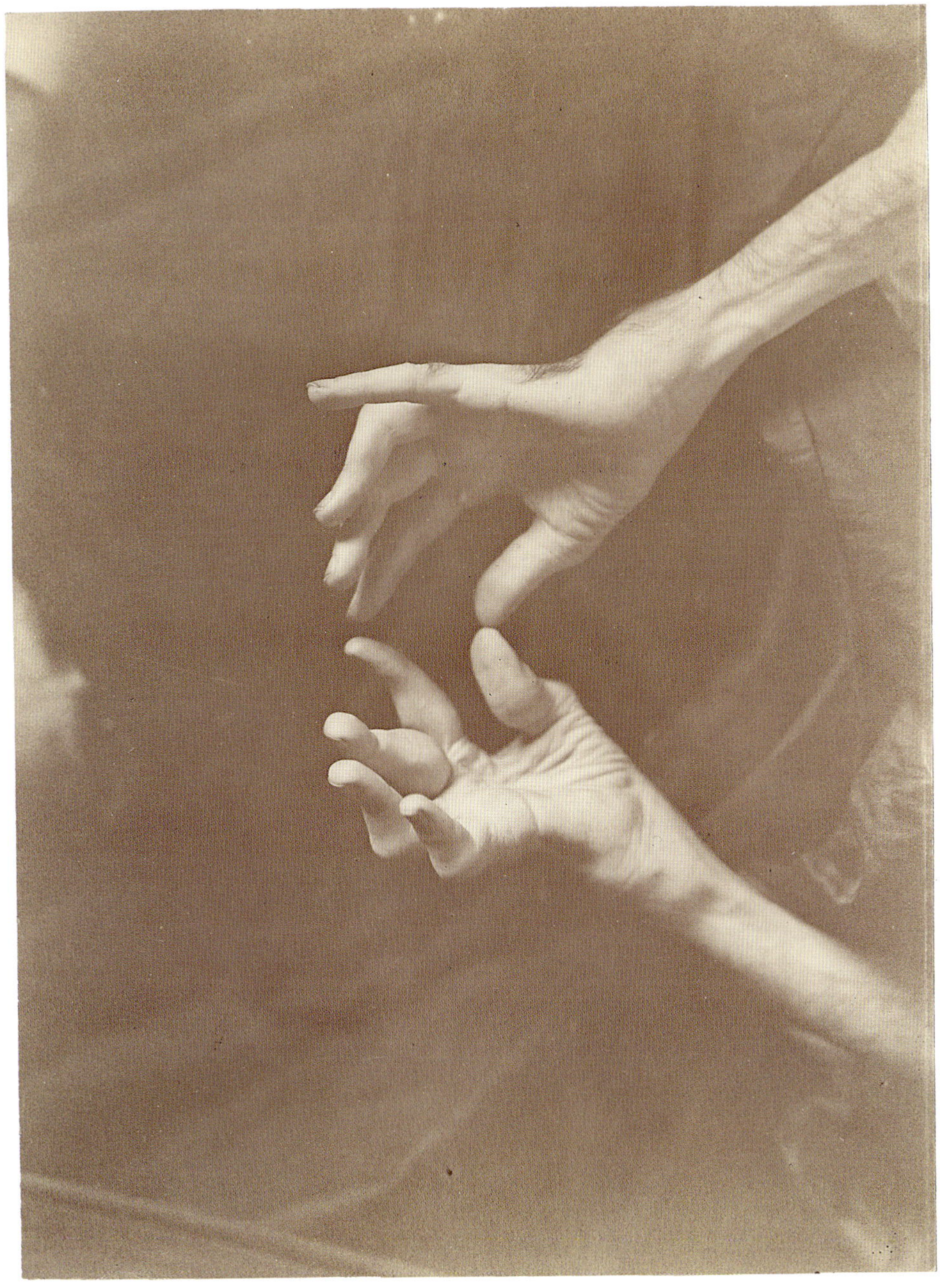

Unidentified disorder. Patient of James Hendrie Lloyd, M.D. (1853–1932), neurologist to the Philadelphia Hospital and author of "Diseases of the Cerebrospinal and Sympathetic Nerves" (*Twentieth Century Practice of Medicine*, vol. 11, ed. Thomas L. Stedman, 1897) and others. Photograph by James F. Wood, from the album of photographs by Wood presented to the Mütter Museum in 1898, ca. 1892–1900.

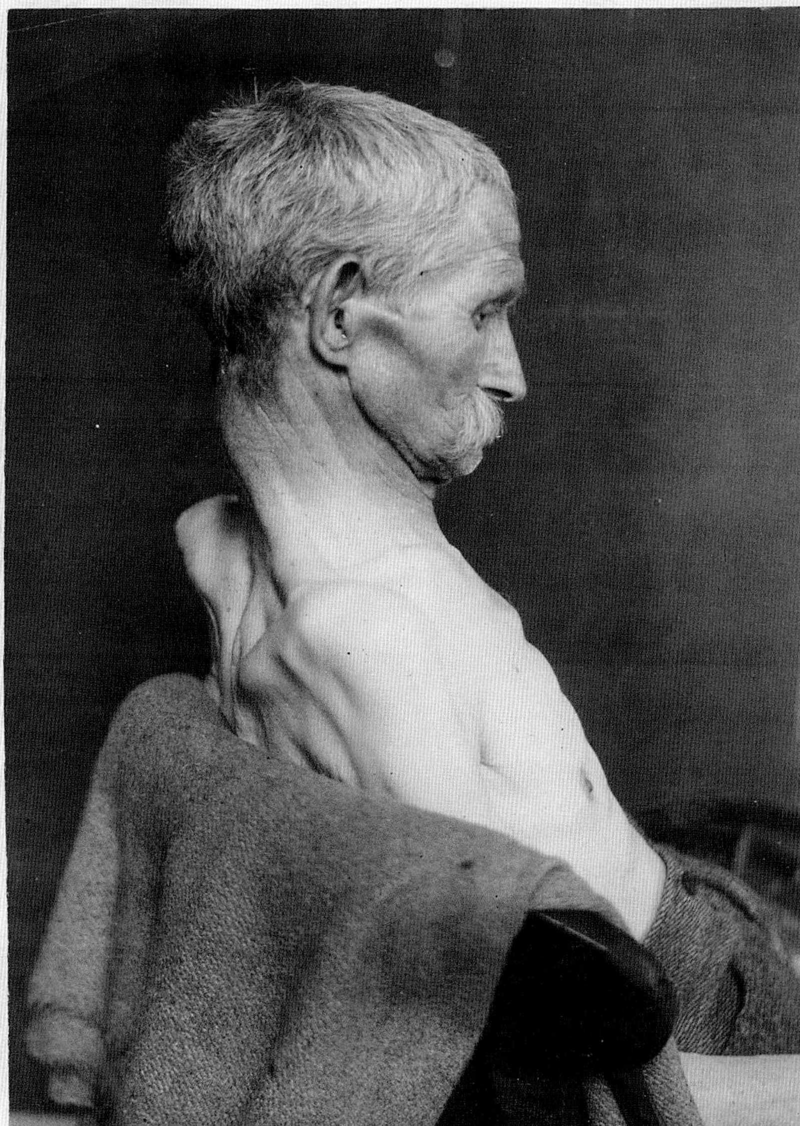

Lloyd

Unidentified disease or disorder of jaw. Photographs by Herman H. Henrici, Philadelphia, ca. 1888–99.

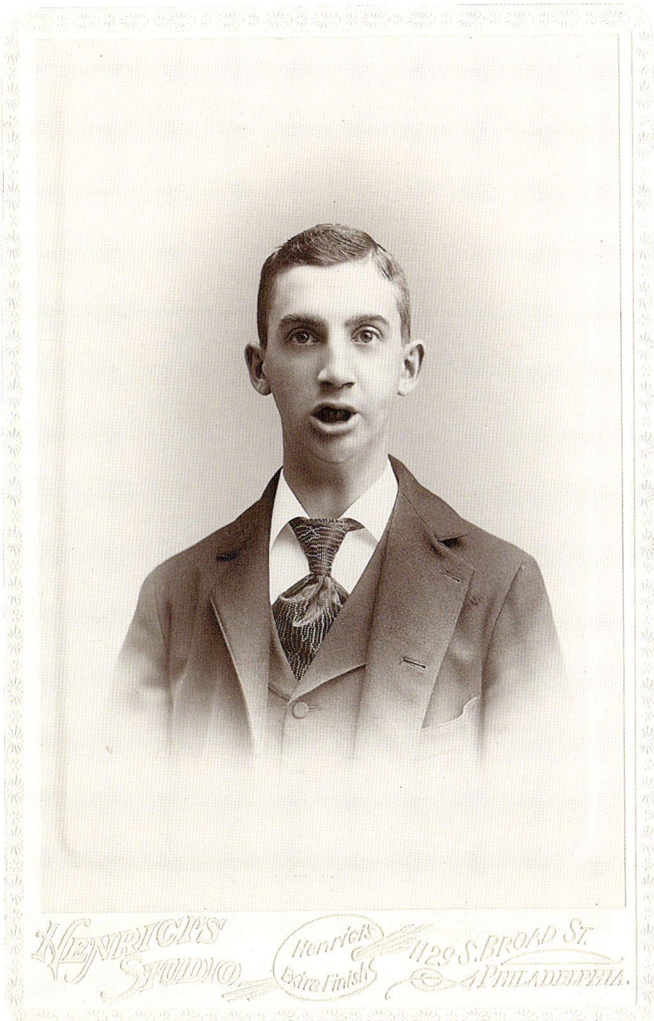
HENRICI'S STUDIO
Henrici's Extra Finish
1129 S. BROAD ST.
PHILADELPHIA.

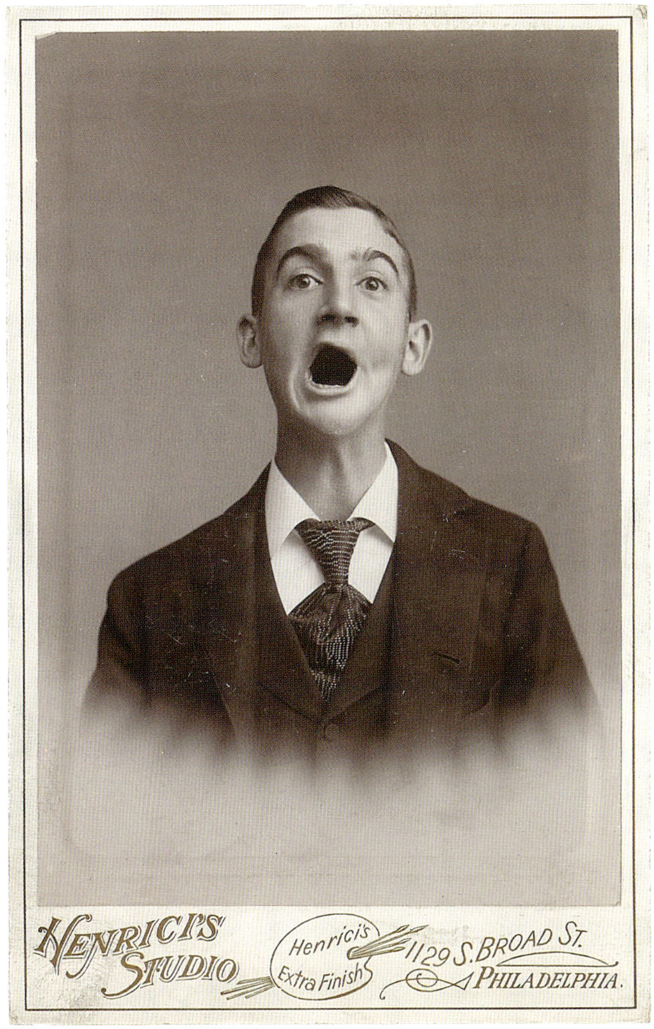
HENRICI'S STUDIO
Henrici's Extra Finish
1129 S. BROAD ST.
PHILADELPHIA.

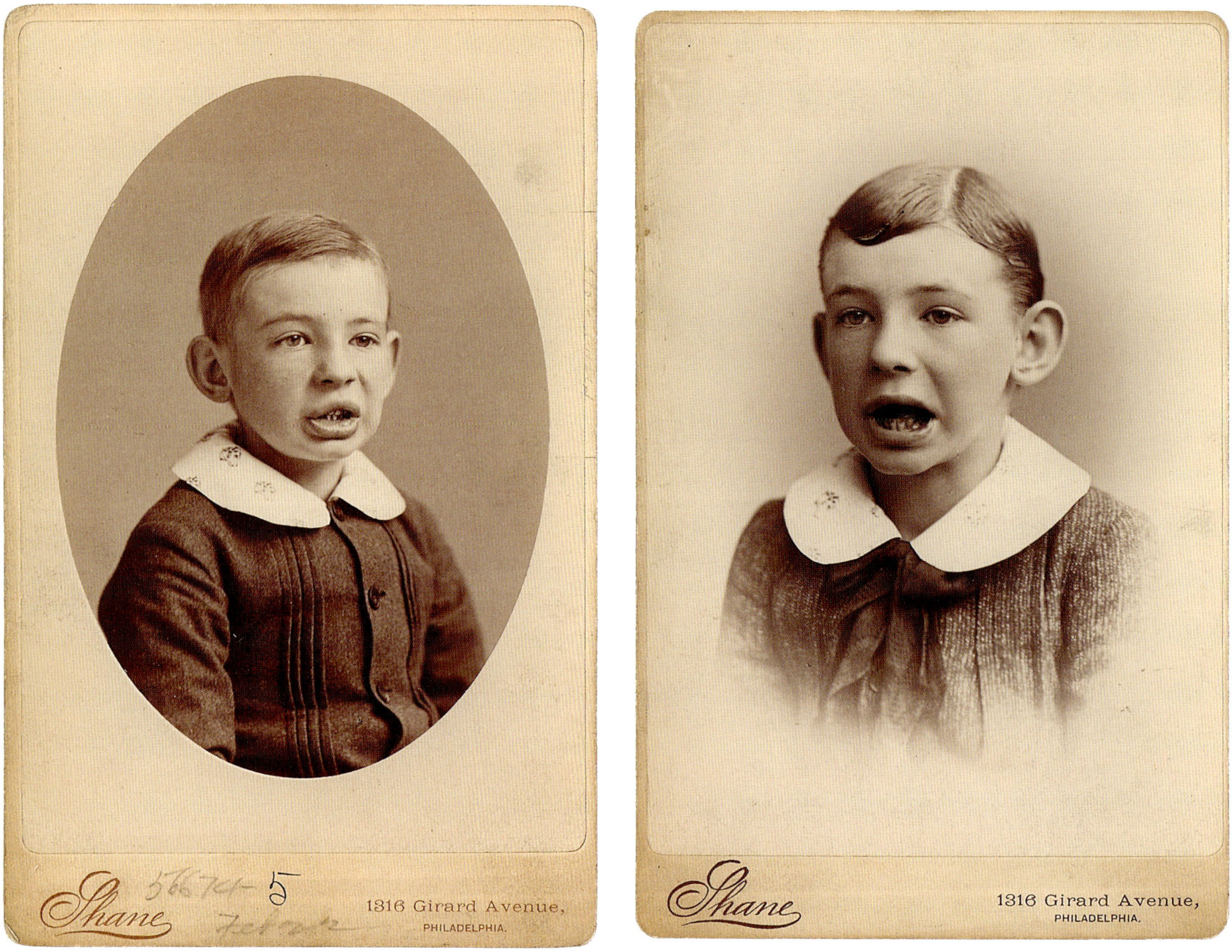

Unidentified disease or disorder of jaw. Photographs by William Shane, Philadelphia, ca. 1881–1900.

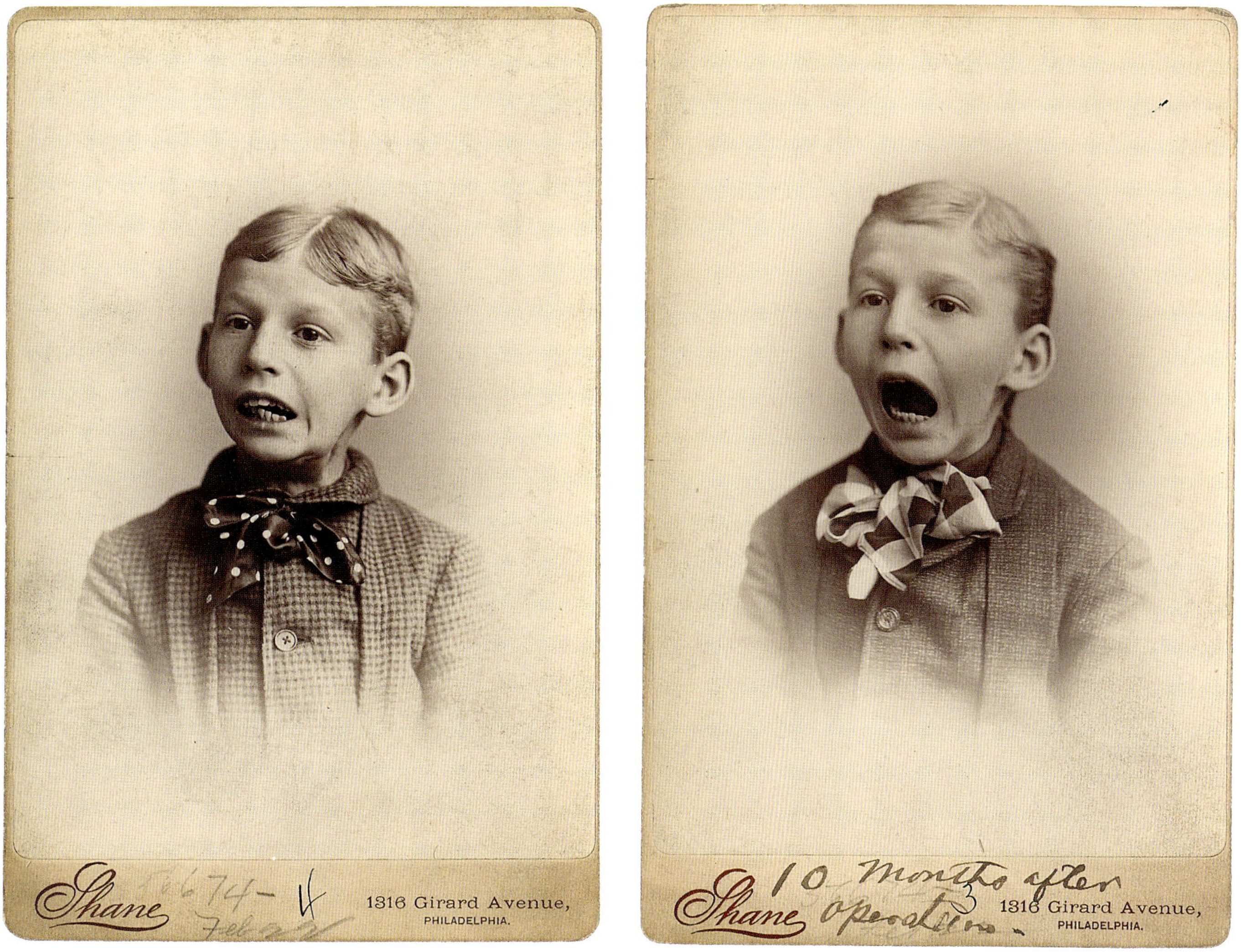

Unidentified disease or disorder of jaw. Photograph on right ten months after operation. Photographs by William Shane, Philadelphia, ca. 1881–1900.

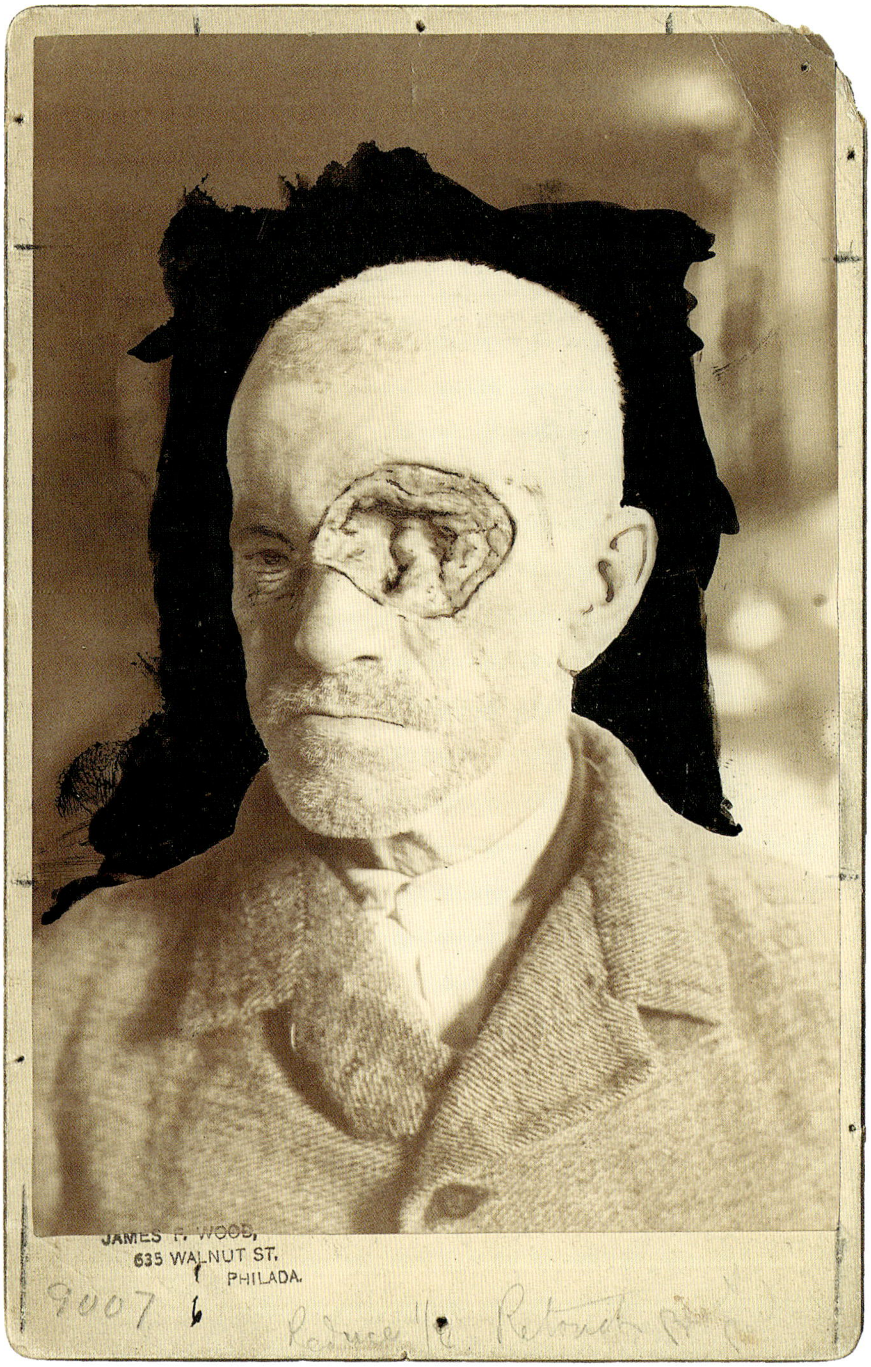

Inscription on photograph: “Kennedy, age sixty +. Disease began sixteen years ago in the form of a pimple at inner margin of eyelid. The eyeball was still in place five years ago. This and the entire contents of orbit was then removed. Scraped and cauterized with zinc chloride six weeks from date of photograph.” The appearance is consistent with a basal cell carcinoma of the skin. Photograph by James F. Wood, Philadelphia, ca. 1892–1900. Opaqued for reproduction. Patient of Dr. George Edmund de Schweinitz (1858–1938), Philadelphia Hospital. Donor: Dr. John Ashhurst, M.D. (1839–1900).

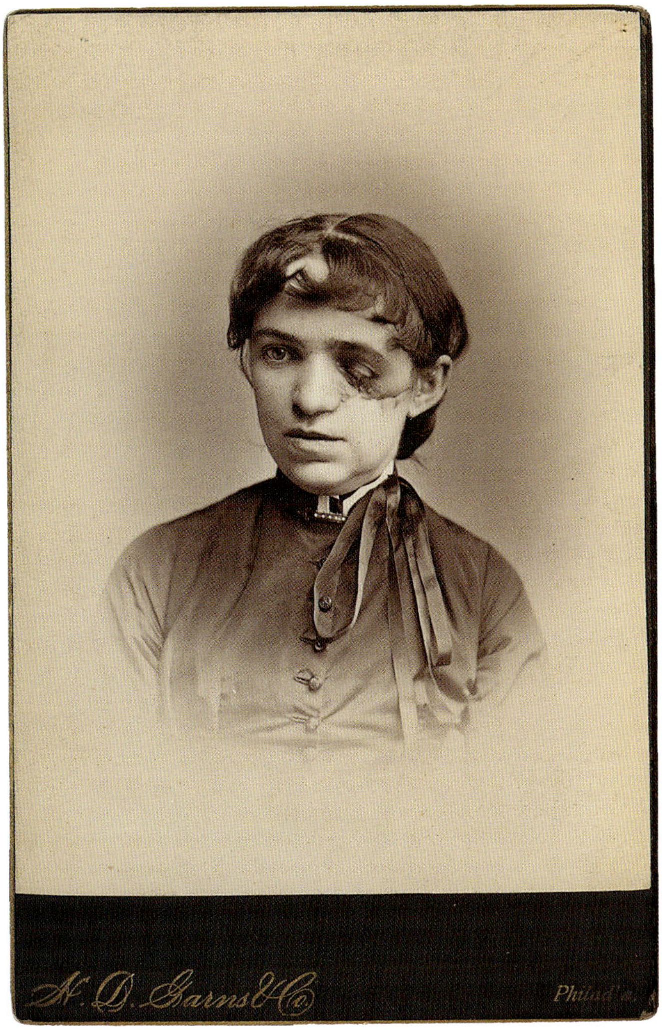

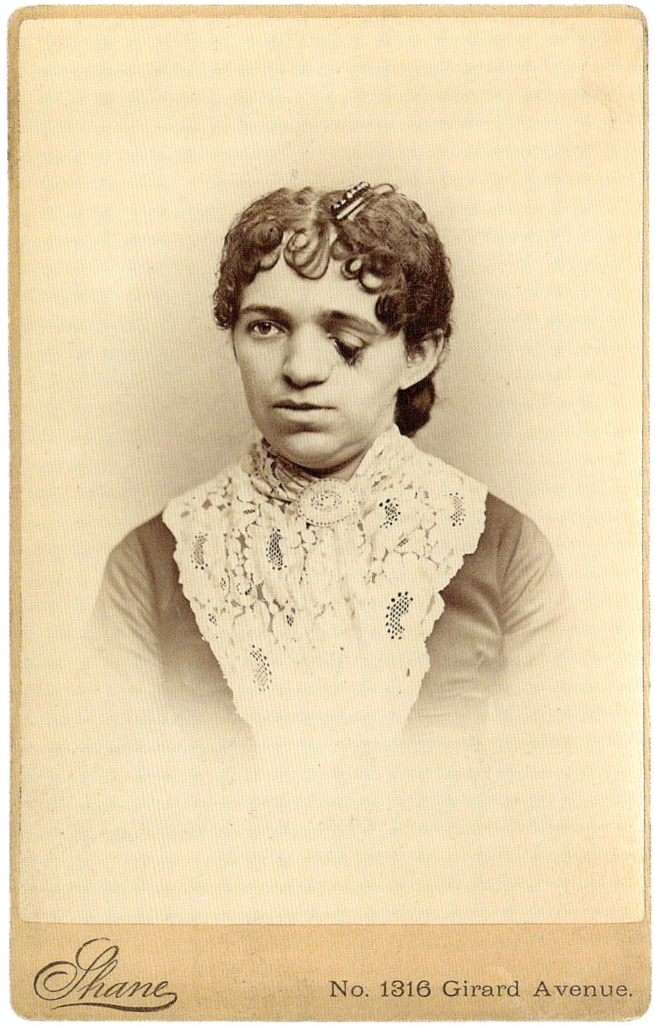

Unidentified condition of the left eye, cause unknown, leading to ptosis (drooping) of the eyelid. Left photograph by Henry D. Garns & Co., Philadelphia, ca. 1877–81; right photograph by William Shane, Philadelphia, ca. 1881–1900.

Dermatological Disorder

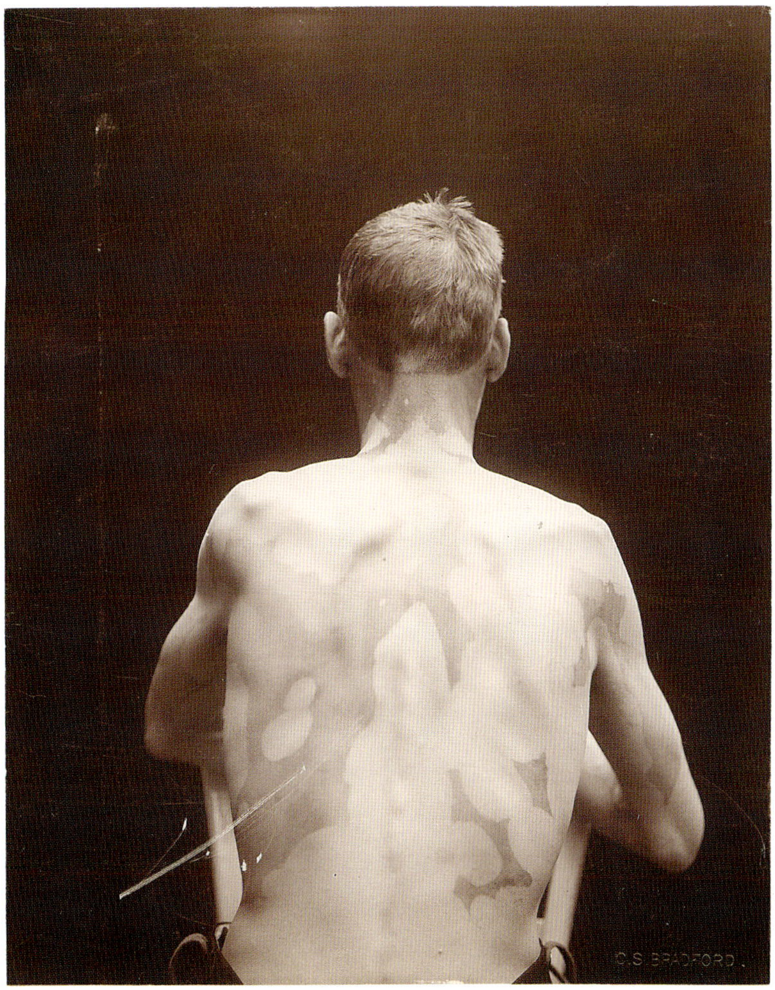

Pernicious anemia with vitiligo, a pigmentation disorder in which melanocytes are destroyed, causing white patches of skin to appear on the body. Patient, Harvey Hosier, admitted to Pennsylvania Hospital May 2, 1901. Silver gelatin print. Photograph by C. S. Bradford, ca. 1901.

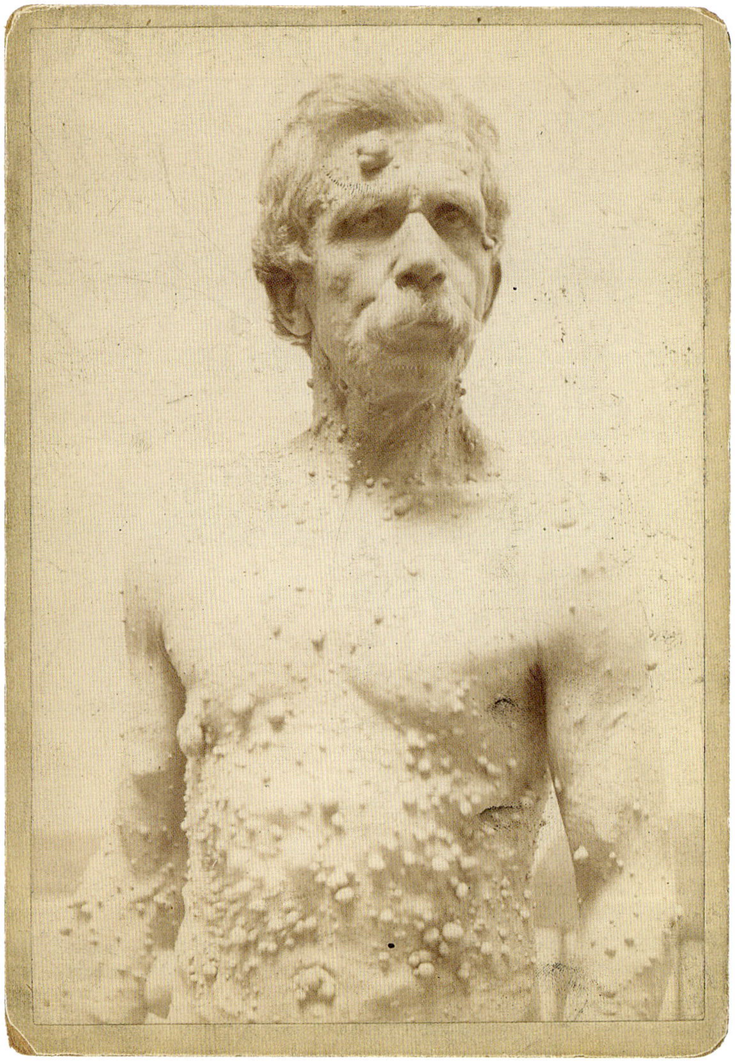

ABOVE AND OPPOSITE: Von Recklinghausen's disease (neurofibromatosis), a hereditary disorder in which many neurofibromas are present chiefly in the subcutaneous tissues. Reported at the Philadelphia Academy of Surgery, June 5, 1893, by Addinell Hewson, Jr., M.D. (1855–1938). Photographer unidentified, ca. 1893.

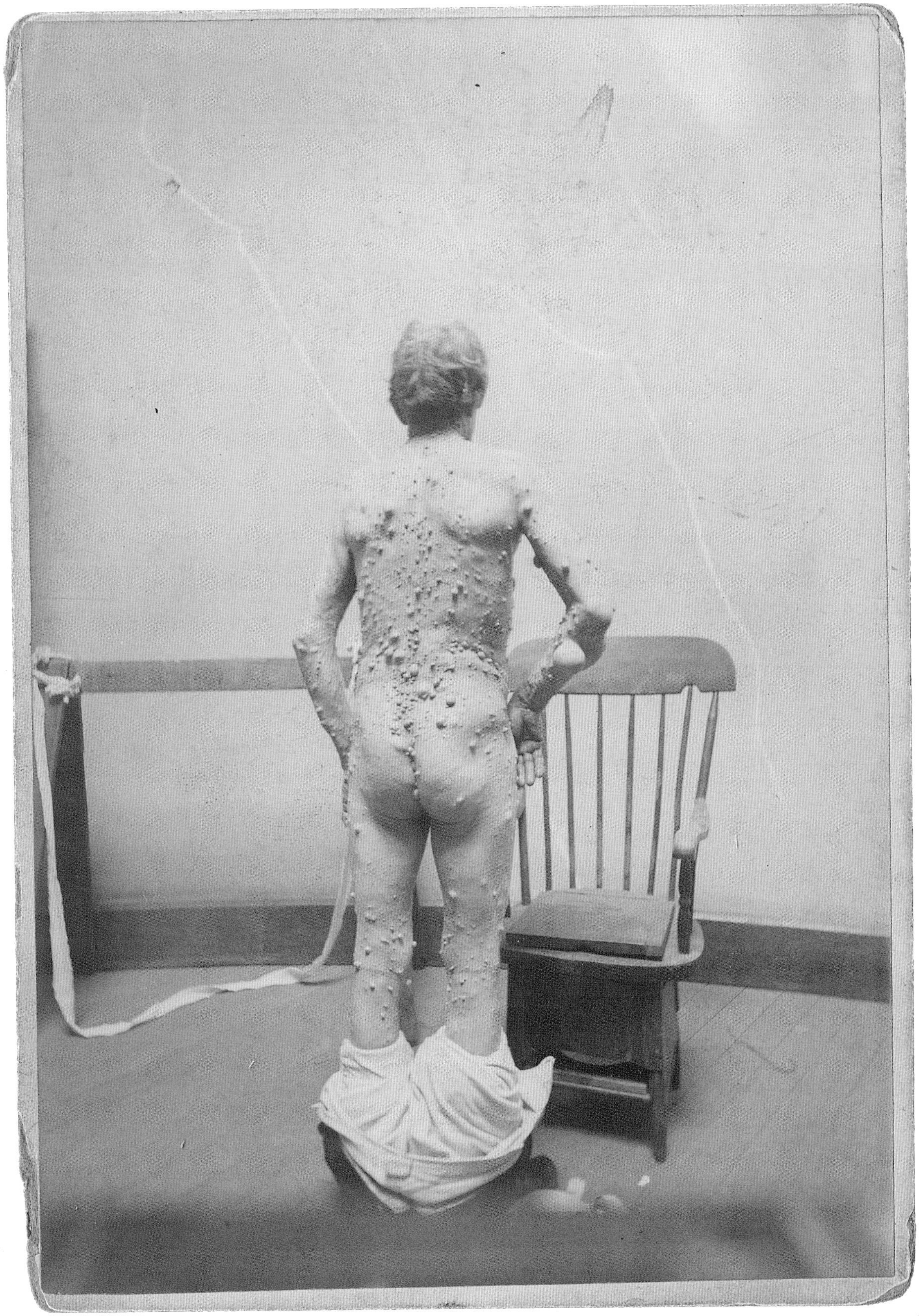

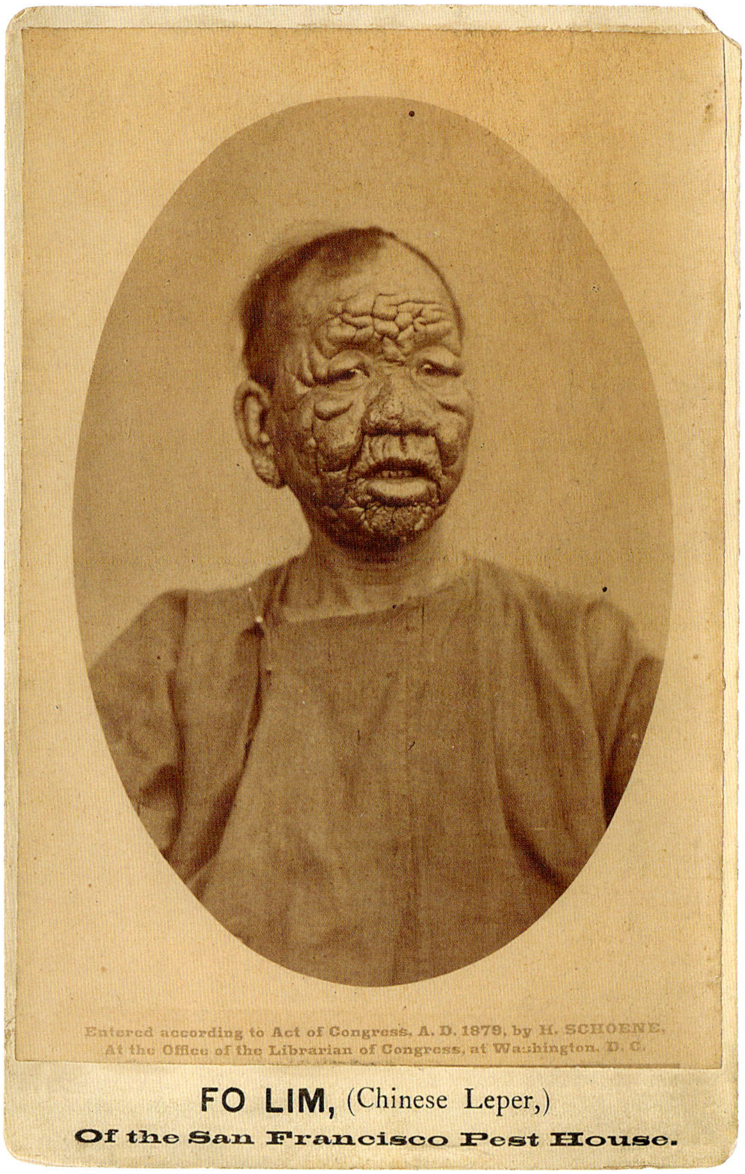

Leonine facies of leprosy (Hansen's disease). Fo Lim, San Francisco Pest House. Albumen print, photograph by H. Schoene, Santa Clara, California, 1879.

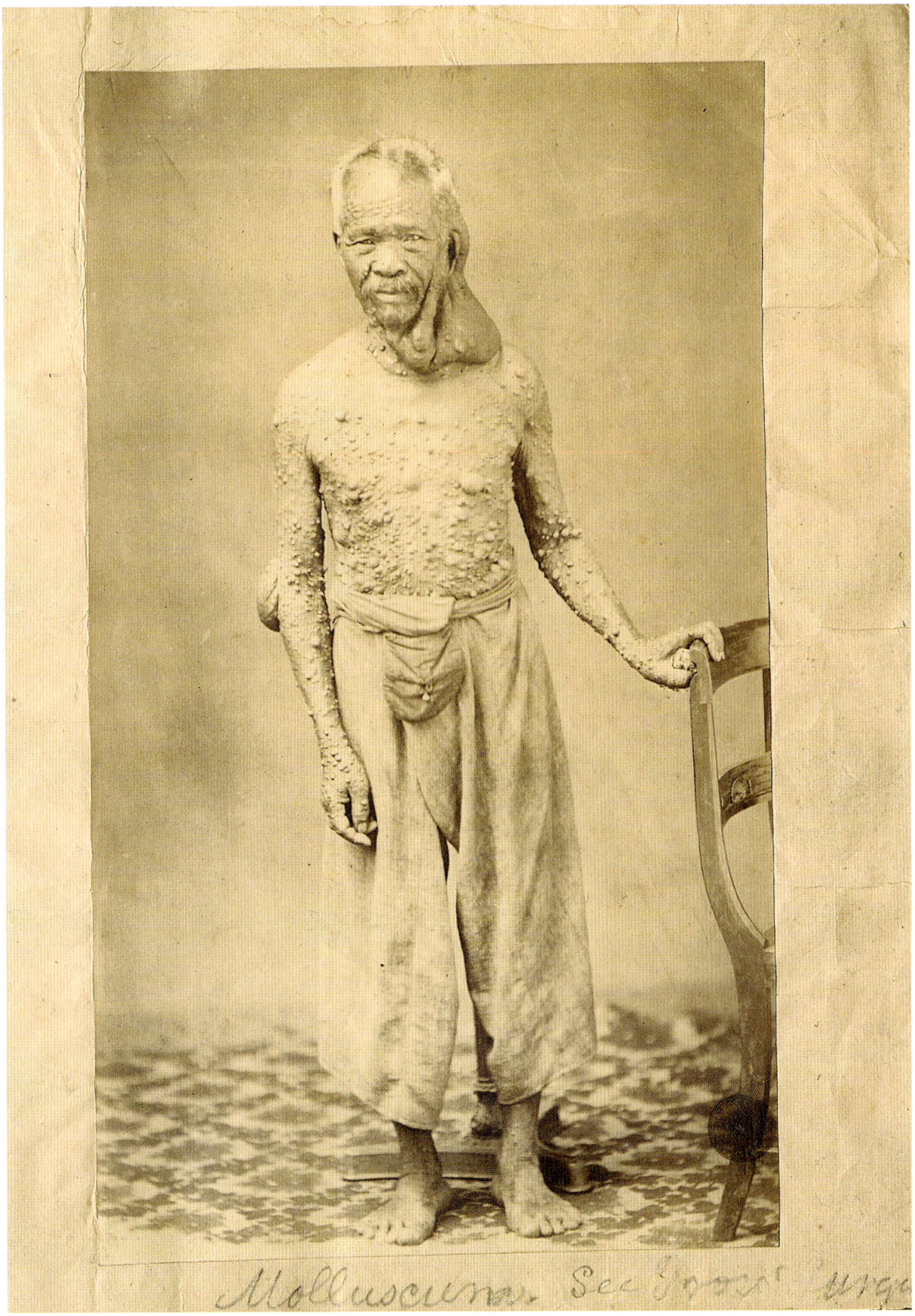

Von Recklinghausen's disease (neurofibromatosis), labeled as molluscum on photograph. From an album by John Glasgow Kerr, M.D. (1824–1901), of photographs of his practice in Canton, China.

Ringworm, a common contagious skin disorder caused by a superficial fungal infection. Photographer and date unidentified.

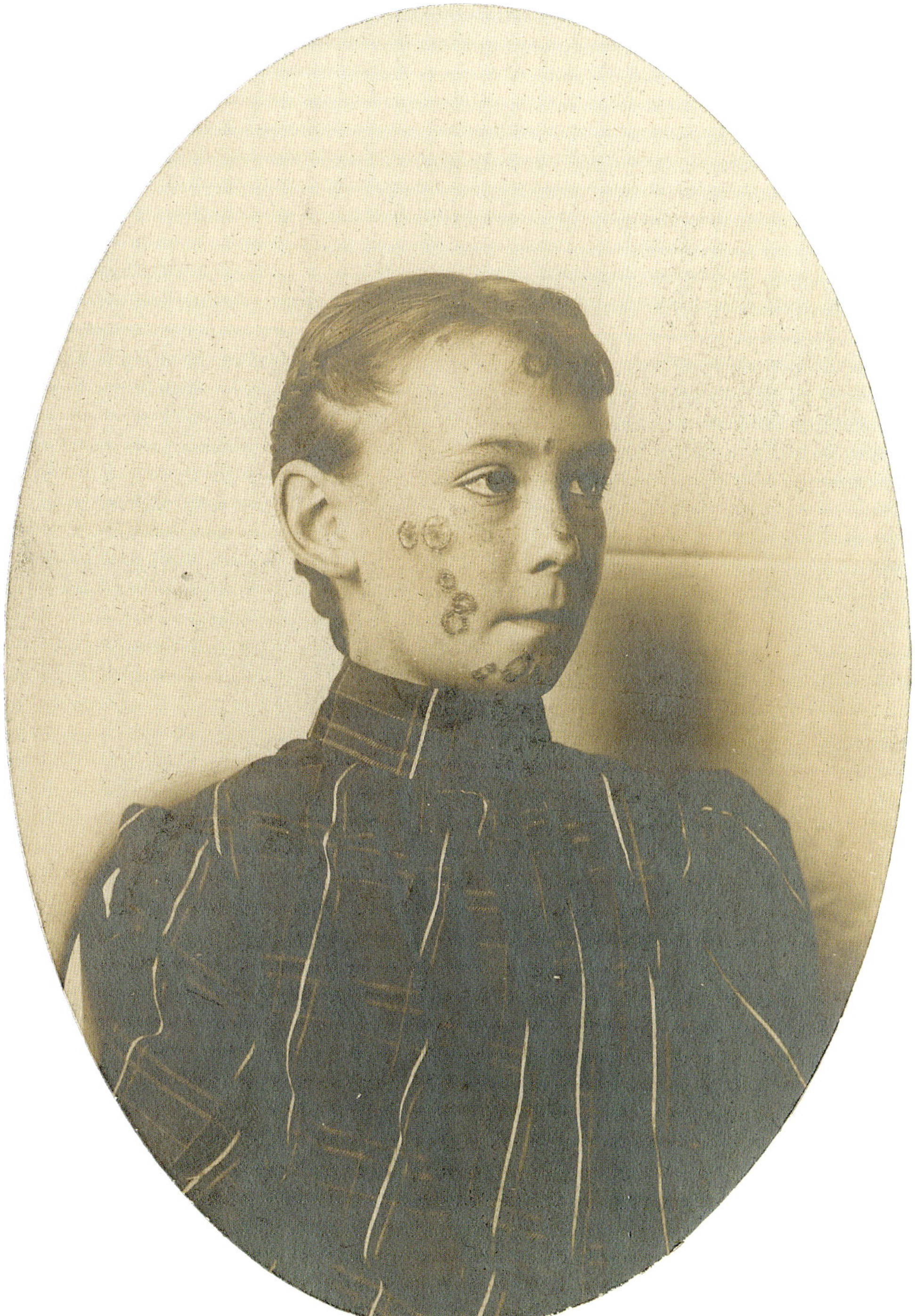

156

Herpes circinatus et iris, lesion characteristic of erythema multiforme (tinea corporis, or ringworm). Photograph by Ambrose H. Lincoln, Boston, ca. 1858–87.

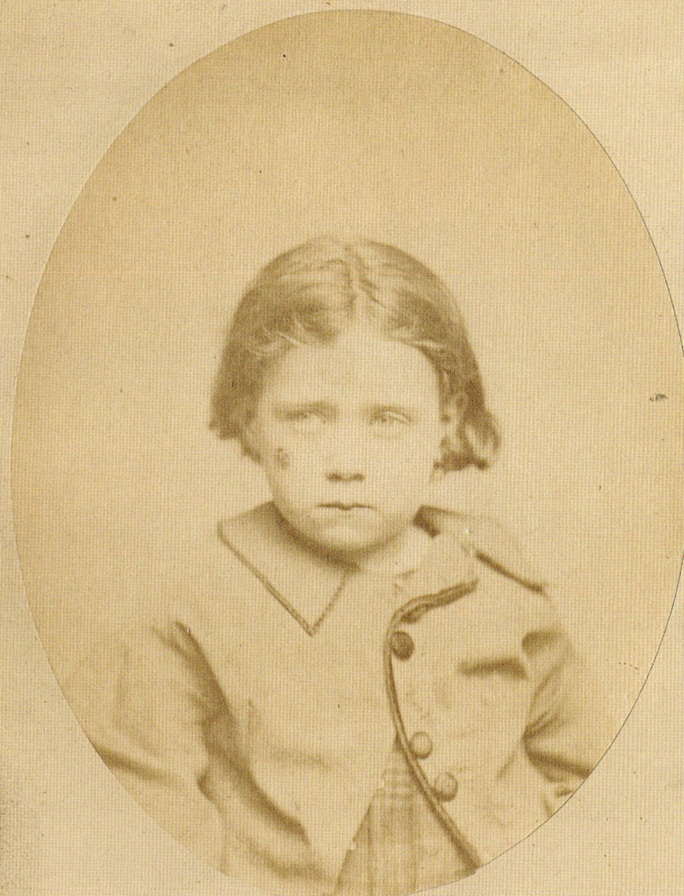

Herpes circinatus et iris.

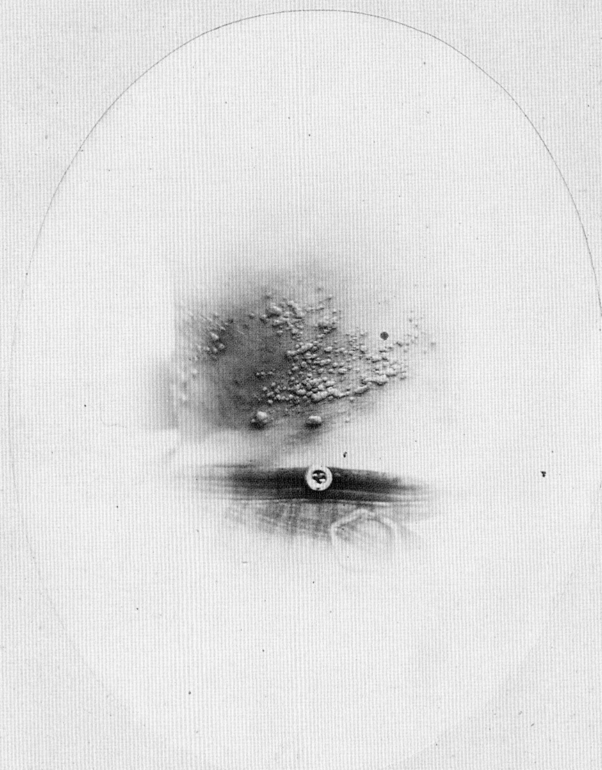

HERPES (ZOSTER).

Publisher,
JAMES CAMPBELL,
18 Tremont St.,
BOSTON.

Photographer,
A. H. LINCOLN,
556 Washington St.,
BOSTON.

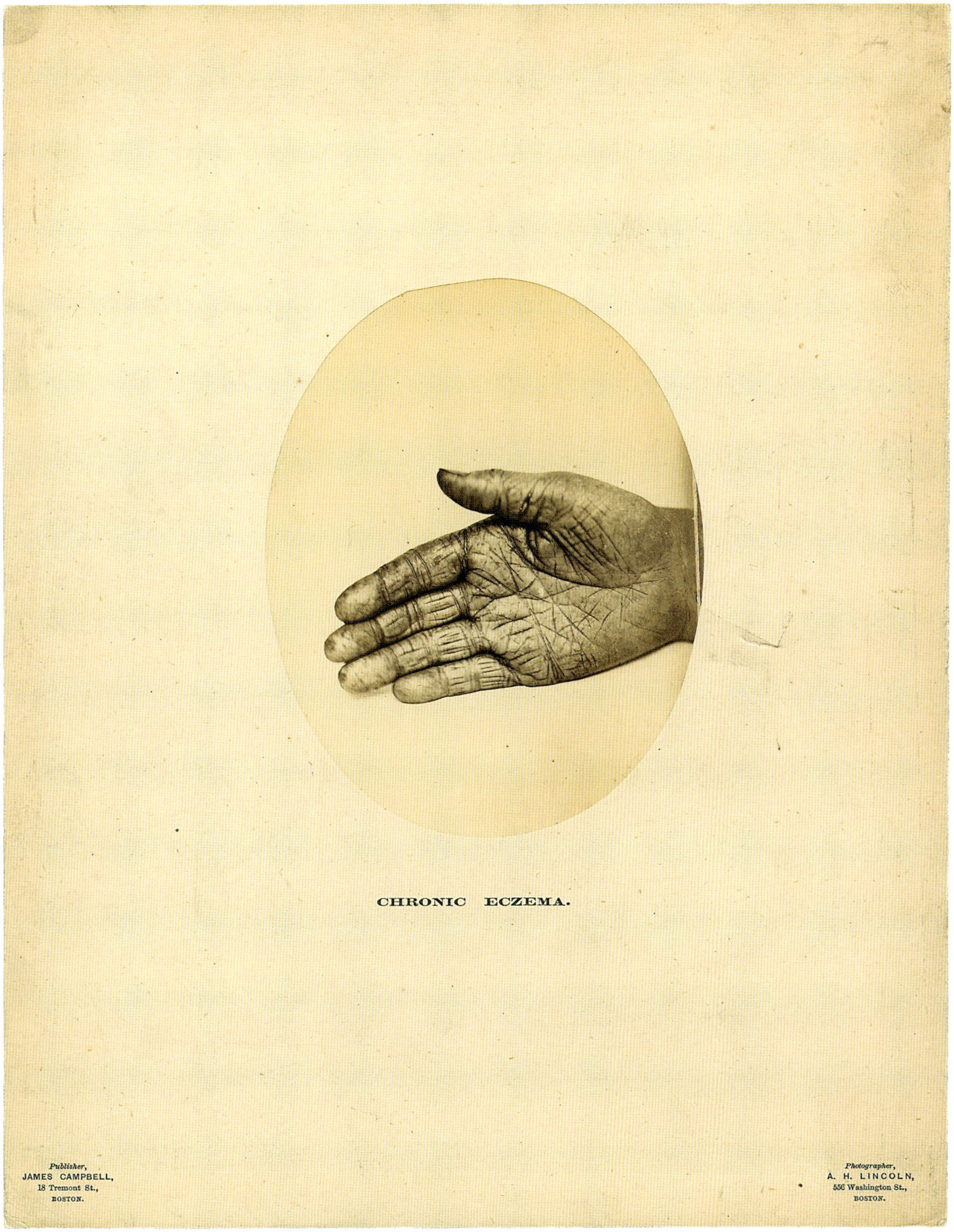

OPPOSITE: Herpes zoster (shingles). Photograph by Ambrose H. Lincoln, Boston, ca. 1858–87, James Campbell, publisher, ca. 1874.

ABOVE: Chronic eczema. Photograph by Ambrose H. Lincoln, Boston, ca. 1858–87, James Campbell, publisher, ca. 1874.

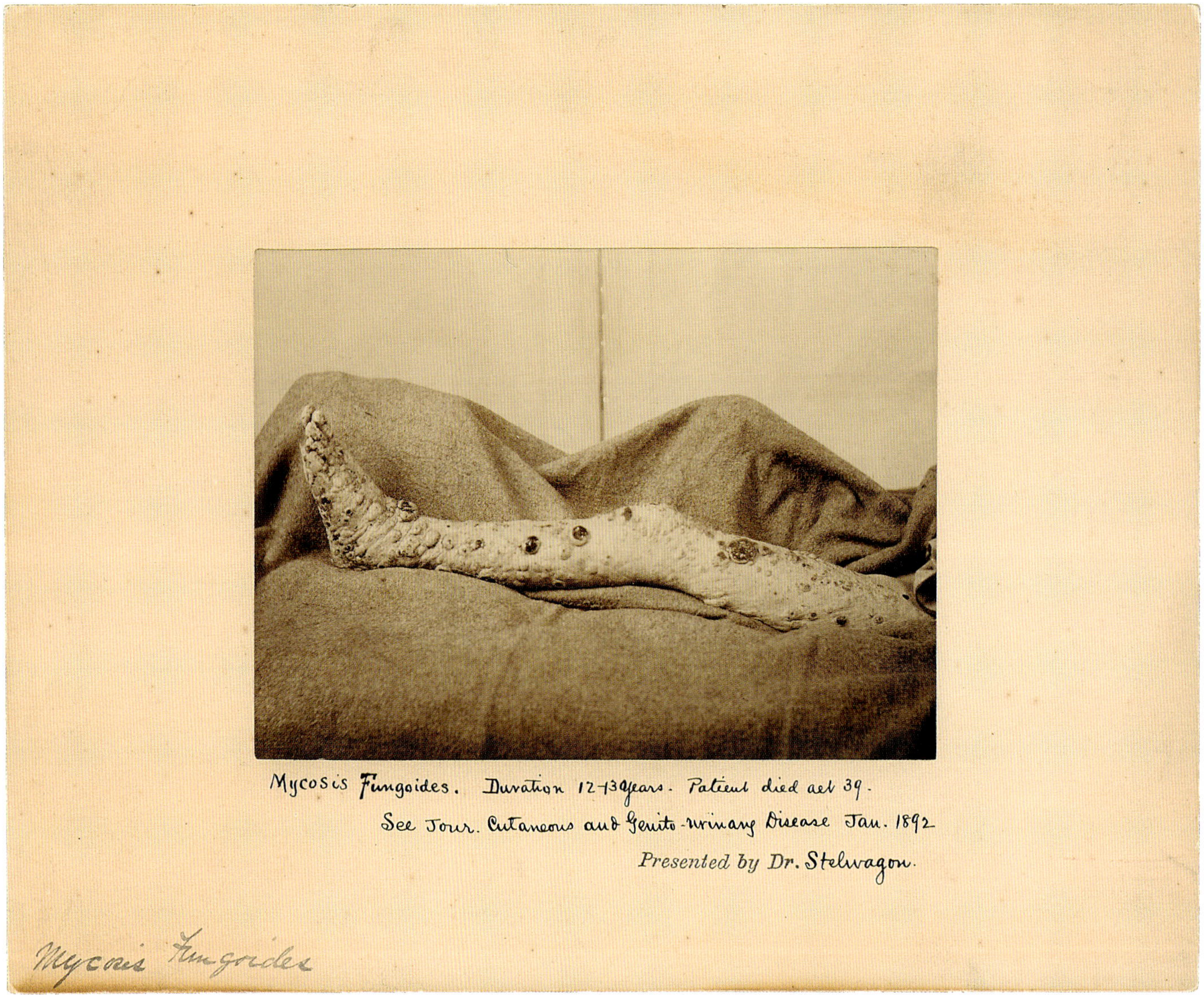

Dr. Stelwagon's case of mycosis fungoides, a disease in which lymphocytes become malignant and affect the skin. The disease may progress, as it has here, from a scaly rash to involve lymph nodes and internal organs and cause death. Case of Morris Petty, first symptoms at age twenty-six or twenty-seven. Patient died at thirty-nine in Philadelphia Hospital. Full report published in the *Journal of Cutaneous and Genito-Urinary Disease*, January 1892. Donor: Dr. Henry Weightman Stelwagon (1853–1919).

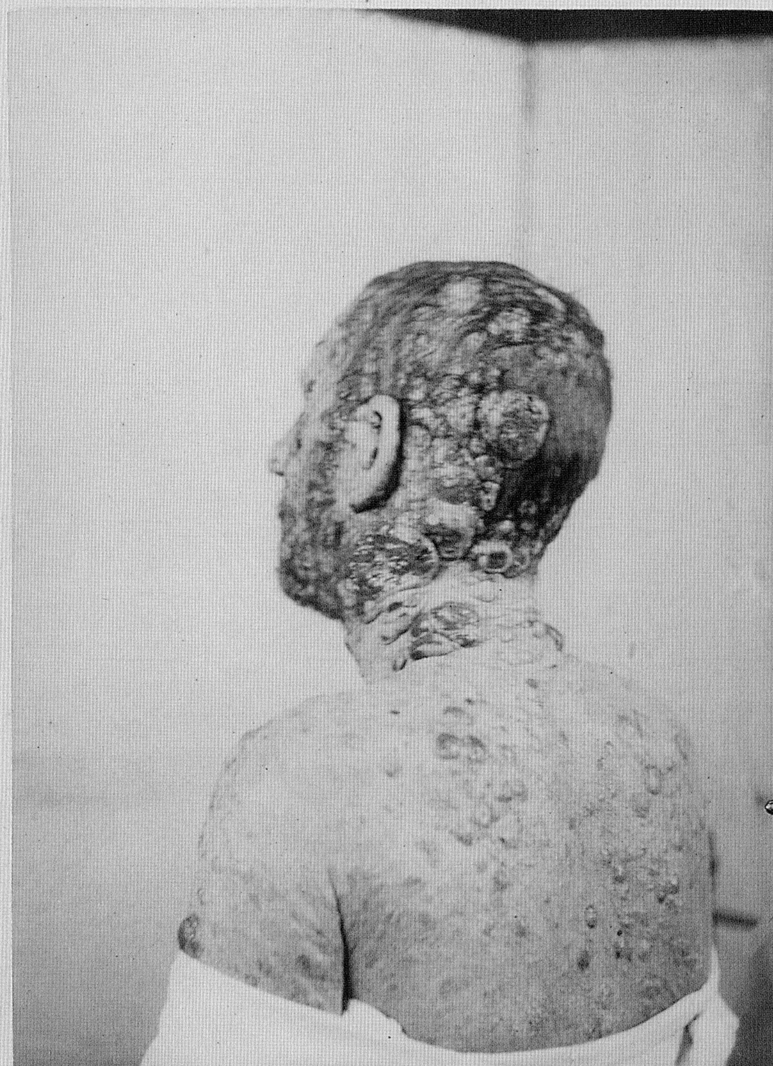

Mycosis Fungoides. Presented by Dr. Stelwagon.

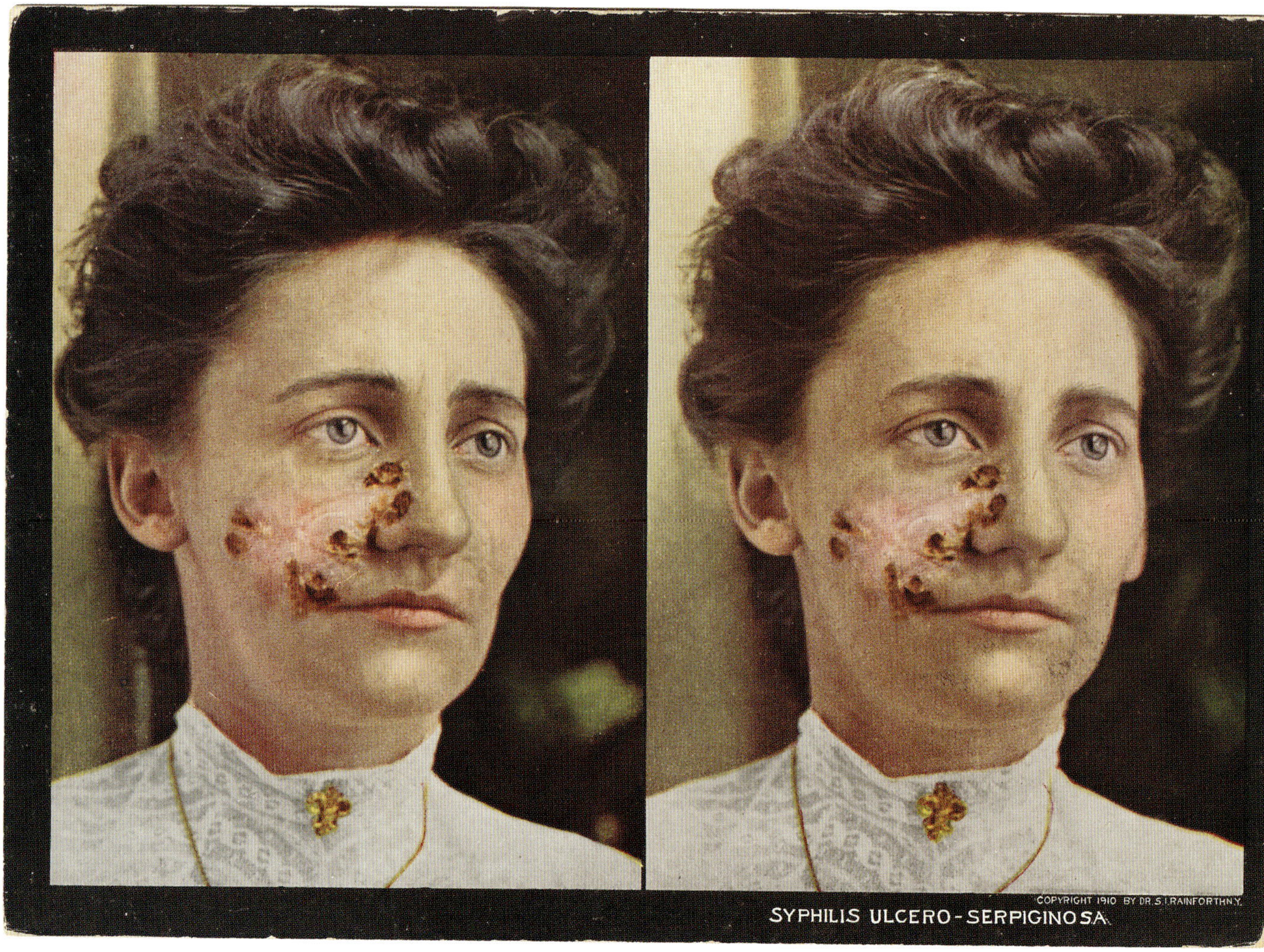

ABOVE, OPPOSITE, AND PAGES 164–65: Stereographic cards from "The Stereoscopic Skin Clinic," 1911, © 1910, Dr. Selden Irwin Rainforth (1879–1960), New York. Donor: Allentown State Hospital.

Syphilis tertiaria showing syphilis ulcero-serpiginosa. The ulcerative tendency of a tubercular syphilid may exist from the earliest appearance of the lesion or show itself only after a group or patch of tubercles has formed and lasted for some time. The ulceration may be deep or shallow, and the ulcers travel slowly over the skin by healing and scarring at one margin and advancing at the other. It is unusual for ulcers to heal spontaneously, although almost invariably they respond rapidly to specific constitutional treatment with mercury and potassium iodid.

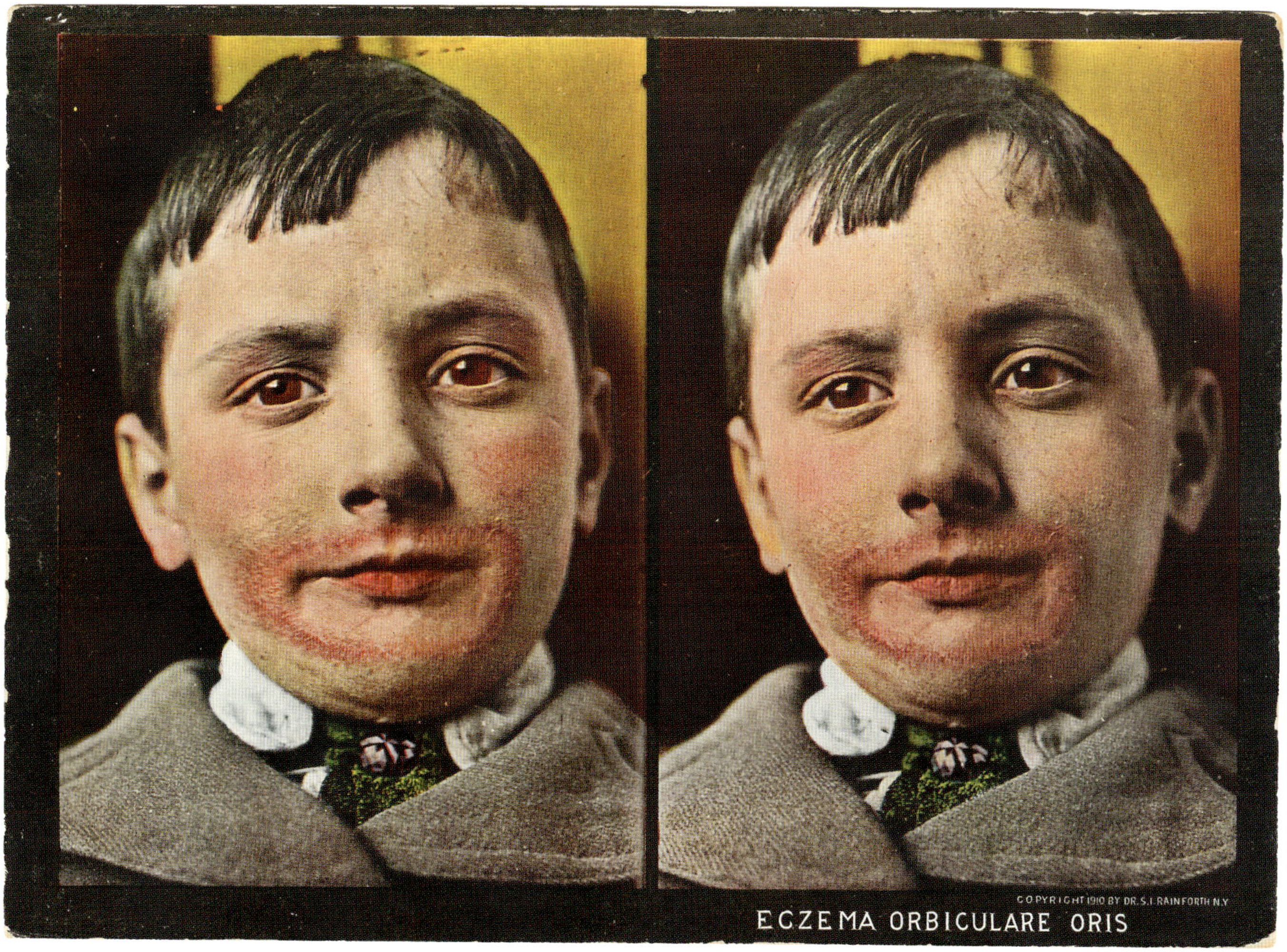

Eczema orbiculare oris. Eczema about the mouth often consists of an orbicular patch with a fairly well marked outer margin that sometimes defines the limits of the area that the tongue can reach. Eczema of the lips may be caused by mucous secretion or by the use of strongly aromatic mouth washes or toothpastes or by tobacco, and it may be protracted to some extent by the movements of the lips in laughing, talking, and eating, but in most instances the pertinacity of the condition is due to the habit of frequently moistening the lips with the tongue. If the habit of moistening the lips can be broken, the condition usually responds readily to treatment with simple remedies.

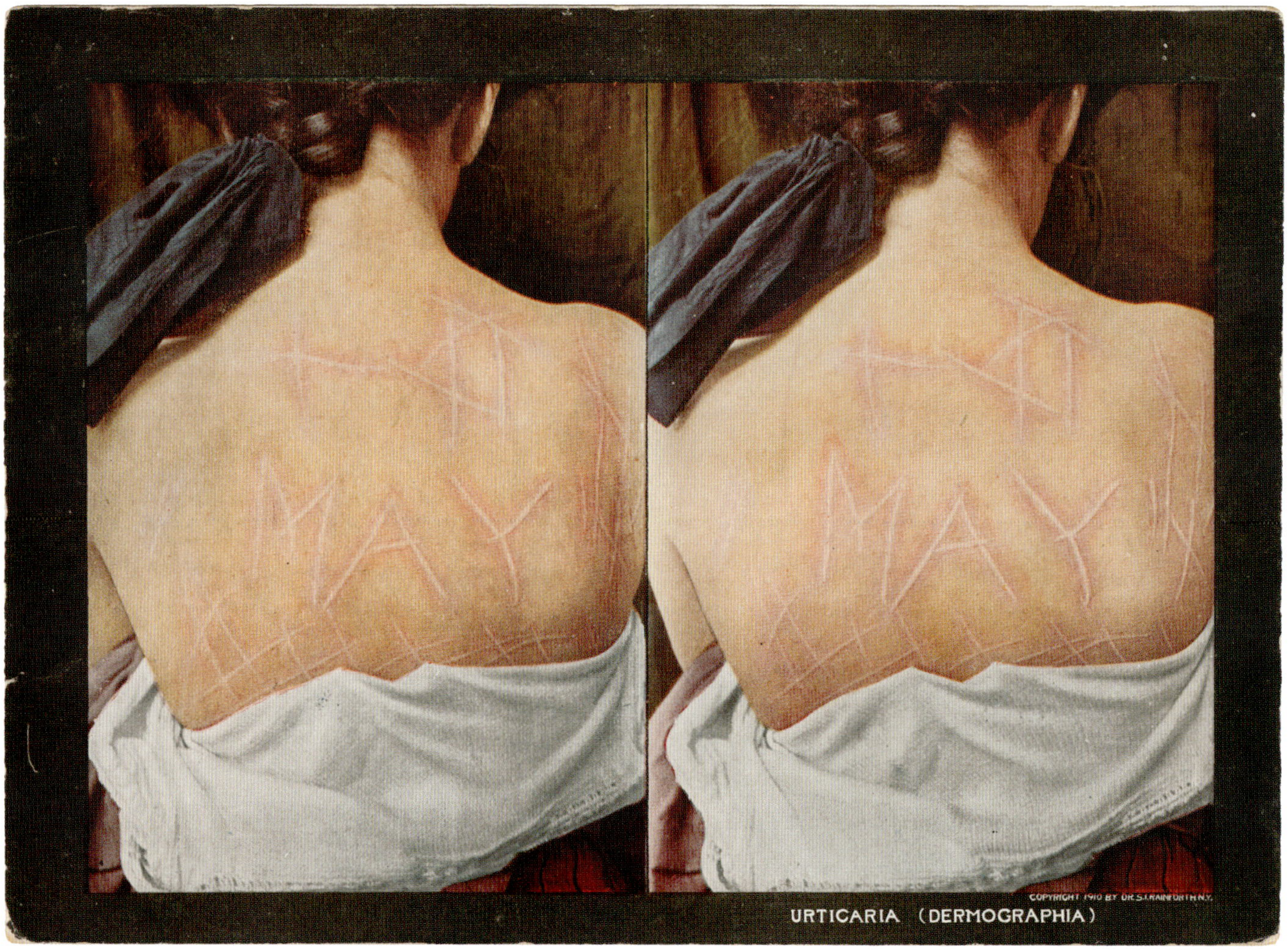

Urticaria (dermographia [hives]). Urticaria is characterized by a particular form of lesion known as the wheal, which is a round, elongate, or irregularly shaped, flat elevation of the skin due to a circumscribed tense edema of the corium. Wheals vary in size; some may be only as large as the head of a pin, others larger than the palm of the hand. To the touch they are moderately firm and cannot be made to disappear or pit on pressure. The wheals appear suddenly and disappear more gradually, persisting from a few minutes to several hours. When the cutaneous response to mechanical stimulation is very pronounced, the condition is often described as urticaria factitia or dermographia.

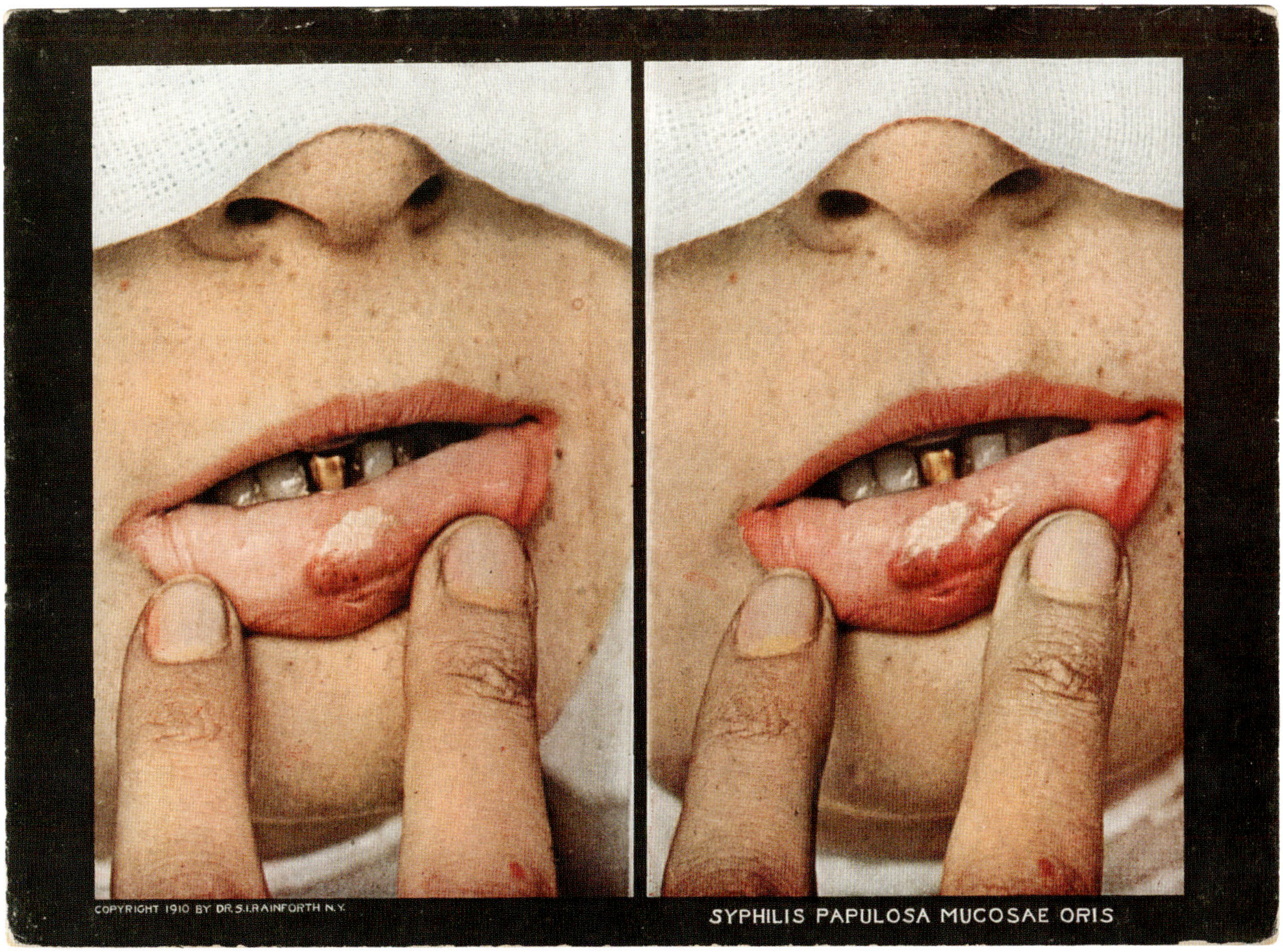

Syphilis secundaria showing syphilis papulosa mucosae oris. Mucous patches are the most constant lesion of secondary syphilis. They may be found upon any part of the oral mucous membrane sometimes in large numbers, though generally there are only two or three. Although they yield readily to constitutional remedies, they are very prone to recur, especially in hard drinkers and inveterate smokers, even in the tertiary period.

Venereal disease. Photographer unidentified, December 9, 1944.

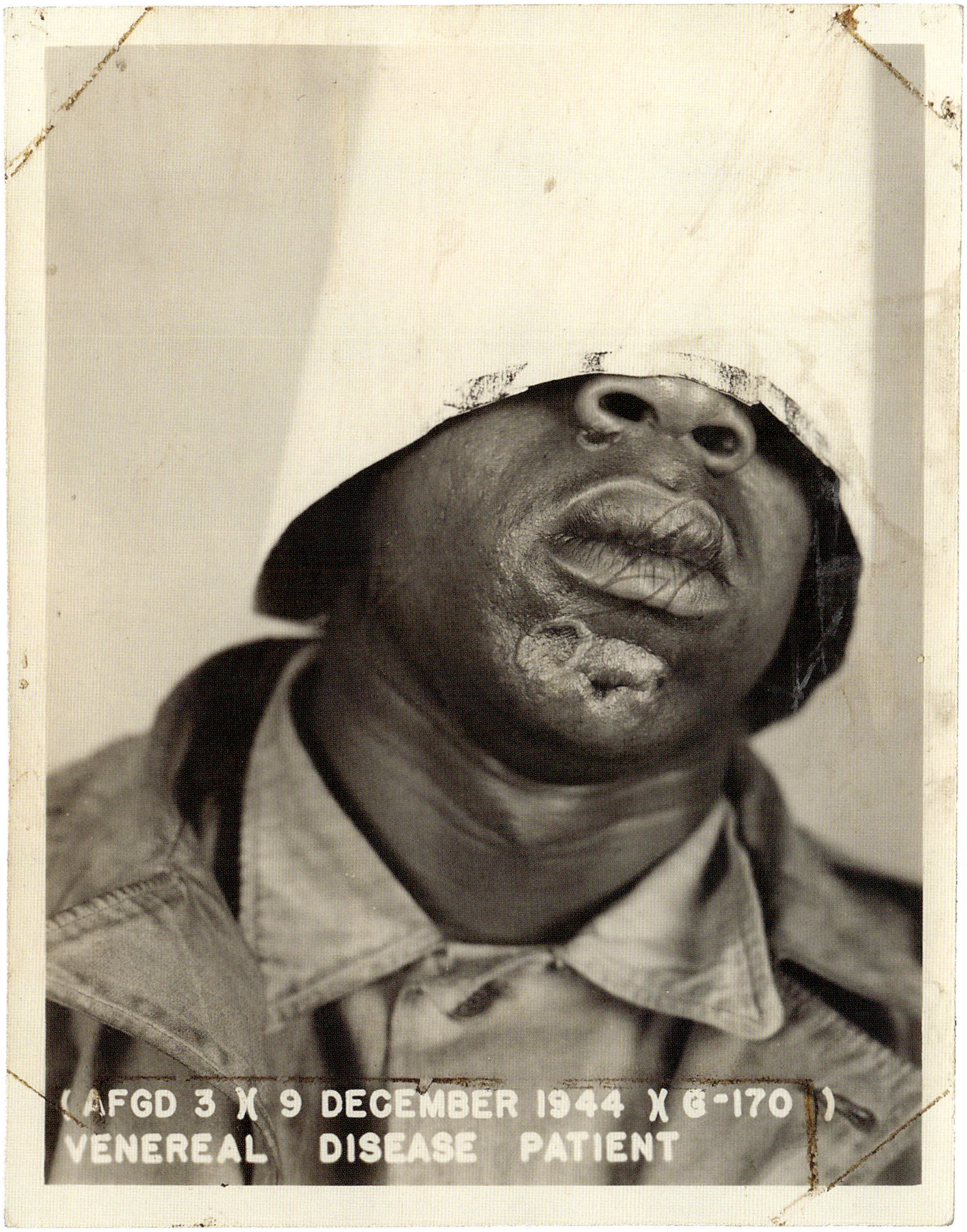
(AFGD 3)(9 DECEMBER 1944)(G-170)
VENEREAL DISEASE PATIENT

Micrography

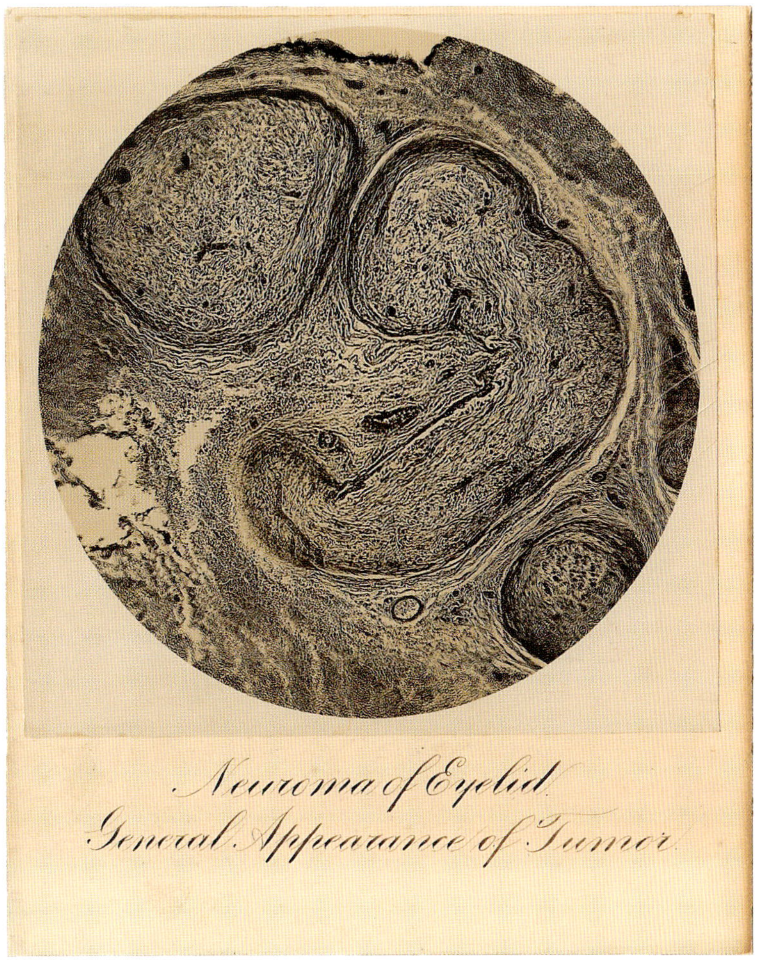

Dr. George Edmund de Schweinitz's (1858–1938) case of neuroma of the eyelid. Photomicrograph by Dr. William M. Gray (1877–1954) of the Army Medical Museum, ca. 1893.

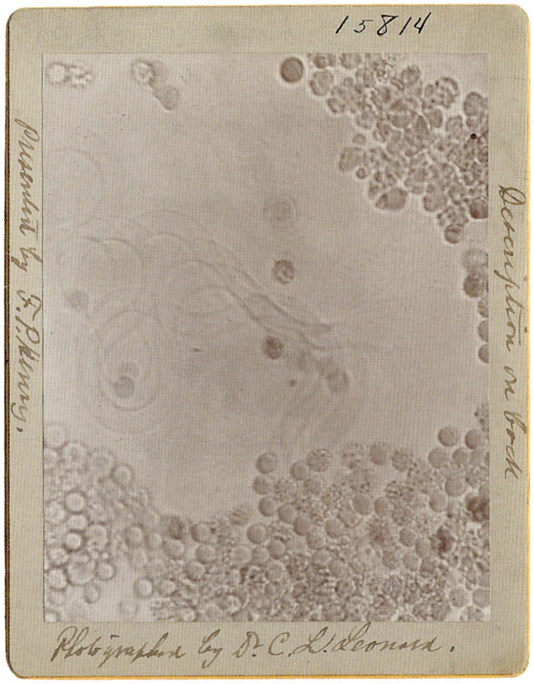

1

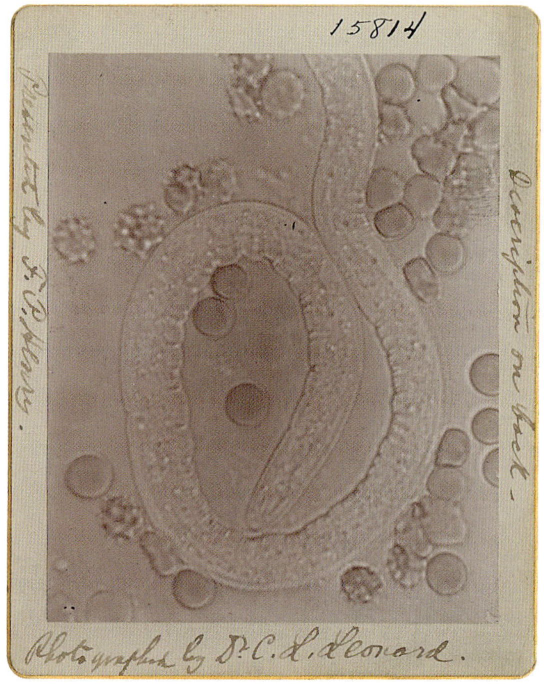

2

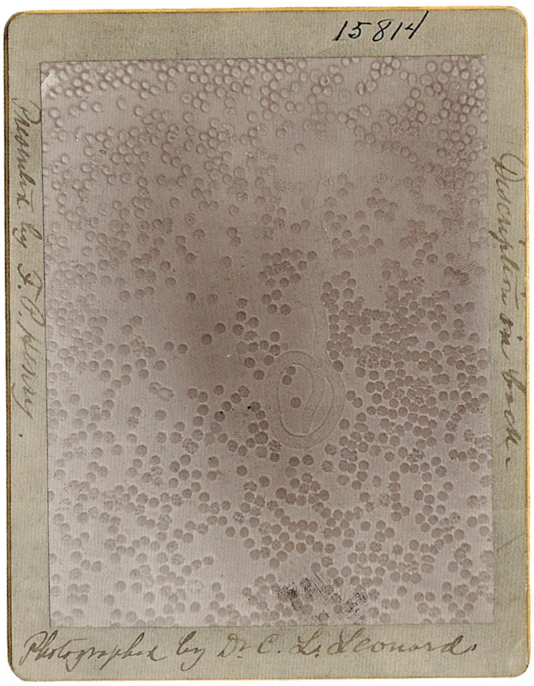

3

1. Shows the movements of a single filaria during a series of four successive instantaneous exposures. The length of each exposure was one-fifth of a second, the entire series occupying less than five seconds. The magnification is to 800 diameters with a Zeiss immersion lens.
2. Filaria alive in the blood. Instantaneous photomicrograph 400 diameters, 4 millimeters Zeiss apochromatic.
3. Same as no. 2, magnified to 1500 diameters, showing structure and commencing granular degeneration.
4. Tail of filaria showing sheath extending beyond the apparent end of the tail, 800 diameters.
5. Head of living filaria.

Filaria sanguinis hominis nocturnia. Case reported in *Medical News*, May 2, 1896. Filaria (*Wuchereria bancrofti*) is a long, threadlike parasitic roundworm that lives in the bodies of humans and animals. It is found mainly in Central Africa, Asia, and the Southwest Pacific. Filarial infection is spread by mosquitoes; adult filaria live in the lymph, causing elephantiasis. Photographs by Dr. Charles Lester Leonard (1861–1913).

A pioneer roentgenologist, Leonard became the foremost authority in the diagnostic application of roentgen rays and was the first in the United States to demonstrate the presence of stones in the kidney. Radiation dermatitis led to ten years of increasing physical distress, the amputation of an arm, and eventually Leonard's death at age fifty-one. Donor: Frederick Porteous Henry (1844–1919).

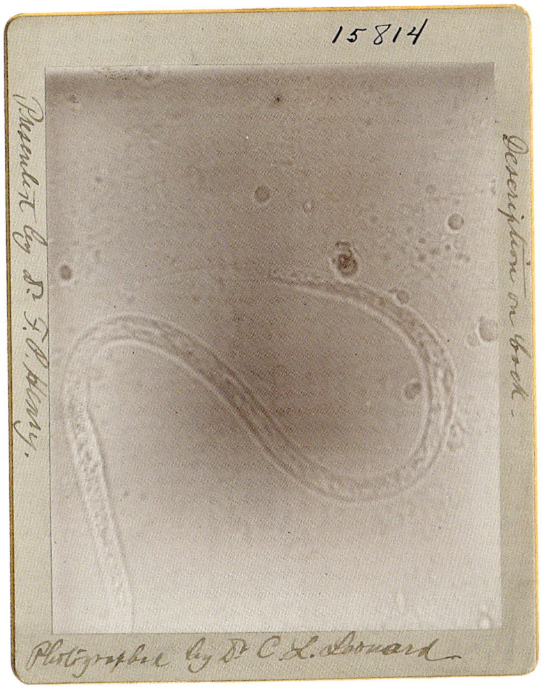
15814
Description on back.
Presented by Dr. F. P. Henry.
Photographed by Dr. C. L. Leonard

4

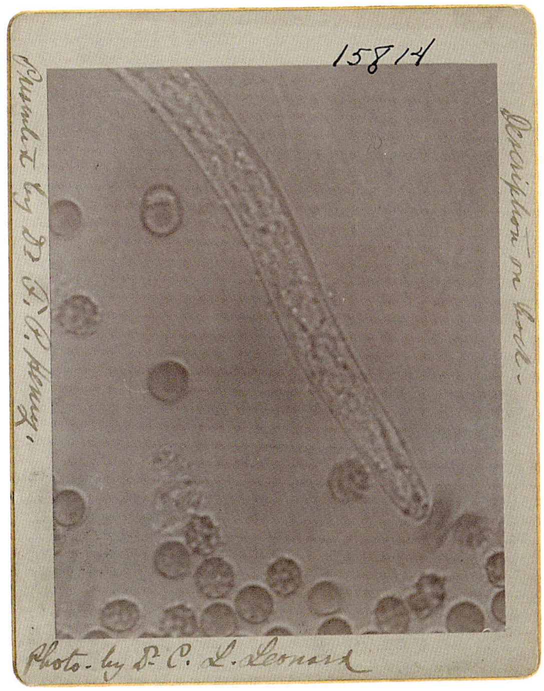
15814
Description on back.
Presented by Dr. F. P. Henry.
Photo. by Dr. C. L. Leonard

5

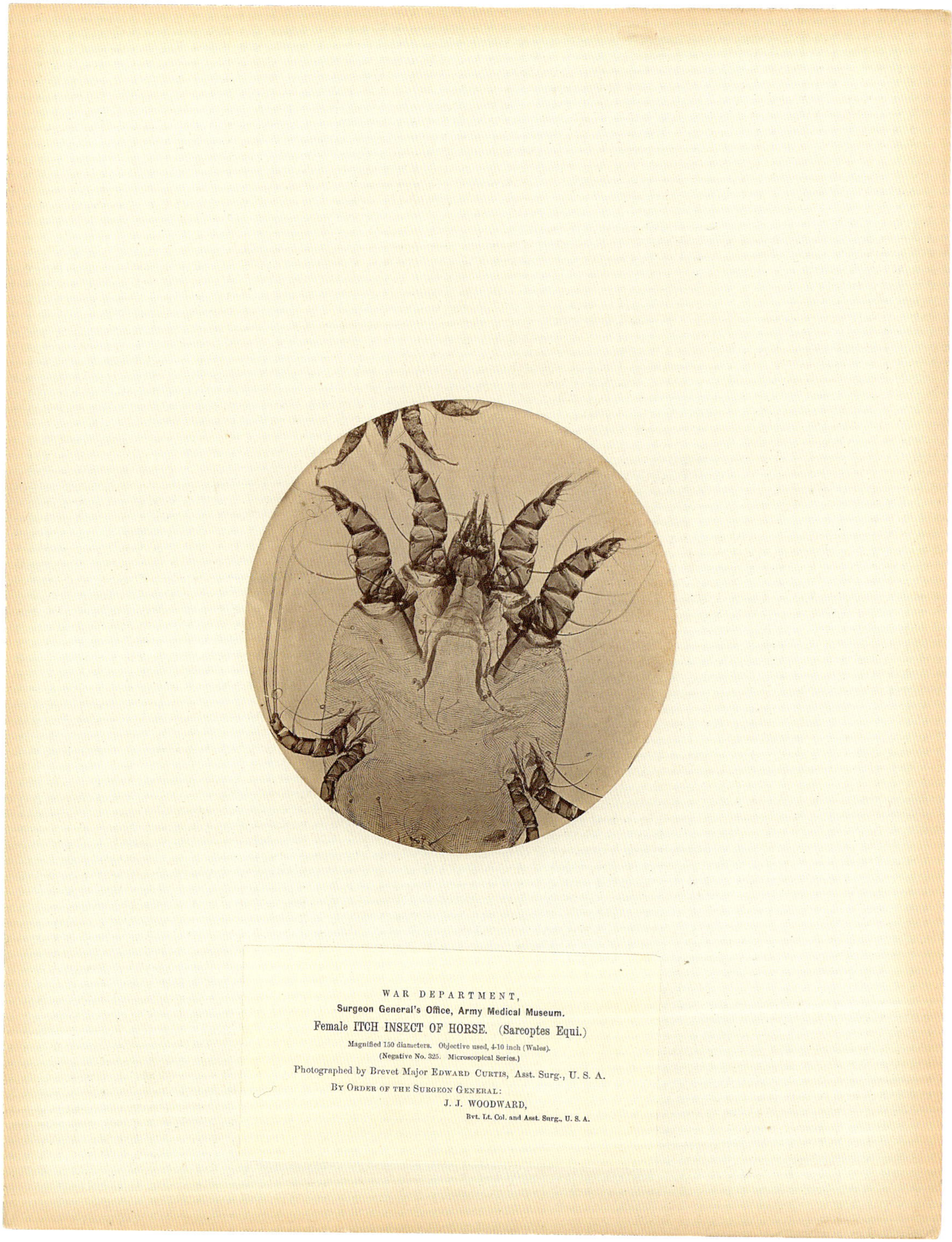

Photomicrograph, female itch insect of horse (*Sarcoptes equi*), magnified 150 diameters. Photograph by Brevet Major Edward Curtis (1838–1912), by order of Surgeon General Joseph Janvier Woodward (1833–1884) for the Army Medical Museum, ca. 1865–67.

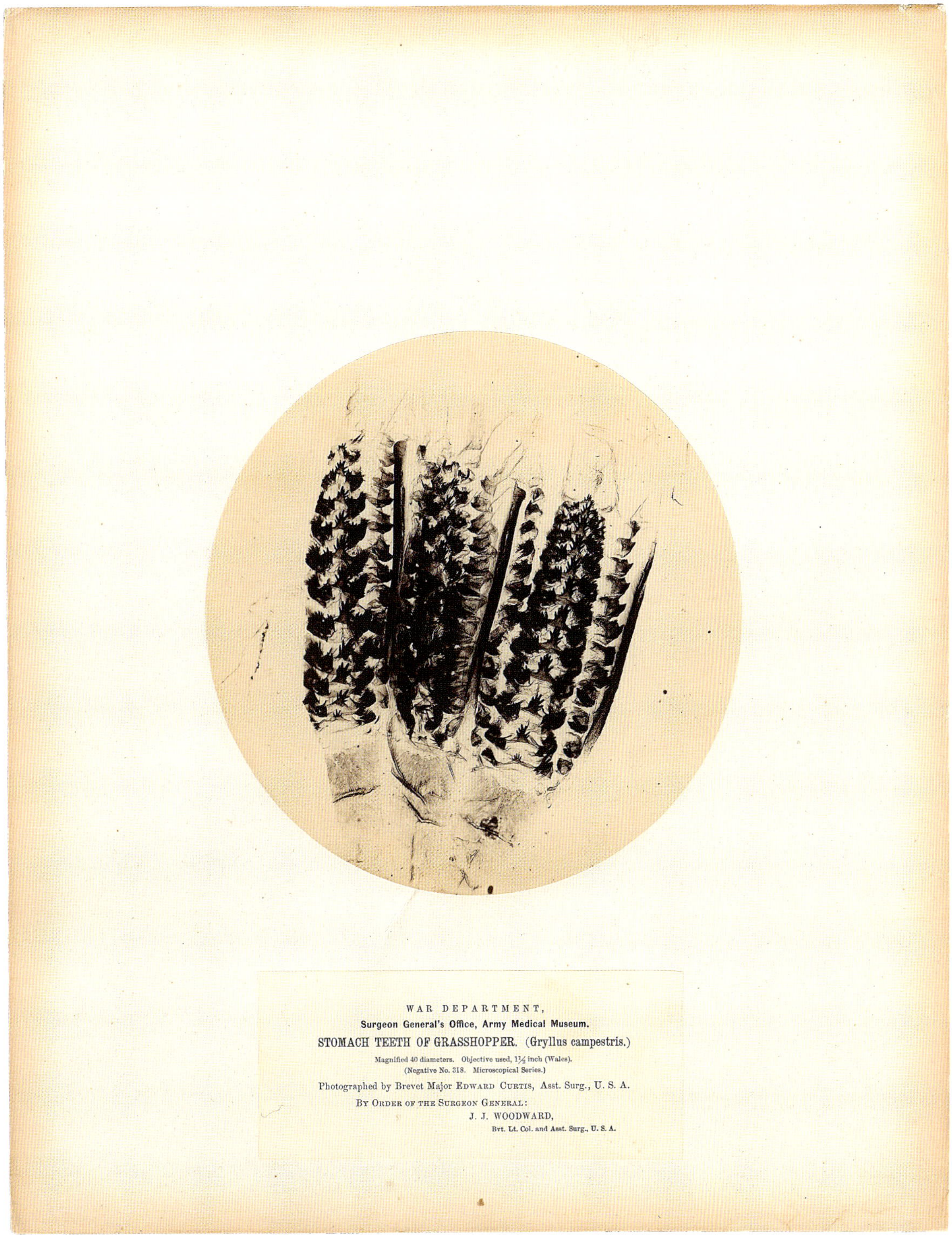
WAR DEPARTMENT,
Surgeon General's Office, Army Medical Museum.
STOMACH TEETH OF GRASSHOPPER. (Gryllus campestris.)
Magnified 40 diameters. Objective used, 1½ inch (Wales).
(Negative No. 318. Microscopical Series.)
Photographed by Brevet Major EDWARD CURTIS, Asst. Surg., U. S. A.
BY ORDER OF THE SURGEON GENERAL:
J. J. WOODWARD,
Bvt. Lt. Col. and Asst. Surg., U. S. A.

Photomicrograph, stomach teeth of grasshopper (*Gryllus campestris*), magnified 40 diameters. Photograph by Brevet Major Edward Curtis, by order of Surgeon General Joseph Janvier Woodward for the Army Medical Museum, ca. 1865–67.

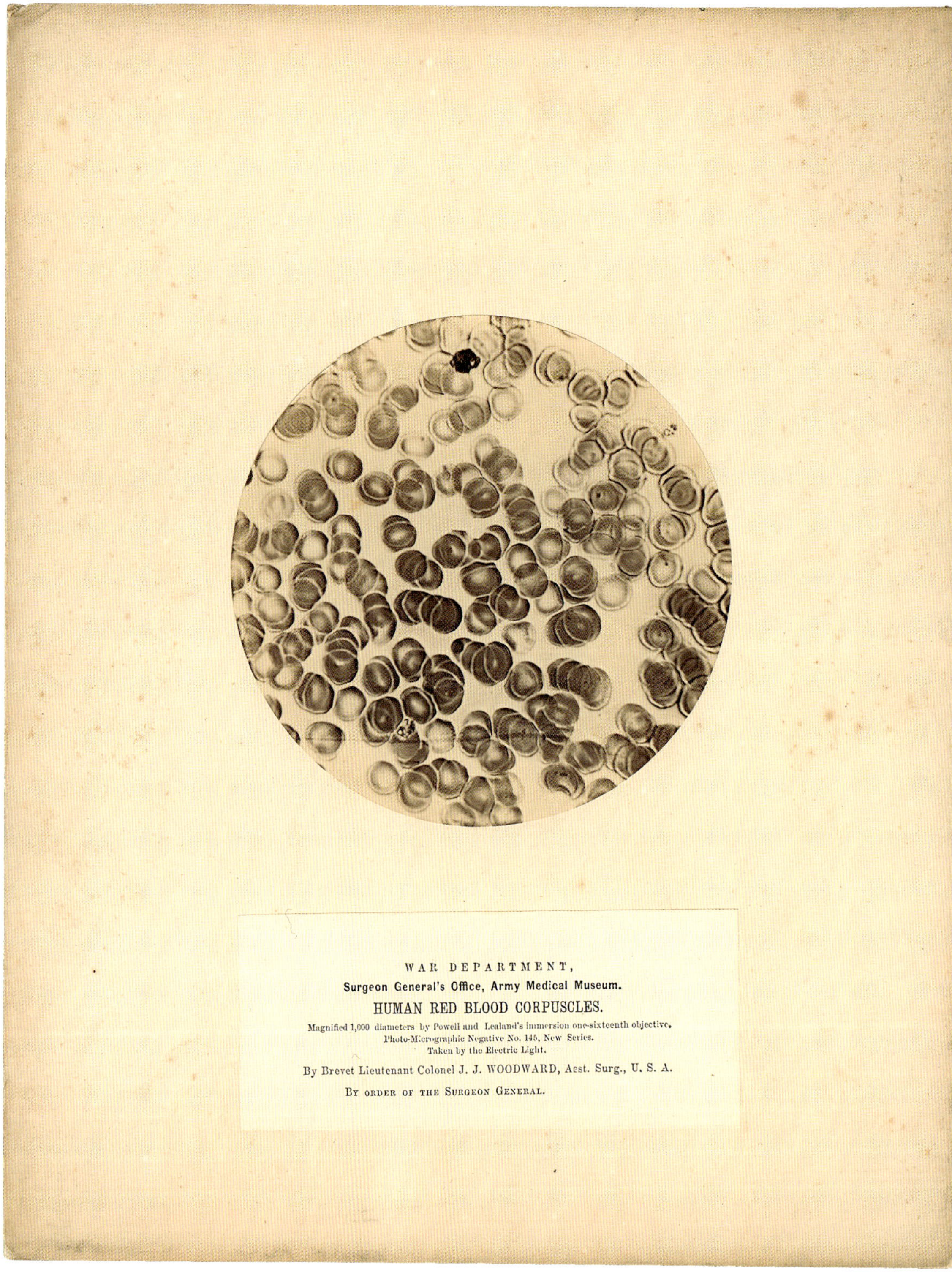

Human red blood corpuscles, magnified 1,000 diameters. Photomicrograph by Brevet Lieutenant Colonel Joseph Janvier Woodward (1833–1884) for the Army Medical Museum, ca. 1865–70.

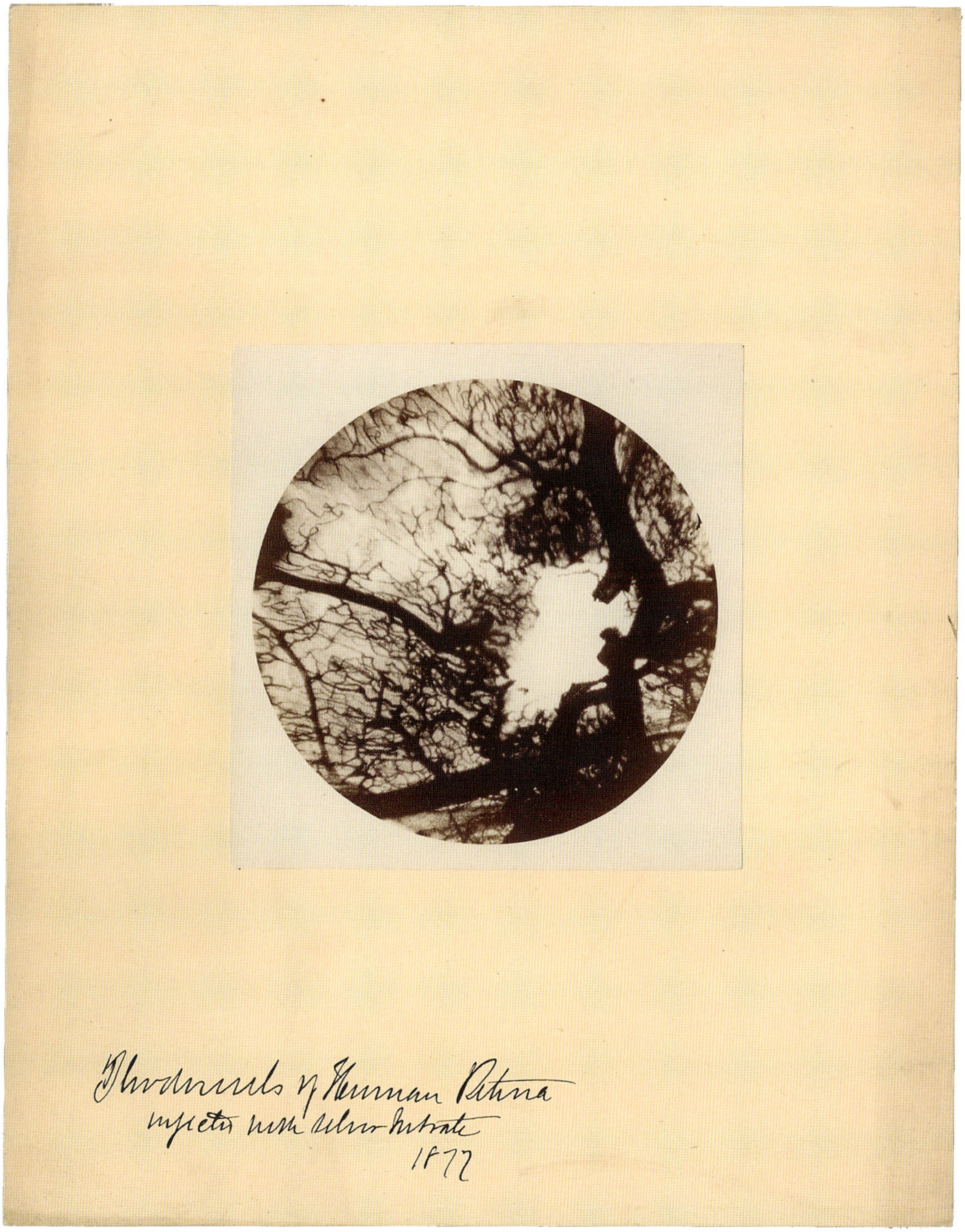

Blood vessels of human retina injected with silver nitrate.
Photomicrograph, 1877, probably by Dr. George Arthur Piersol (1856–1924),
collected by Dr. James Wallace and Dr. William Fisher Norris (1839–1901).

Cysts and Tumors

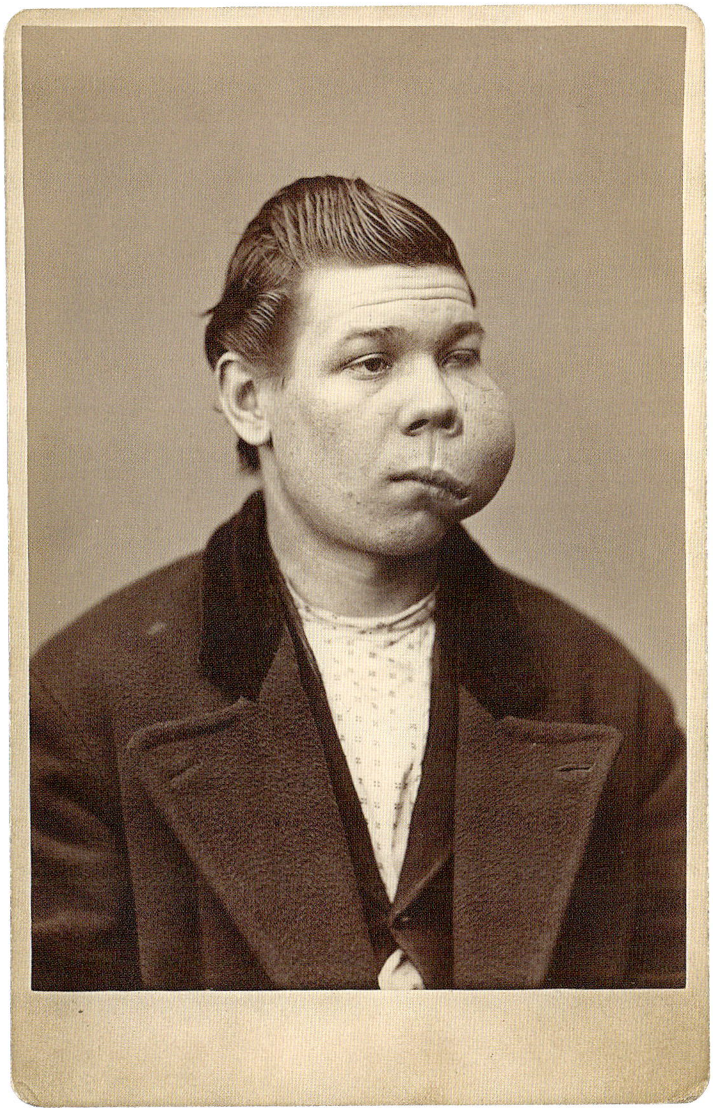

Unidentified disease of jaw, probably tumorous. Photograph by William H. Rhoads, Philadelphia, ca. 1866–98.

Transverse colon with cysts. Heliotype, published in an atlas showing morbid and anatomical lesions of the large and small intestines, photographer unidentified. Published by James R. Osgood (1836–1892) & Co., Boston, publisher of Walt Whitman, Mark Twain, Henry James, et al.

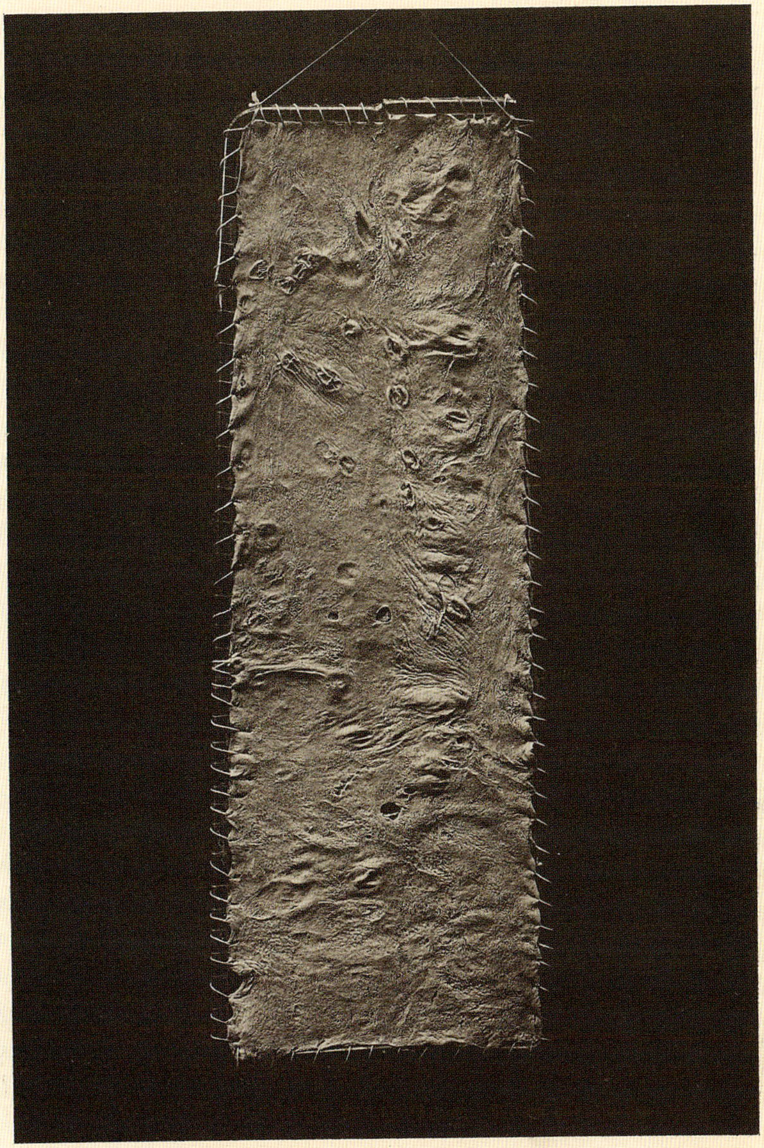

Heliotype. *James R. Osgood & Co., Boston.*

TRANSVERSE COLON WITH CYSTS.

No. 602. MEDICAL SECTION.

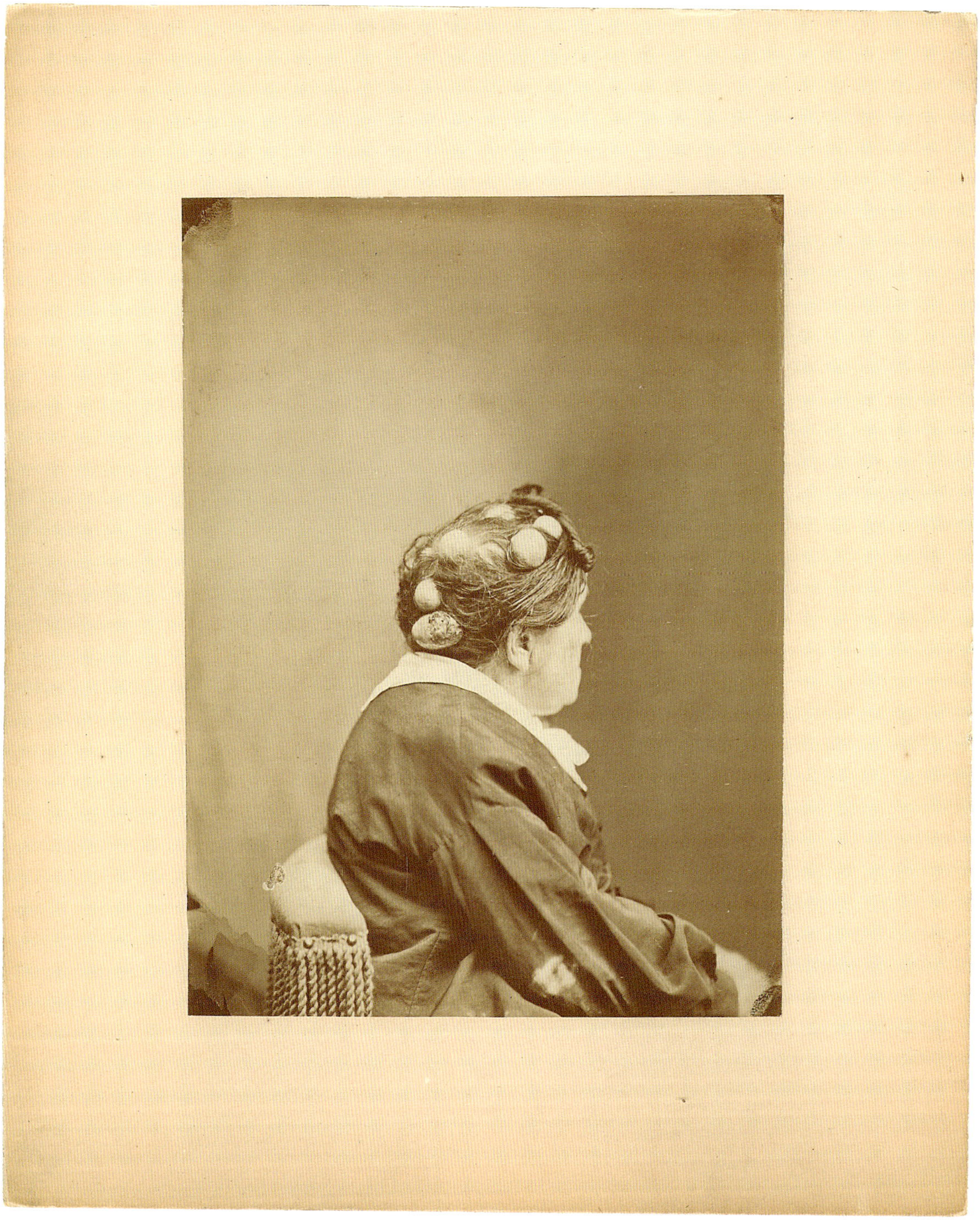

Multiple sebaceous tumors of the scalp. Inscription on photograph: "Patient—a woman nearly eighty years of age—came on nearly forty years ago—the lower, in a state of ulceration, excised—did not interfere with the rest. Jefferson College Clinic, 1875." Albumen print, photographer unidentified.

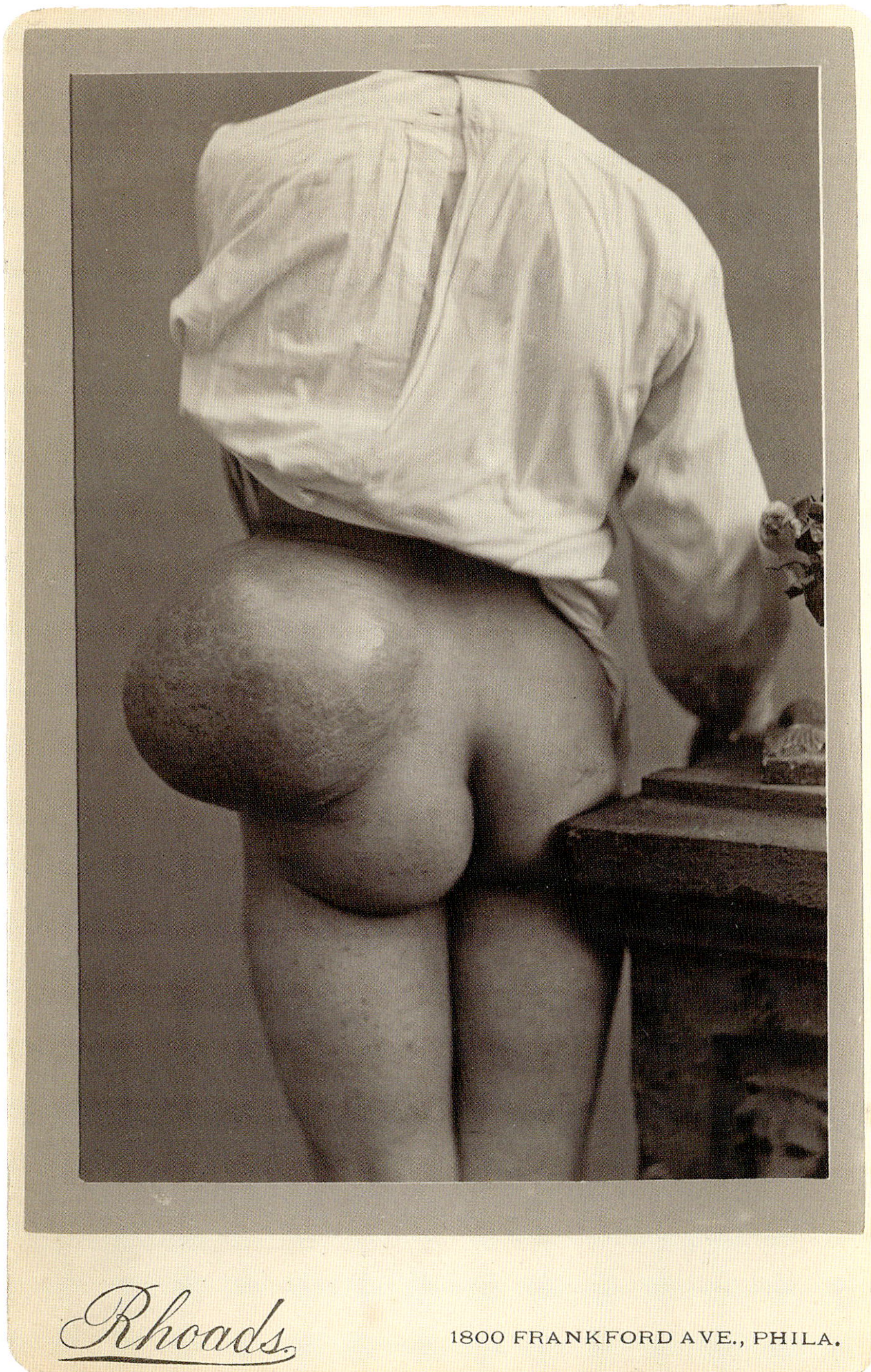

Sarcoma of hip. Albumen print, photograph by William H. Rhoads, Philadelphia, ca. 1866–98.

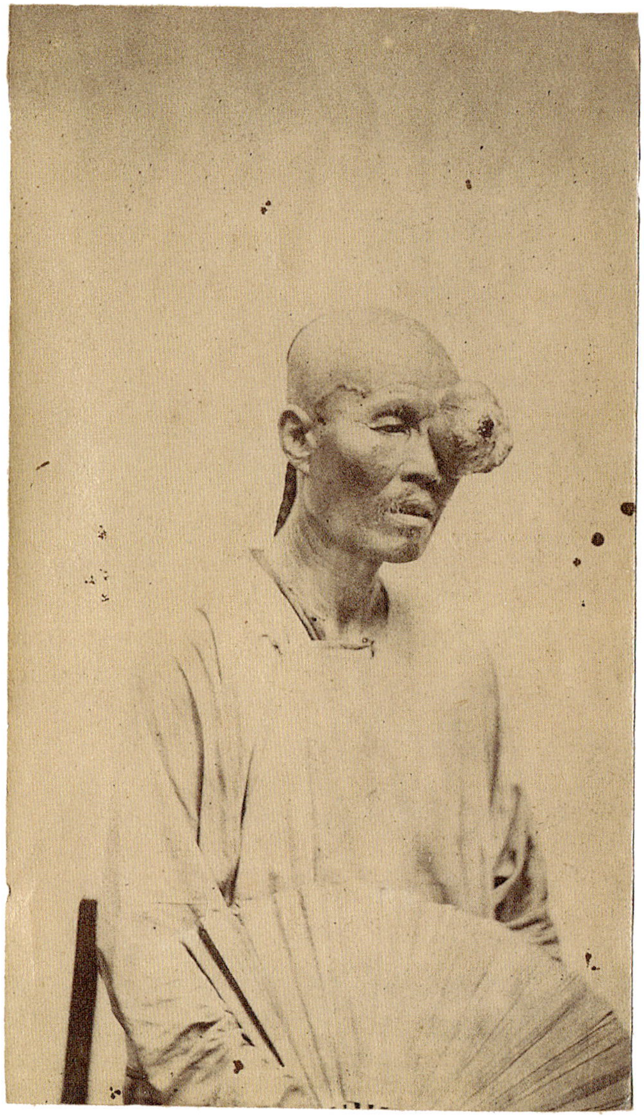

Cancer of eye. Excised. From an album by John Glasgow Kerr, M.D. (1824–1901), of photographs of his practice in Canton, China.

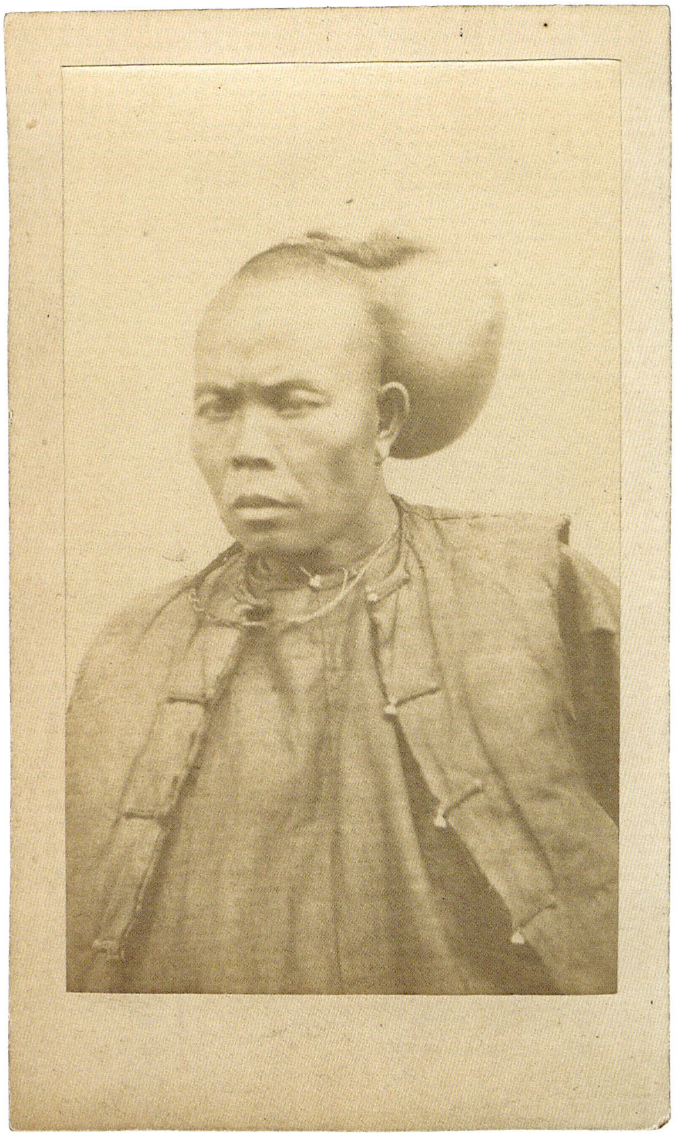

Tumor of scalp. Excised. From an album by John Glasgow Kerr, M.D. (1824–1901), of photographs of his practice in Canton, China.

Sarcoma. Photographer and date unidentified.

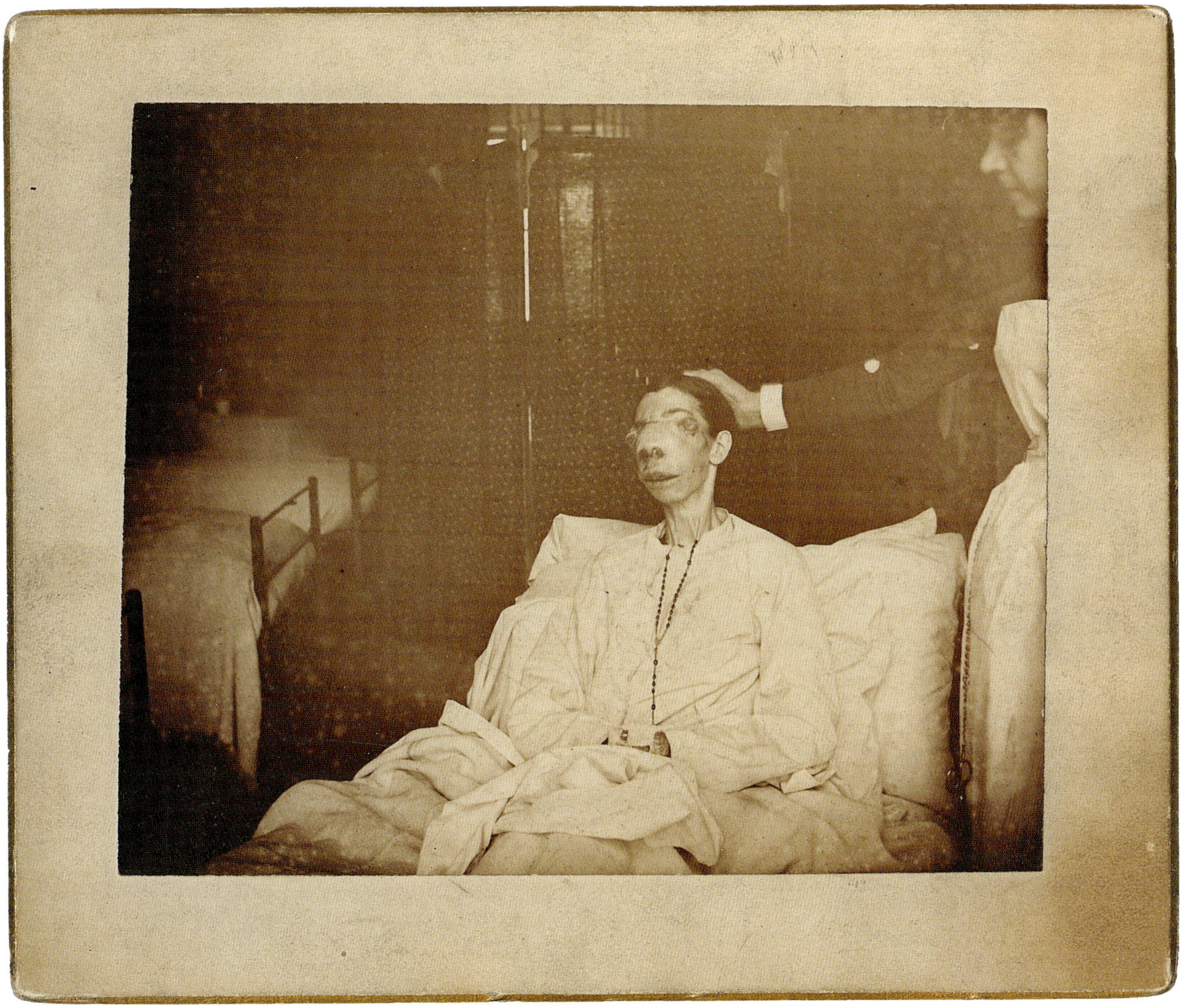

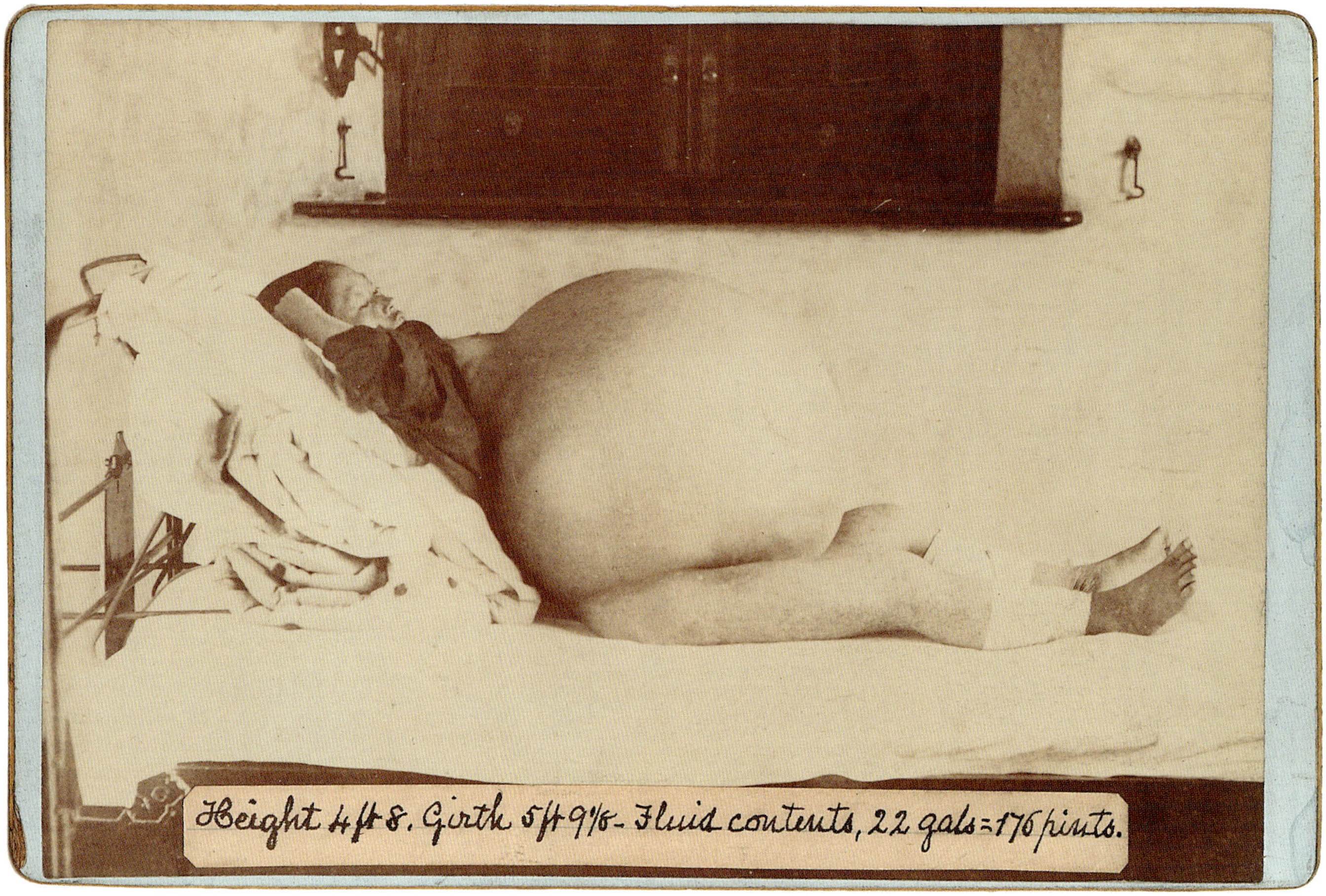

ABOVE AND OPPOSITE: Operation for removal of enormous cyst of left ovary. Yu Yung Lan, a Chinese woman of twenty-five, married, no children, 4' 8". Circumference of tumor 5' ⅛". Tumor of six years' growth, weight of cyst 6½ pounds and weight of whole tumor 182½ pounds, fluid content 22 gallons. Operation of ovariectomy by Elizabeth Reifsnyder, M.D. (1858–1922), on November 1, 1894, at the Margaret Williamson Hospital, Shanghai. Dr. Reifsnyder, a graduate of Women's Medical College, Philadelphia, was the first woman medical missionary to China and she founded the Margaret Williamson Hospital, the first Western hospital in China. Opposite, photographed two months after operation. Photographs by Pow Kee & Co., Shanghai. Donor: Robert P. Harris, M.D. (1822–1899), 1895.

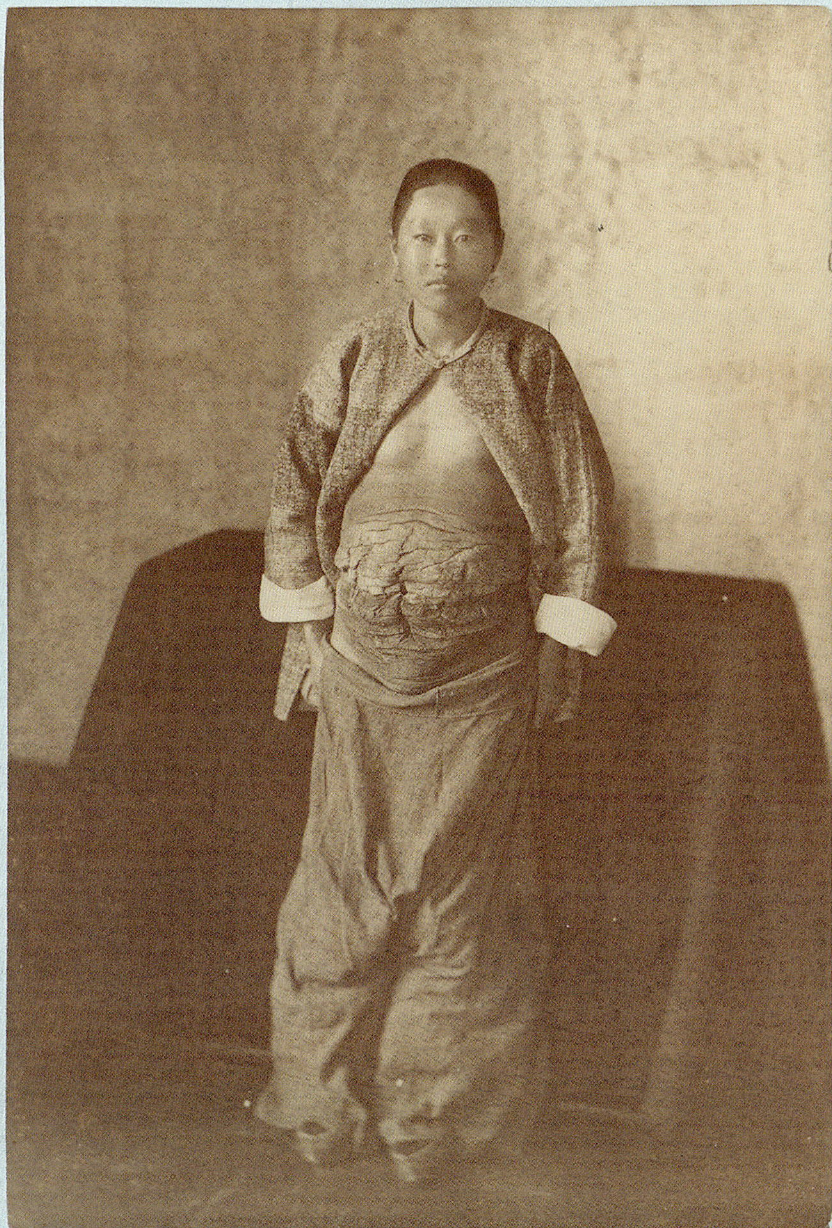

Yu Yung Lau. 4 ft 8.. 2 months after operation

Myo-cysto sarcoma of uterus, with polypoid growths expelled during life ($^1/_2$ natural size). 1. Uterus laid open. a) polypus inside uterus; b) submucous fibroids; c) intra-mural growths; d) subperitoneal fibroids; e) cyst. 2. Polypoid fibroids spontaneously expelled. Largest 7 inches long, weighs 10 oz. Presented June 1876, by his pupil Henry T. Bahuson, Salem, North Carolina, to Professor David Hayes Agnew (1818–1892), a surgeon at Philadelphia Hospital and author of *Lacerations of the Female Perineum and Vesico-Vaginal Fistula* (1873), among many other contributions to the literature of his profession. Agnew attended as operating surgeon after President Garfield was shot by Charles Guiteau in 1881.

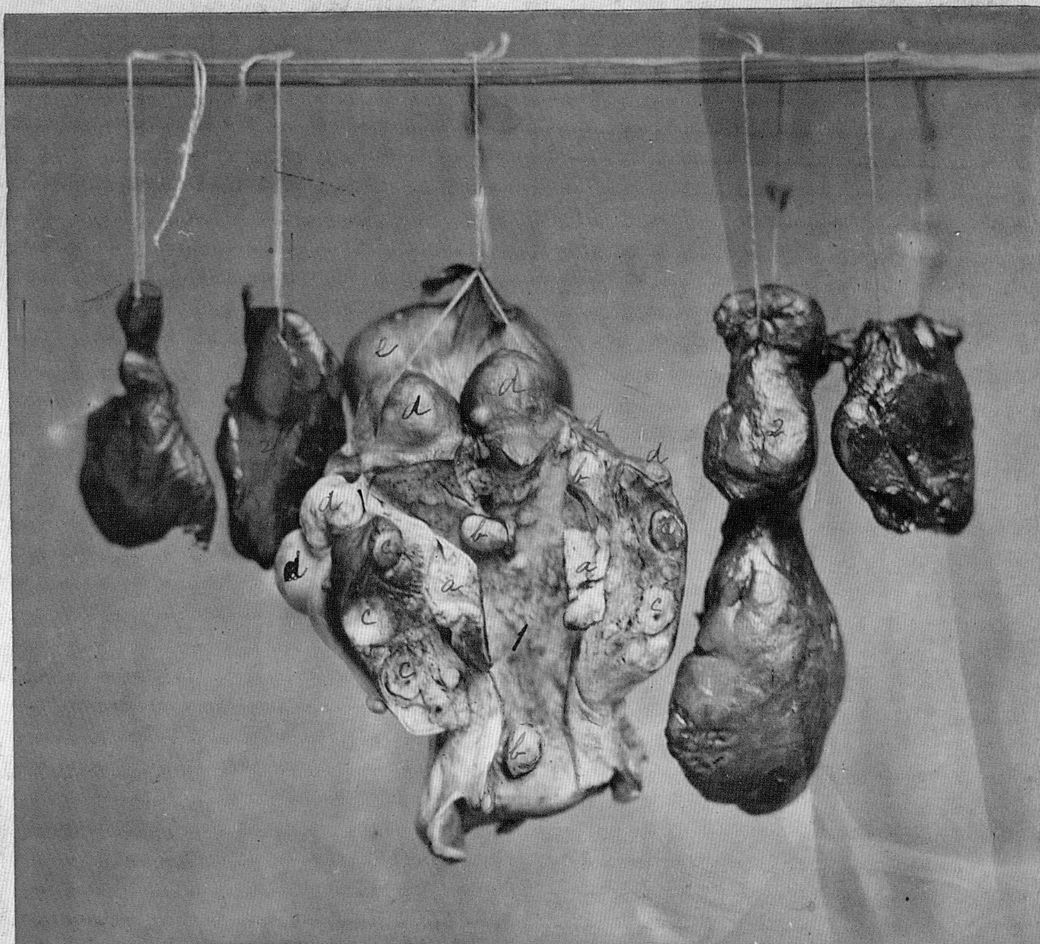

Myo-cysto-Sarcoma of Uterus, with Polypoid growths expelled during life.

(1/2 natural size.

1. Uterus laid open. a. polypus inside uterus. b, submucous fibroids. c, intra-mural growths d, sub-peritoneal fibroids. e, cyst

2. Polypoid fibroids spontaneously expelled. Largest, 7 inches long, weighs 10 oz.

Presented to Prof. D. Hayes Agnew, by his grateful pupil

Henry T. Bahnson Salem N.Ca.

June 1876.

Psychological Disorder

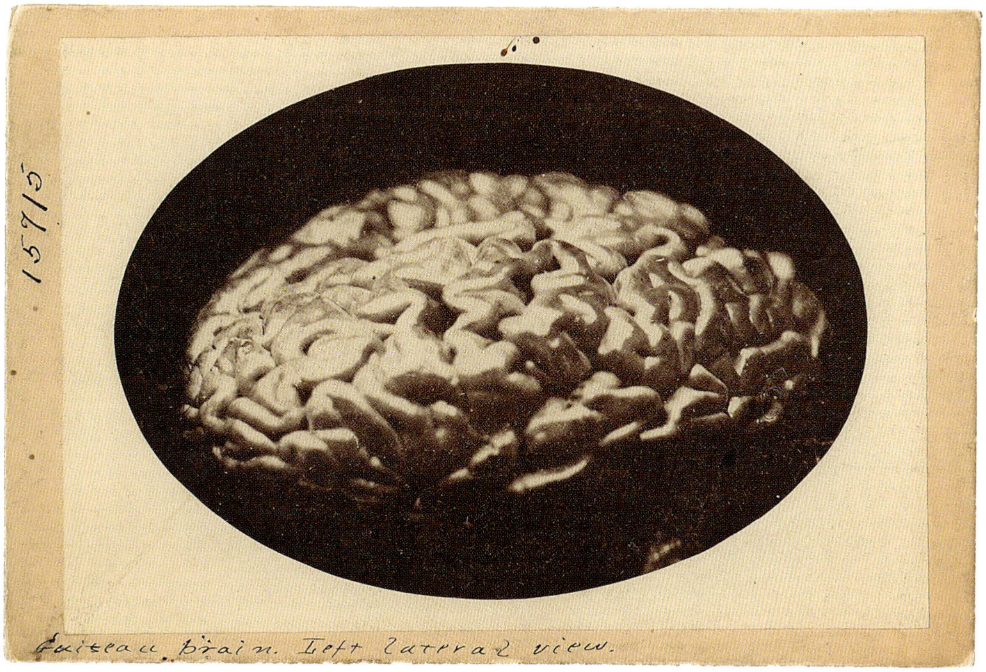

Left lateral view of brain of Charles Julius Guiteau, who shot President James Garfield on July 2, 1881. The president died September 19, 1881. Photograph given by Dr. Daniel Smith Lamb (1843–1929) to Hon. Charles O'Neill of Philadelphia. A six-month trial ensued in which Guiteau argued loudly against the attempts by his attorney to use an insanity defense. Guiteau went to the gallows June 30, 1882, deluded that shooting the president was a noble act commanded by God and that he would be freed and applauded by all for his heroic action. A portion of Guiteau's brain is in the collection of the Mütter Museum.

Unidentified mental illness. Patient of Francis Xavier Dercum, M.D. (1856–1931). Early in his career Dr. Dercum worked as a pathologist at the State Hospital for the Insane in Norristown, Montgomery County, Pennsylvania. One of the founders of the Philadelphia Neurological Society in 1884, Dercum later headed the department of nervous and mental diseases at Jefferson Medical College. Dercum had Eadweard Muybridge make the first pictures to document neurological diseases. Photograph by James F. Wood, from the album of photographs by Wood presented to the Mütter Museum in 1898, ca. 1892–1900.

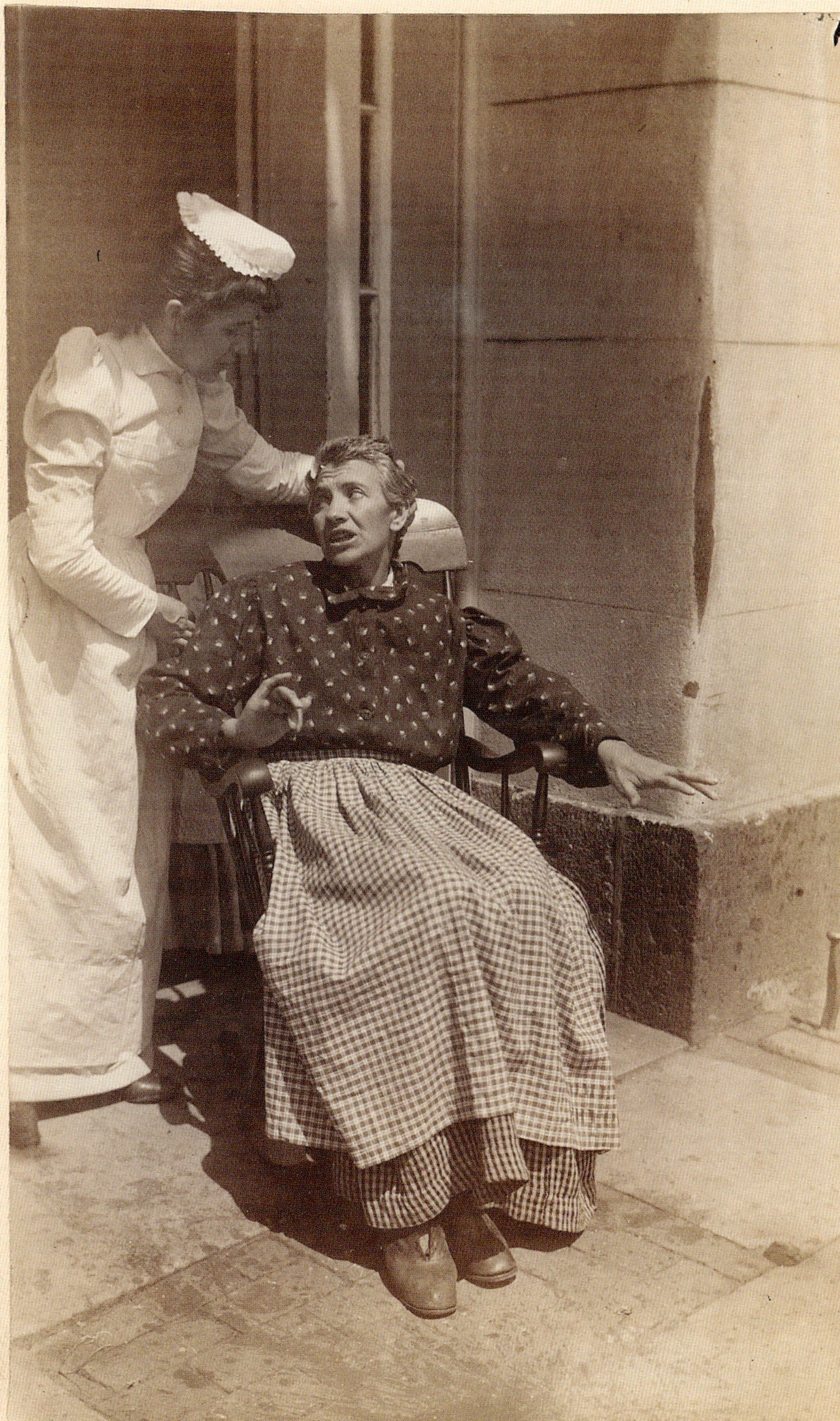

Devaun

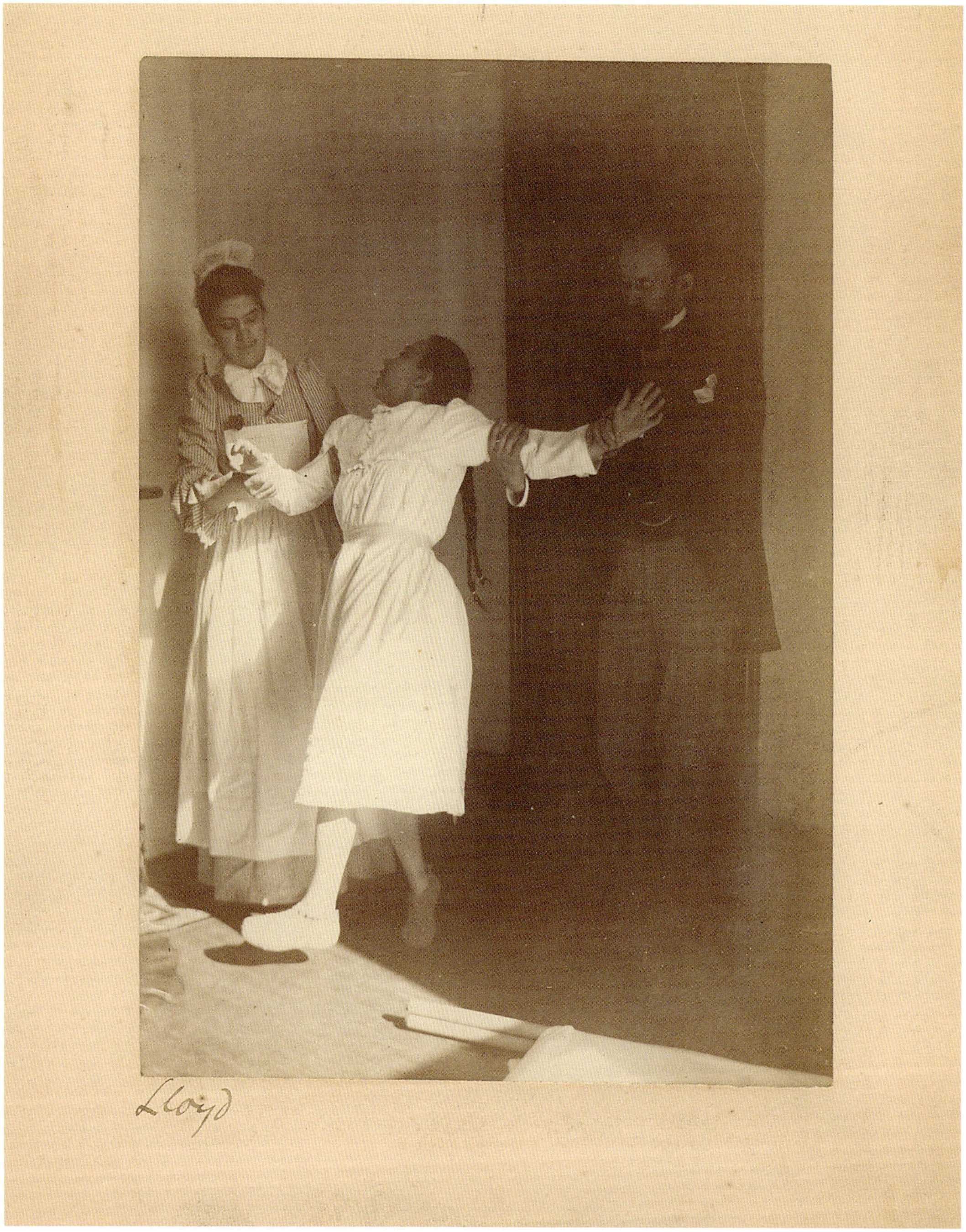

ABOVE AND OPPOSITE: Unidentified mental illness. Patient of James Hendrie Lloyd, M.D. (1853–1932), neurologist to the Philadelphia Hospital, an early member of the Philadelphia Psychiatric Society, and author of "Insanity and Diseases of the Nervous System in the Child-Bearing Woman" (*A System of Obstetrics*, vol. 2, ed. Barton Cooke Hirst, 1888) and others. Photograph by James F. Wood, from the album of photographs by Wood presented to the Mütter Museum in 1898, ca. 1892–1900.

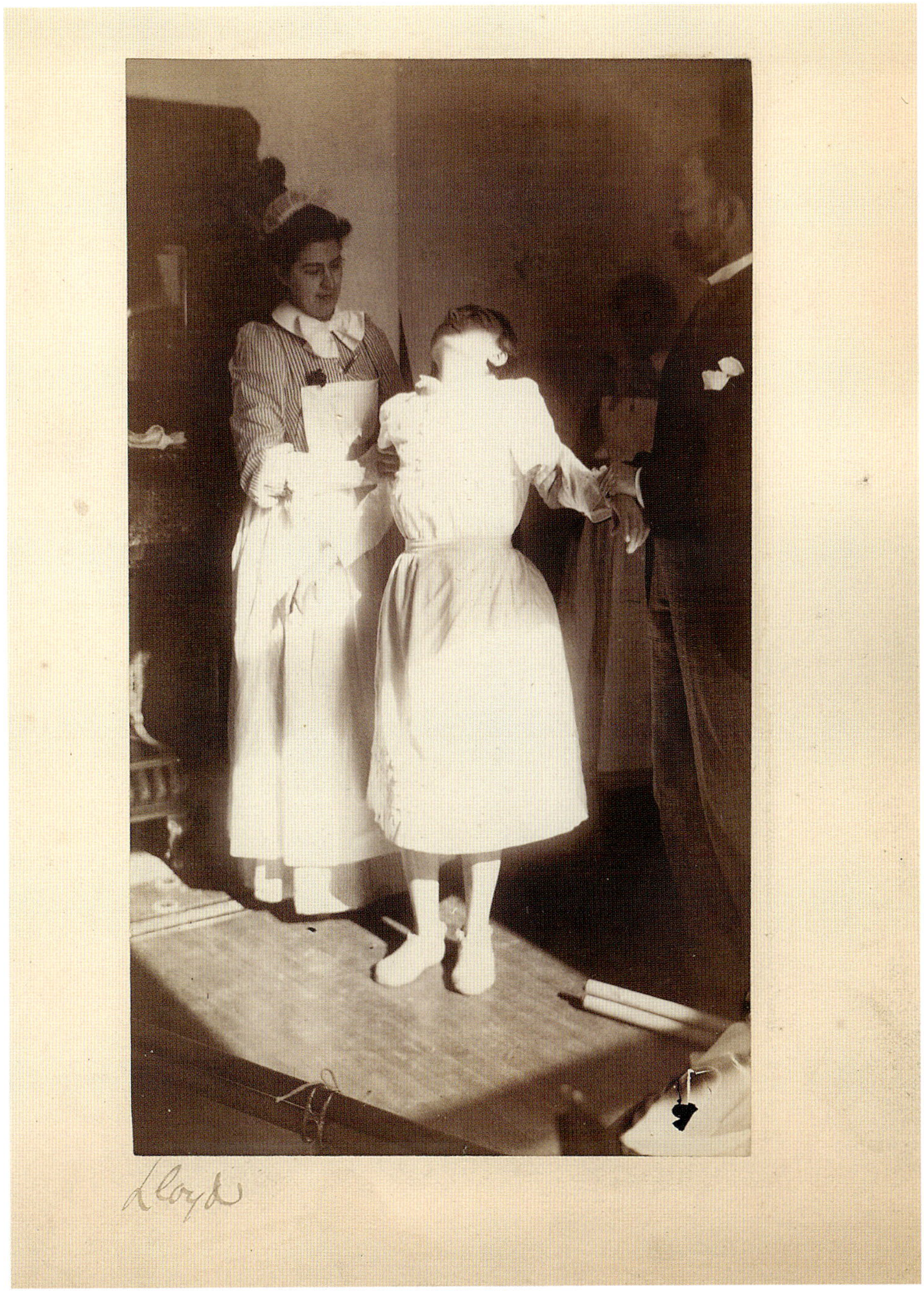
Lloyd

Teratology

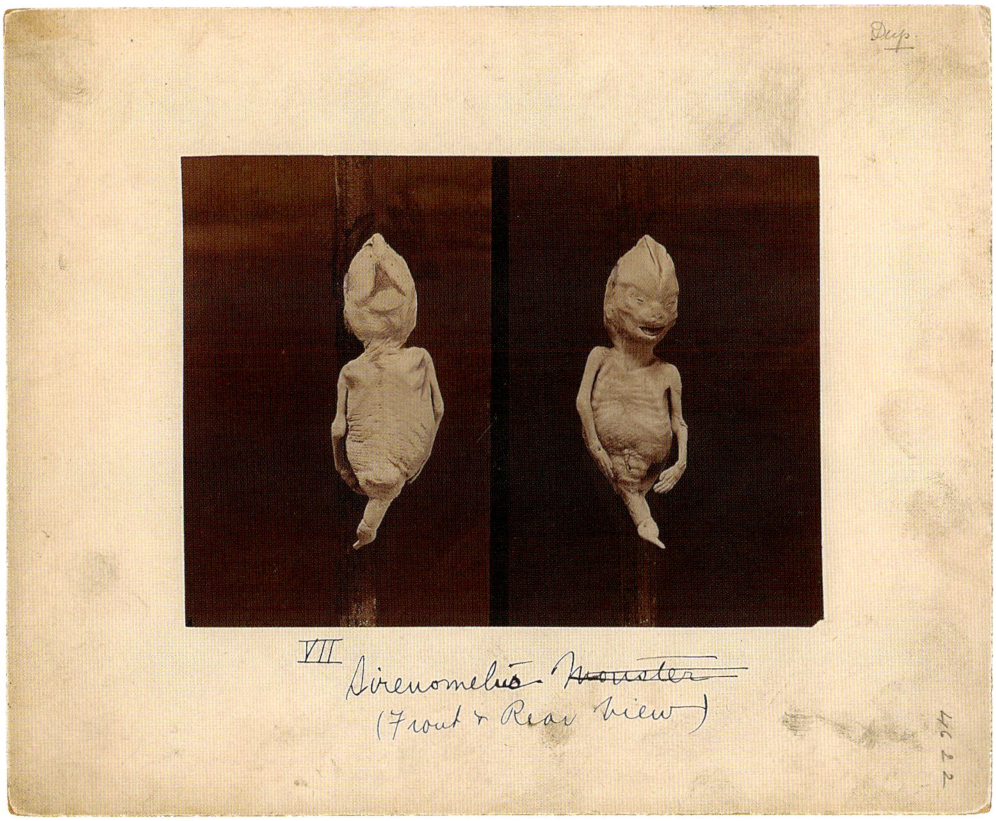

Sirenomelus (front and rear view). Sirenomelia is a very rare, lethal congenital anomaly caused by a disruptive vascular defect and characterized by fusion of the lower extremities. From Part I of the collection of pictures of congenital abnormalities that form the basis of the four-volume atlas *Human Monstrosities*, by Barton Cooke Hirst (1861–1935) and George Arthur Piersol (1856–1924), published 1891–93. Donor: Dr. B. C. Hirst.

Spina bifida, a neural tube defect caused by the failure of a foetus's spine to close properly in the first month of pregnancy, with large spinal meningocele. From Part I of the collection of pictures of congenital abnormalities that form the basis of the four-volume atlas *Human Monstrosities*, by Barton Cooke Hirst (1861–1935) and George Arthur Piersol (1856–1924), published 1891–93. Donor: Dr. B. C. Hirst.

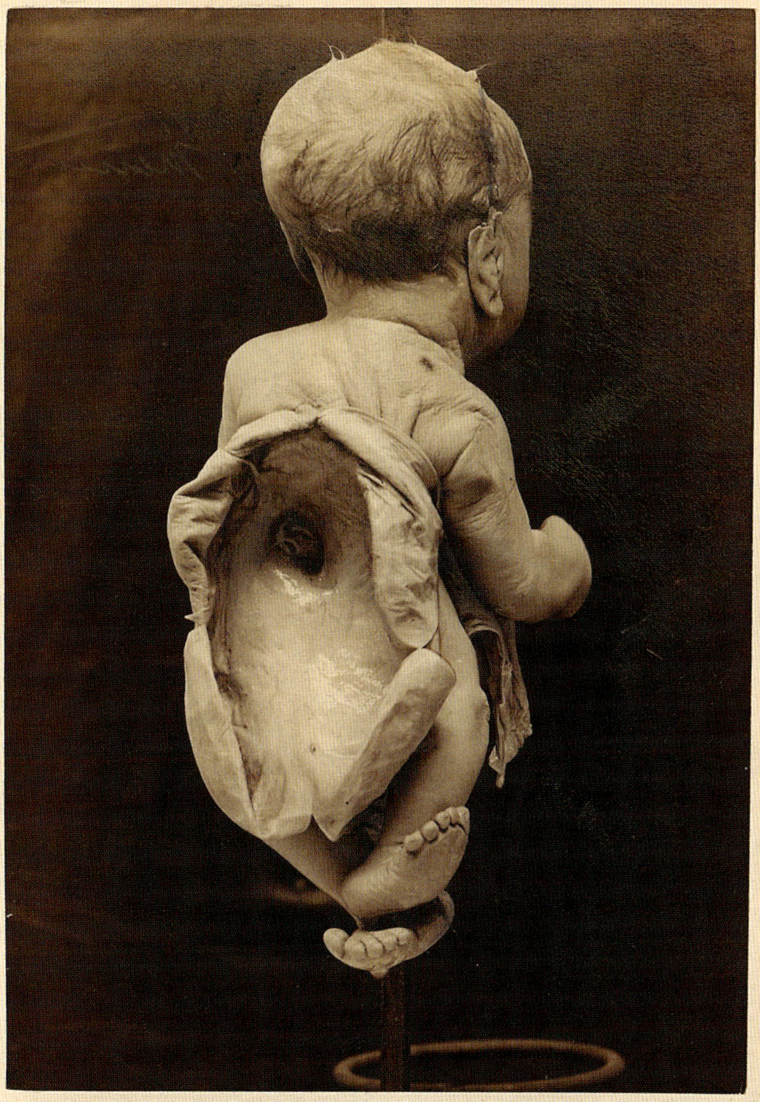

4622

II

Spina bifida with ~~Large~~ Enormous Spinal Meningocele

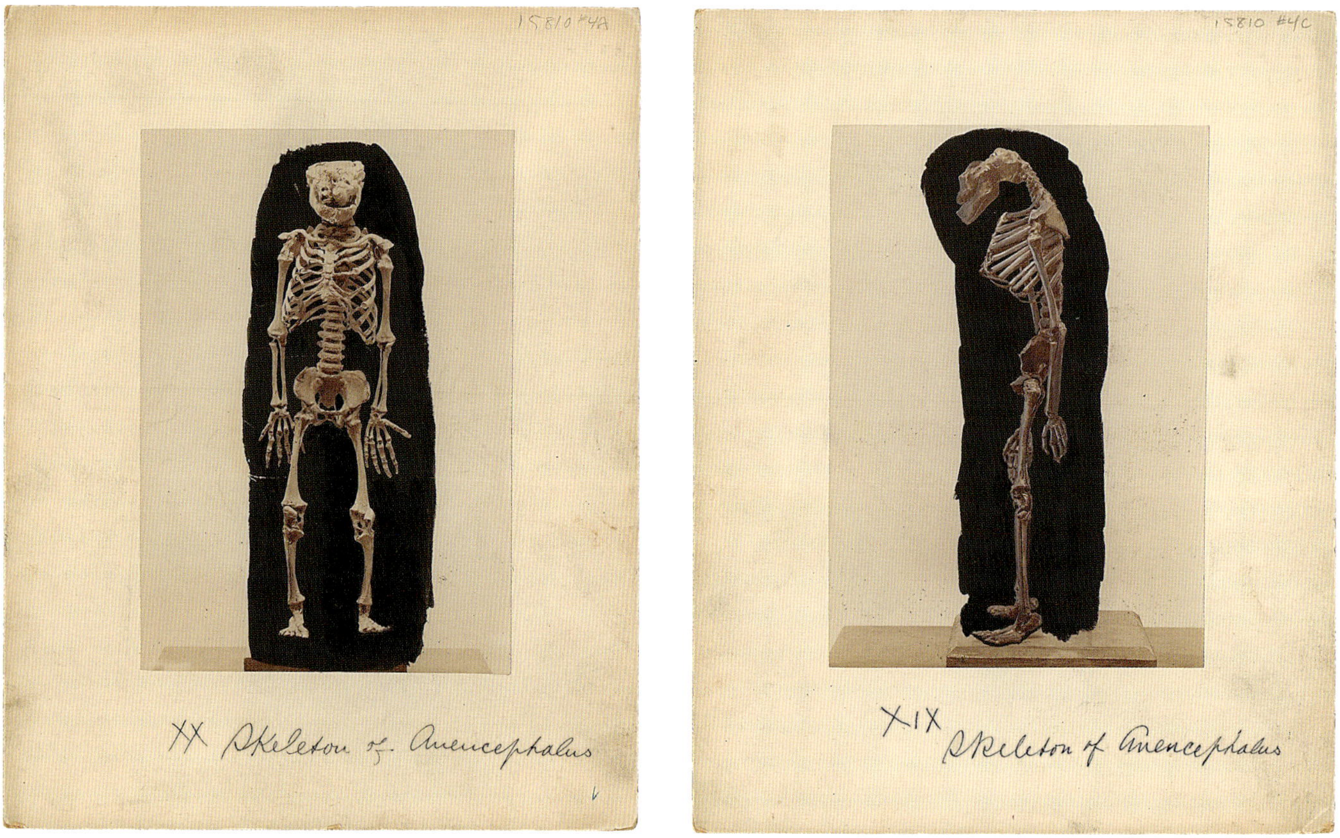

ABOVE: Skeleton of anencephalus (front and side view). Anencephaly is a neural tube defect that occurs when the cephalic end of the neural tube fails to close, resulting in the absence of a major portion of the brain, skull, and scalp. From Part II of the collection of pictures of congenital abnormalities that form the basis of the four-volume atlas *Human Monstrosities*, by Barton Cooke Hirst (1861–1935) and George Arthur Piersol (1856–1924), published 1891–93. Photographs opaqued for reproduction. Donor: Dr. B. C. Hirst.

OPPOSITE: Anencephalus, photographer and date unidentified.

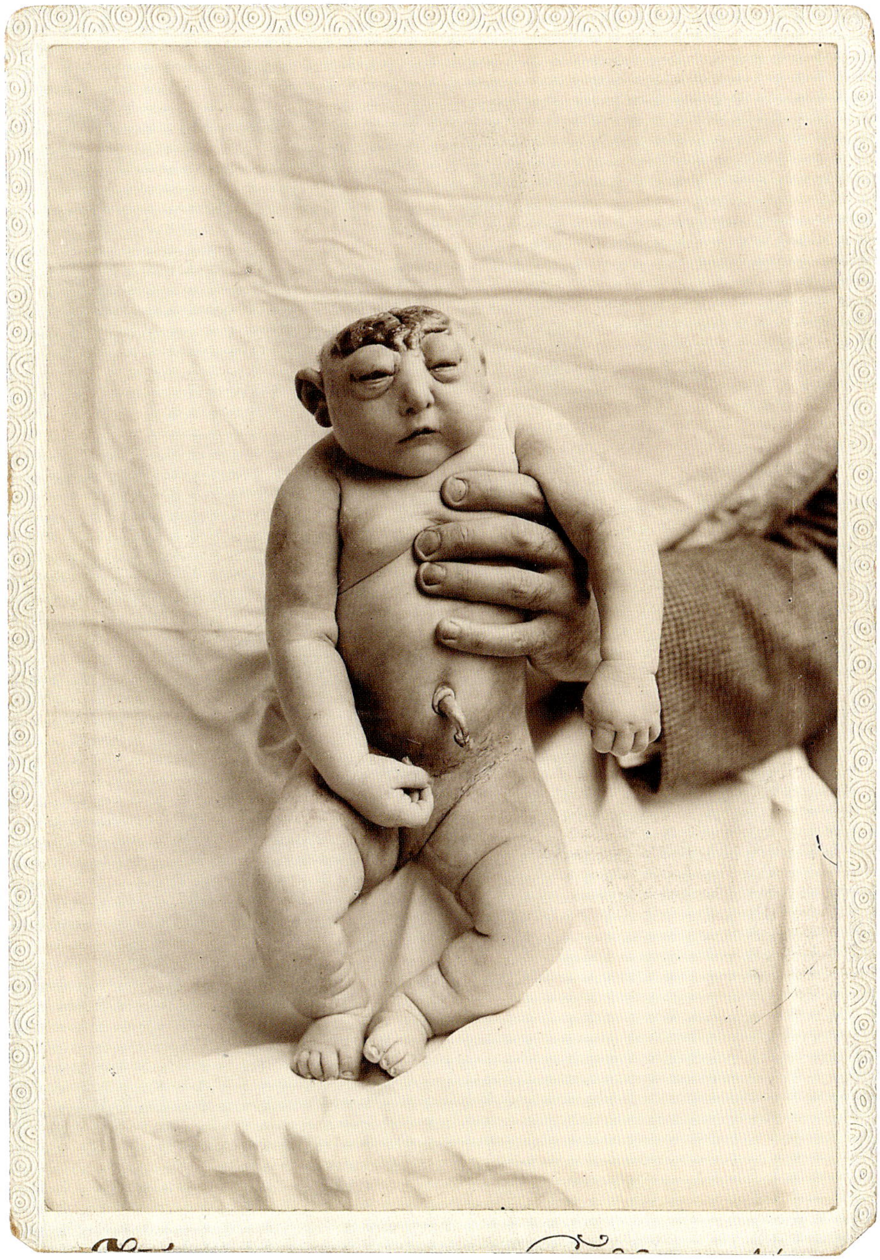

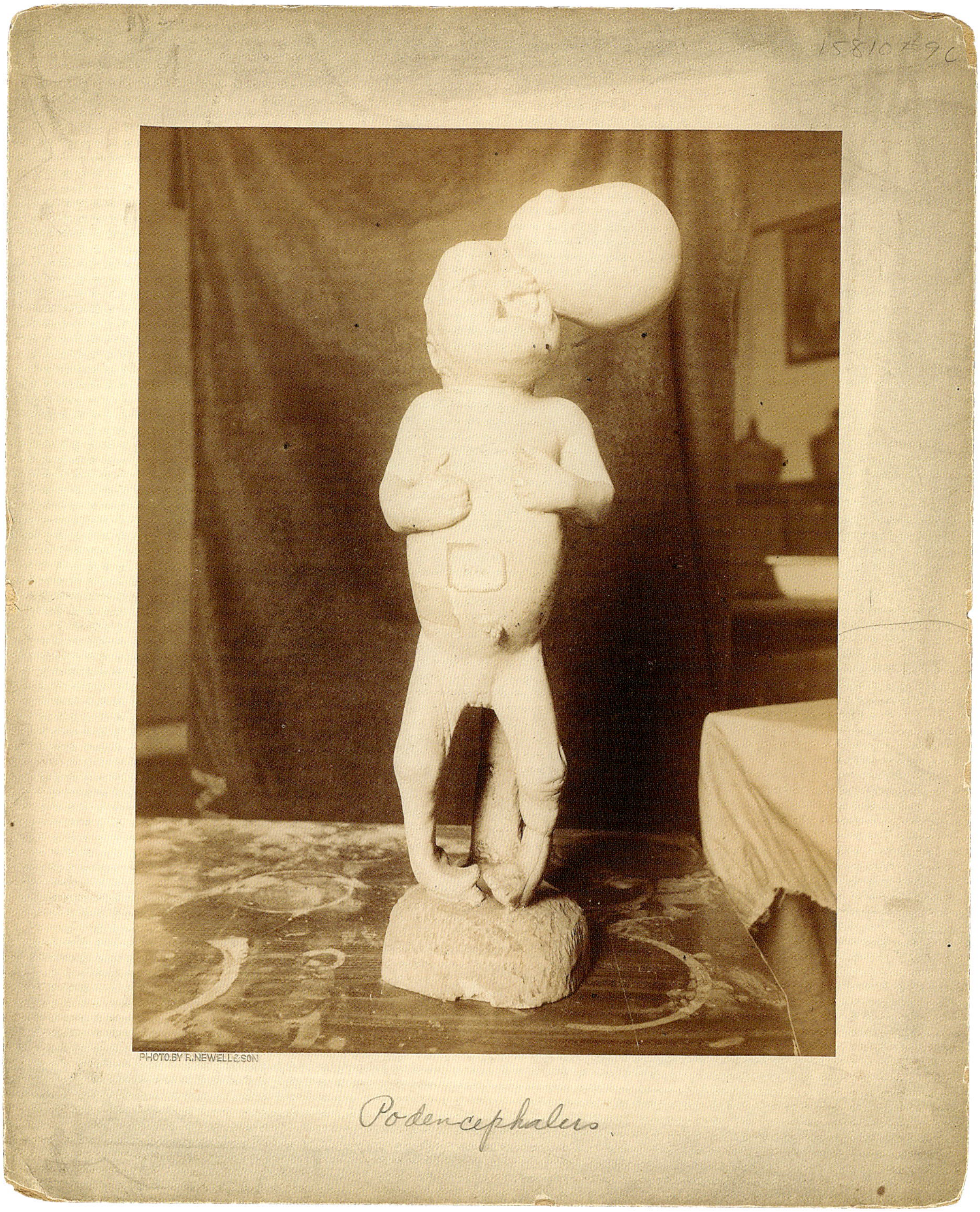

Podencephalus (meningoencephalocele), a protrusion of the meninges and the brain through a congenital defect in the cranium. Plaster model donated by Dr. Mütter. Photograph by R. Newell & Son, Philadelphia, ca. 1873–1900.

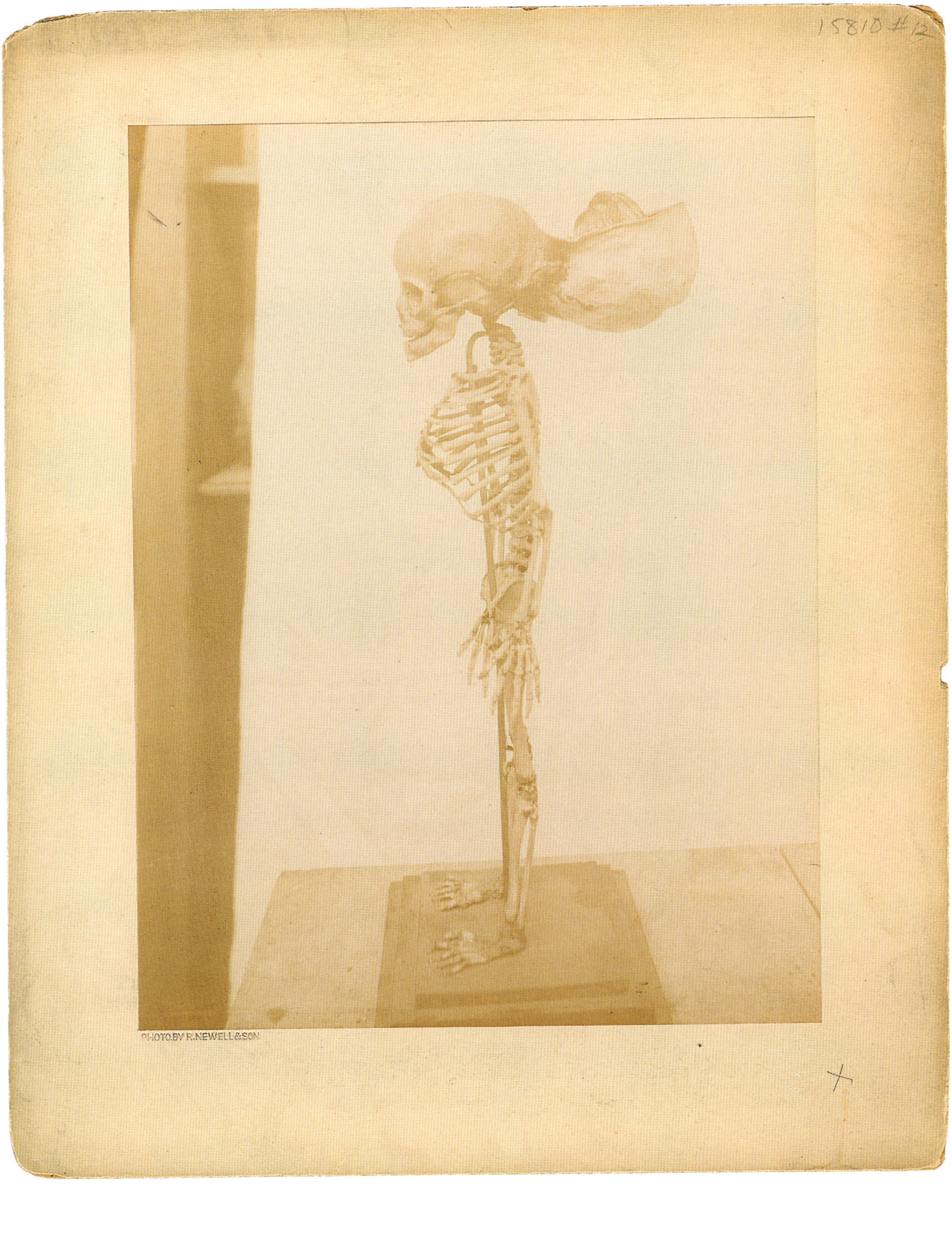

Encephalocele, a congential gap in the skull resulting in a protrusion of brain material. Photograph by R. Newell & Son, Philadelphia, ca. 1873–1900.

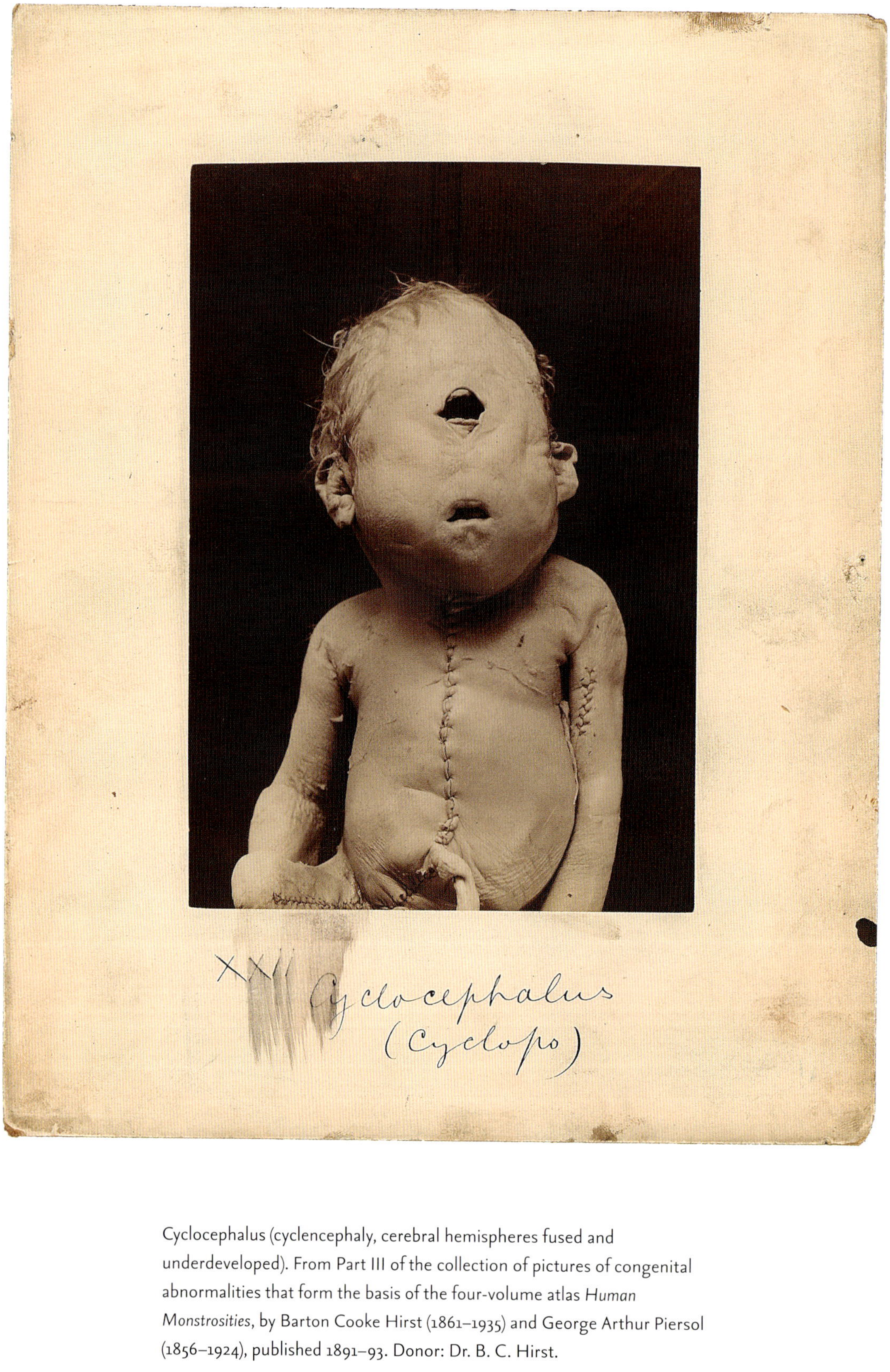

Cyclocephalus (cyclencephaly, cerebral hemispheres fused and underdeveloped). From Part III of the collection of pictures of congenital abnormalities that form the basis of the four-volume atlas *Human Monstrosities*, by Barton Cooke Hirst (1861–1935) and George Arthur Piersol (1856–1924), published 1891–93. Donor: Dr. B. C. Hirst.

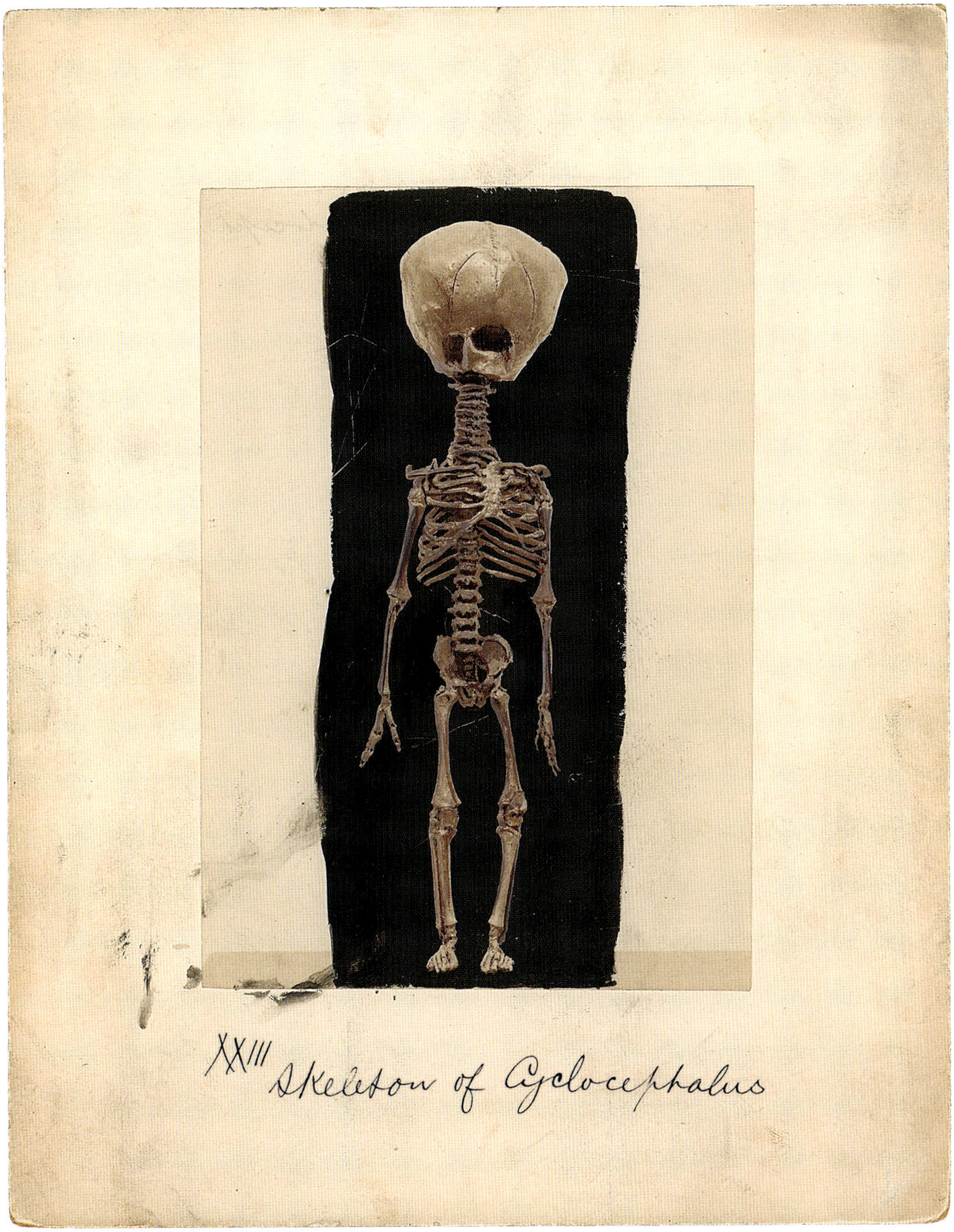

Skeleton of cyclocephalus in the Wistar Museum of the University of Pennsylvania. From Part III of the collection of pictures of congenital abnormalities that form the basis of the four-volume atlas *Human Monstrosities*, by Barton Cooke Hirst (1861–1935) and George Arthur Piersol (1856–1924), published 1891–93. Photograph opaqued for reproduction. Donor: Dr. B. C. Hirst.

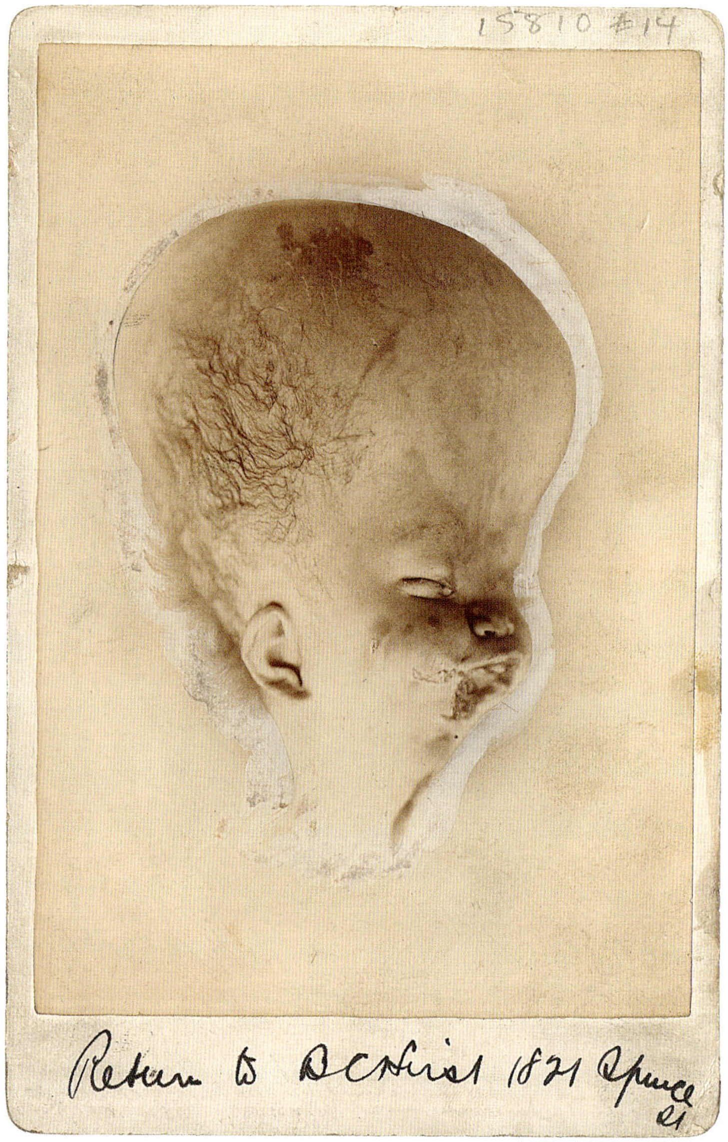

Hydrocephaly, caused by an accumulation of cerebrospinal fluid in the ventricles of the brain due to a narrowing or obstruction of the drainage leading to the spinal cord. Photograph for memorandum by Alexander Fulton, M.D. (1855–1898), in an issue of *University Medical Magazine* (1895–96), opaqued for reproduction. Photographer and date unidentified. Donor: Dr. B. C. Hirst (1861–1935).

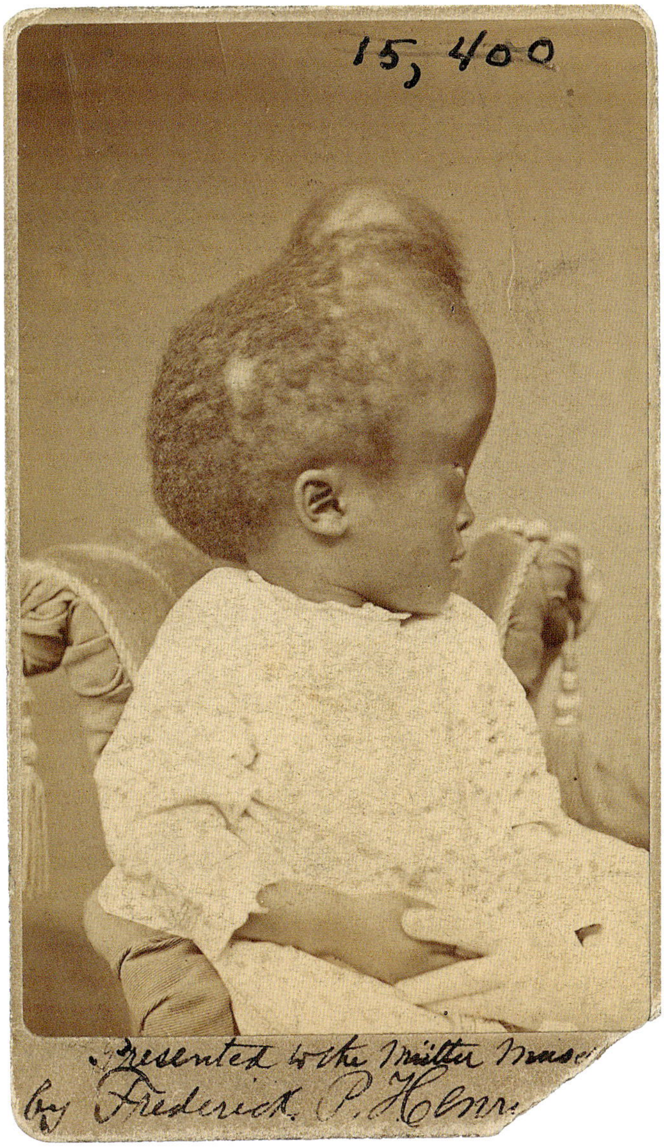

Case of hydrocephaly. Thomas Jeff, a seven-year-old male who died in 1882. Skeleton donated 1882 to the Mütter Museum by Richard Hickman Harte, M.D. (1855–1925). Photograph by William H. Rhoads, Philadelphia, ca. 1882. Donor: Frederick Porteous Henry, M.D. (1844–1919), Honorary Librarian to the College of Physicians of Philadelphia from 1890–1919.

Ectopagus (laterally conjoined) dicephalus dibrachius tripus twins. From Part IV of the collection of pictures of congenital abnormalities that form the basis of the four-volume atlas *Human Monstrosities*, by Barton Cooke Hirst (1861–1935) and George Arthur Piersol (1856–1924), published 1891–93. Photograph opaqued for reproduction. Donor: Dr. B. C. Hirst.

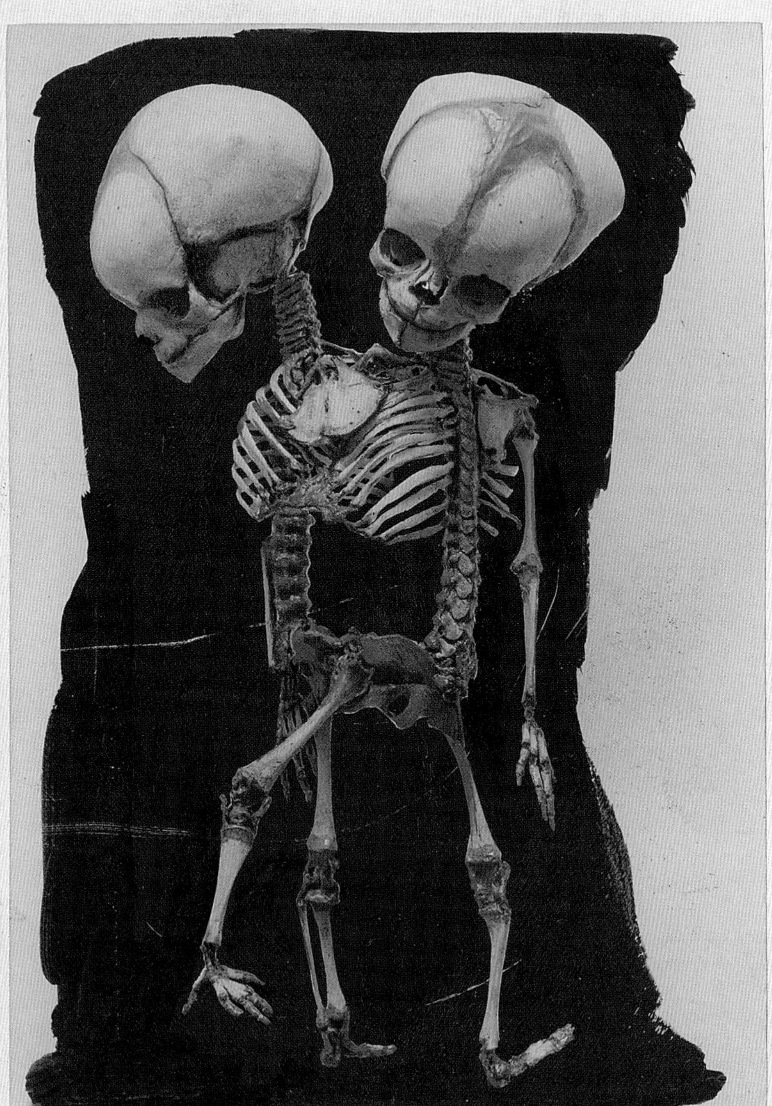

XXXIII Ectopagus

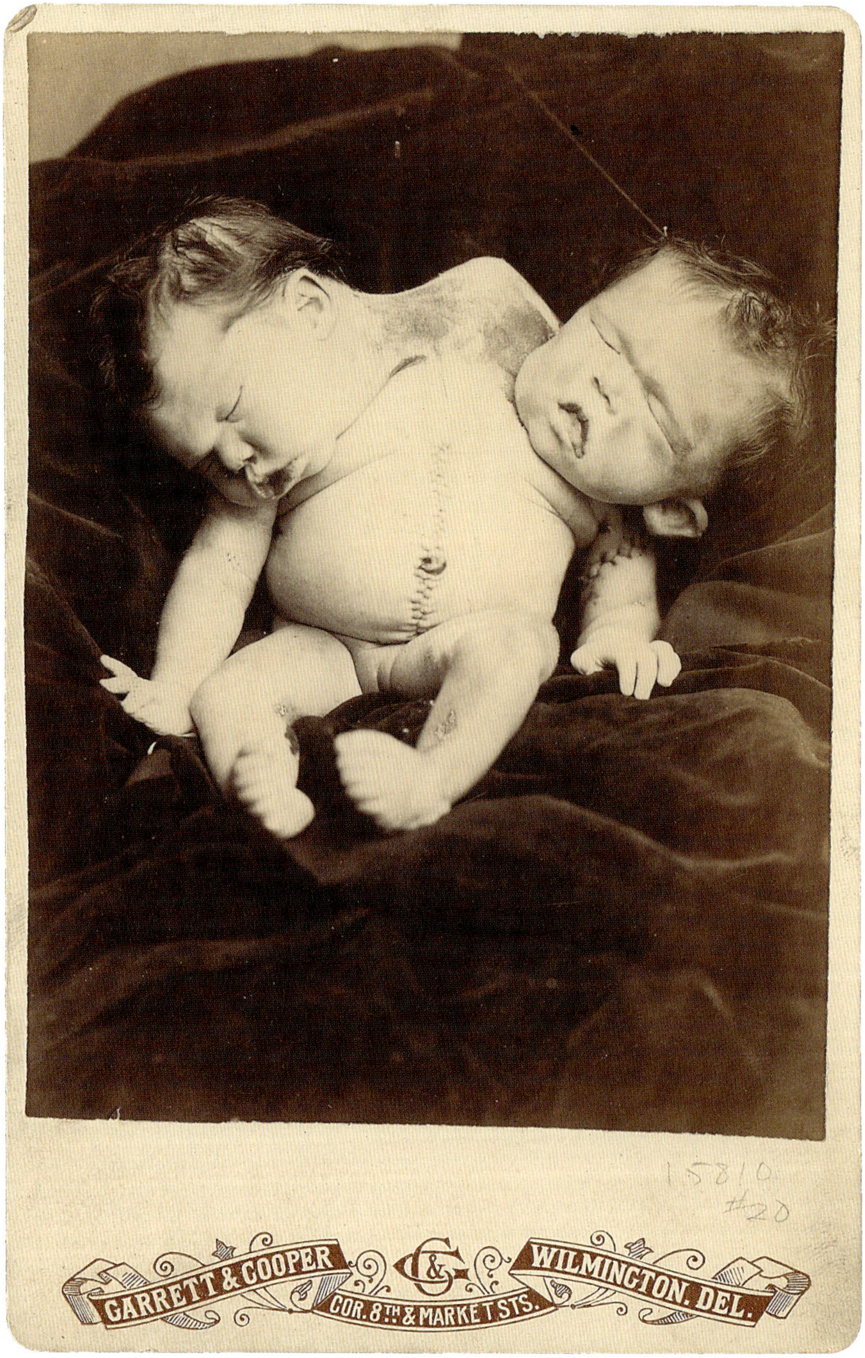

Bicephalus (symmetric conjoined twins with two separate heads).
Photograph by Garrett & Cooper, Wilmington, Delaware, November 1889.
Donor: A. E. Frantz, M.D., Wilmington, Delaware.

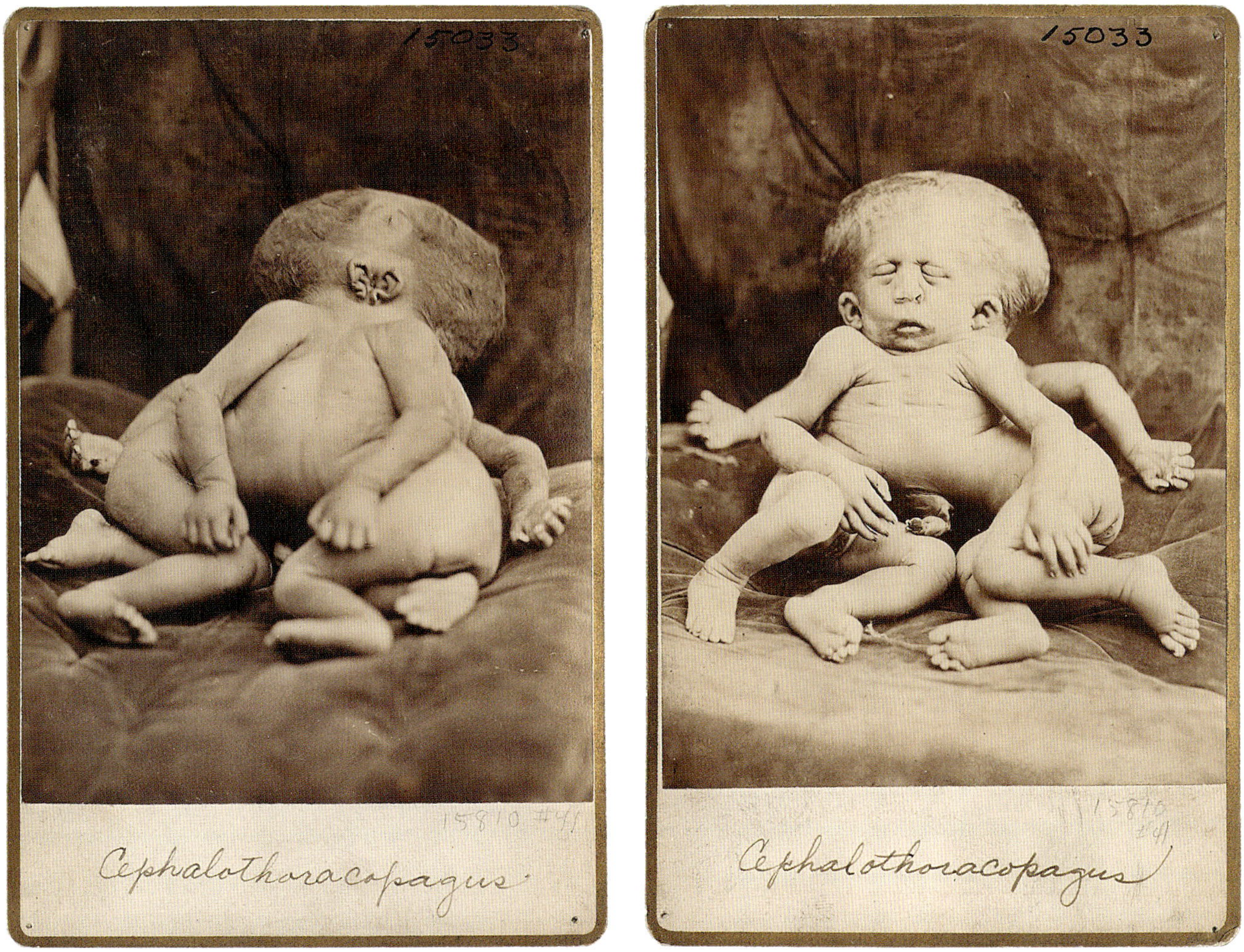

Cephalothoracopagus (conjoined twins with bodies fused in the cephalic and thoracic regions). Inscription on photograph reads: "in possession of Dr. [S. Lewis] Ziegler [1862–1926] of Reading." Photographs by Leaman & Lee, Reading, Pennsylvania, undated.

Autopsy and Dissection

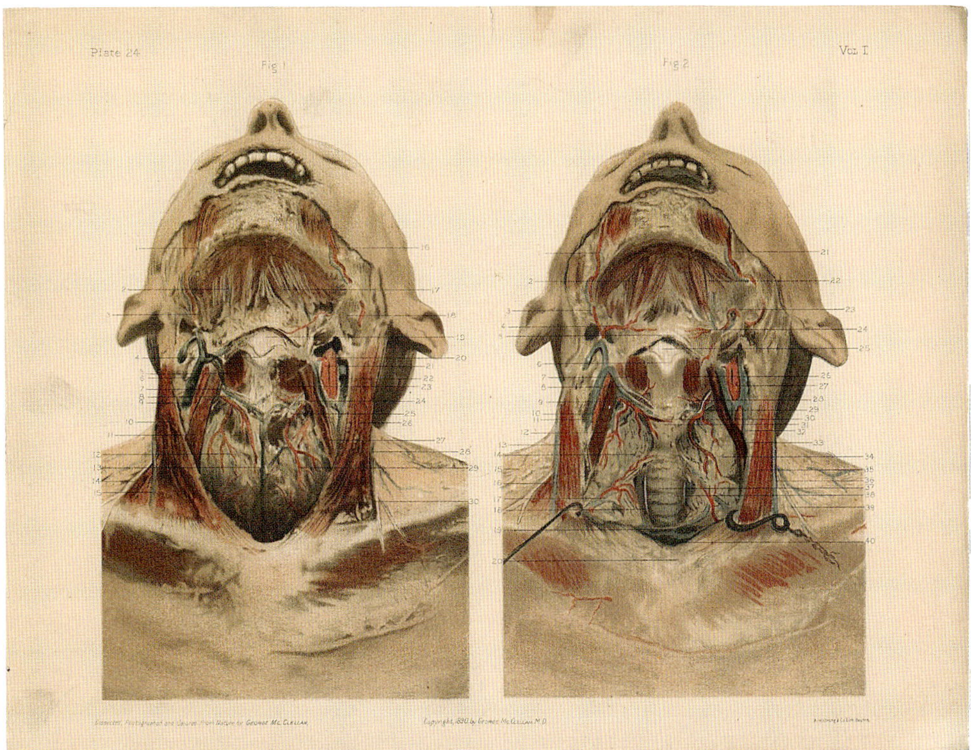

Lithographic plate printed by Armstrong & Co., Lith., Boston, from *Regional Anatomy*, 1892, by George B. McClellan, M.D. (1849–1913). Illustration of anatomical points of the front of the neck. Dissected, photographed, and colored from nature by McClellan. McClellan studied anatomy under Professor Joseph Hyrtl (1810–1894) of Vienna and founded the Pennsylvania College of Anatomy and Surgery in Philadelphia in 1881. He became professor of applied anatomy at Jefferson Medical College (founded by his grandfather) in 1906.

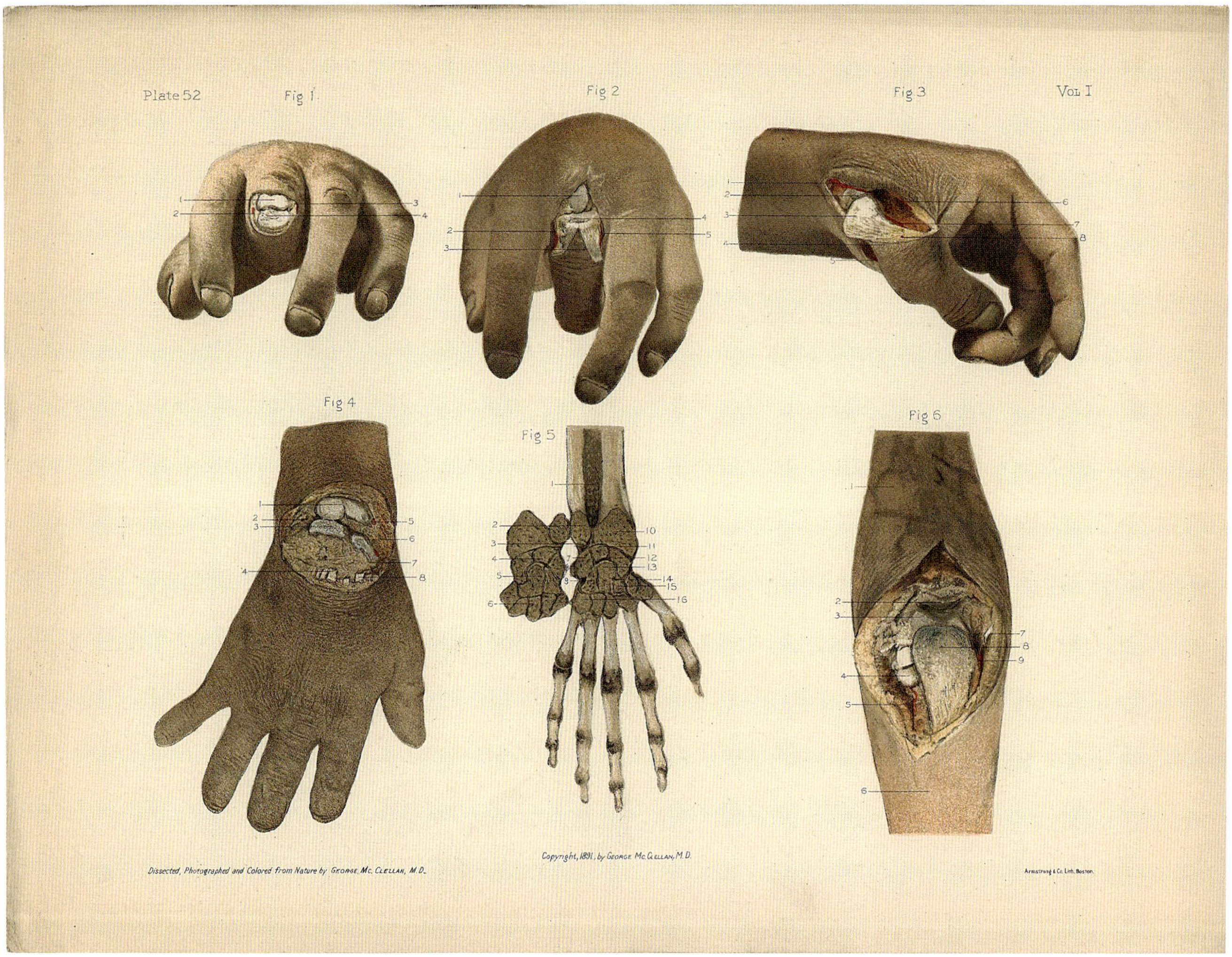

ABOVE AND OPPOSITE: Lithographic plates printed by Armstrong & Co. Lith., Boston, from *Regional Anatomy*, 1892, by George B. McClellan, M.D. (1849–1913). Dissected, photographed, and colored from nature by McClellan.

Illustration of anatomical points of the hand (above); illustration of anatomical points of the anterior thorax and neck (opposite).

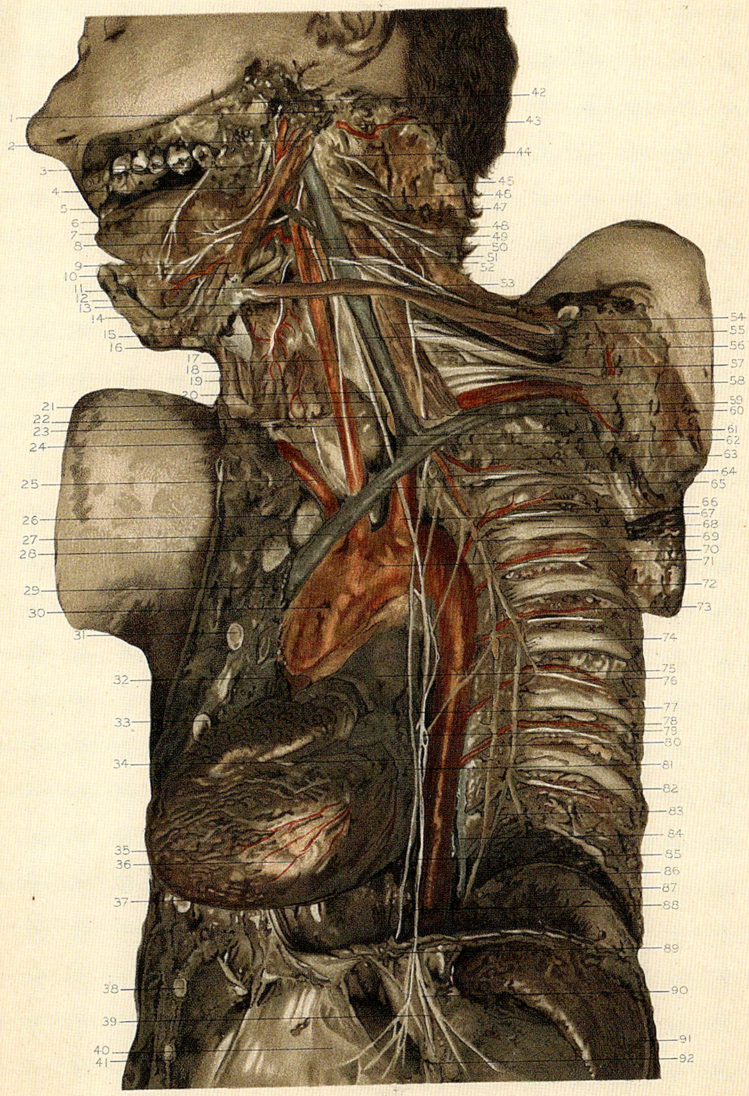

Dissected, Photographed and Colored from Nature by George Mc Clellan, M.D.

Armstrong & Co. Lith. Boston.

Lithographic plate printed by Armstrong & Co. Lith., Boston, from *Regional Anatomy*, 1892, by George B. McClellan, M.D. (1849–1913). Dissected, photographed, and colored from nature by McClellan.

Illustration of anatomical points of the basic structures of the thorax.

Plate 26

Vol. I

Fig 1

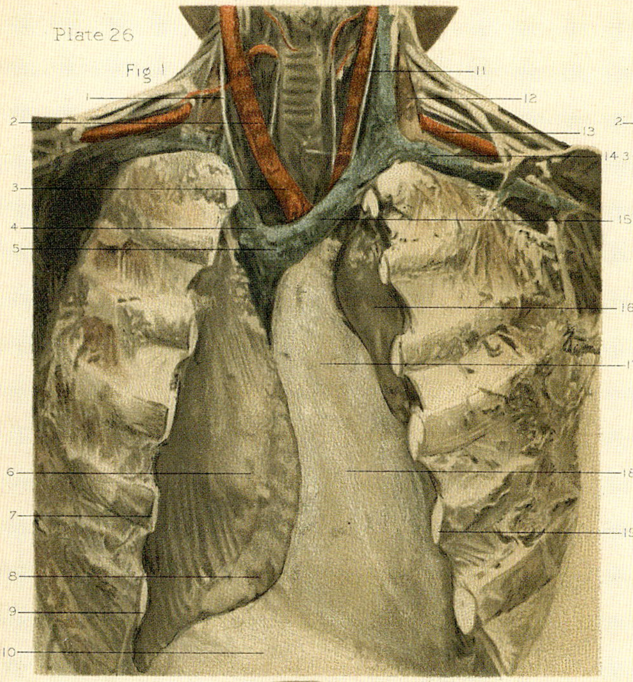

Fig 2

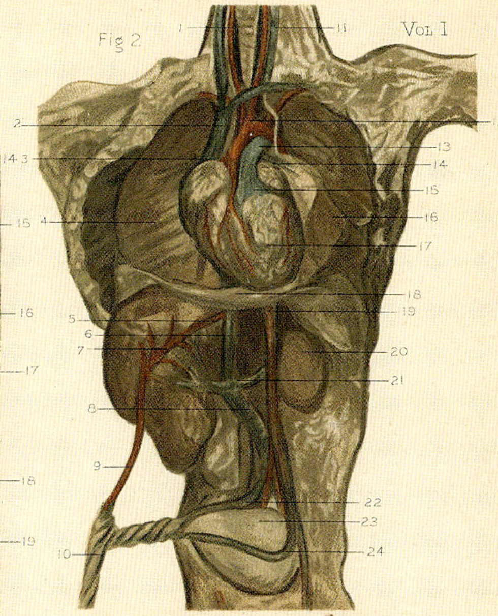

Fig 3

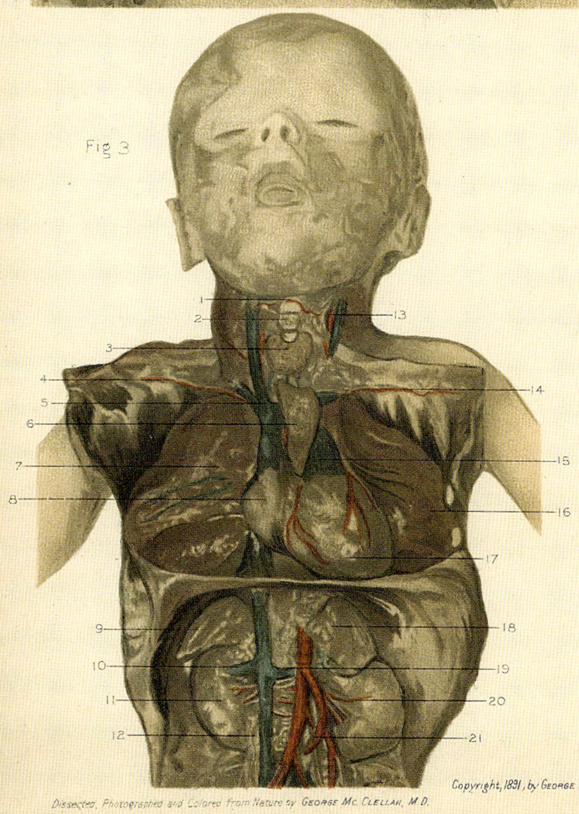

Fig 4

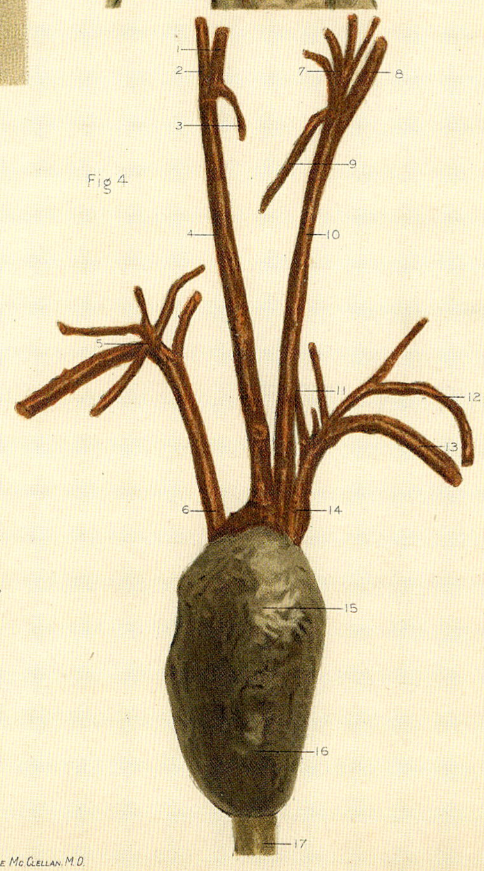

Dissected, Photographed and Colored from Nature by George Mc Clellan, M.D.

Armstrong & Co. Lith. Boston.

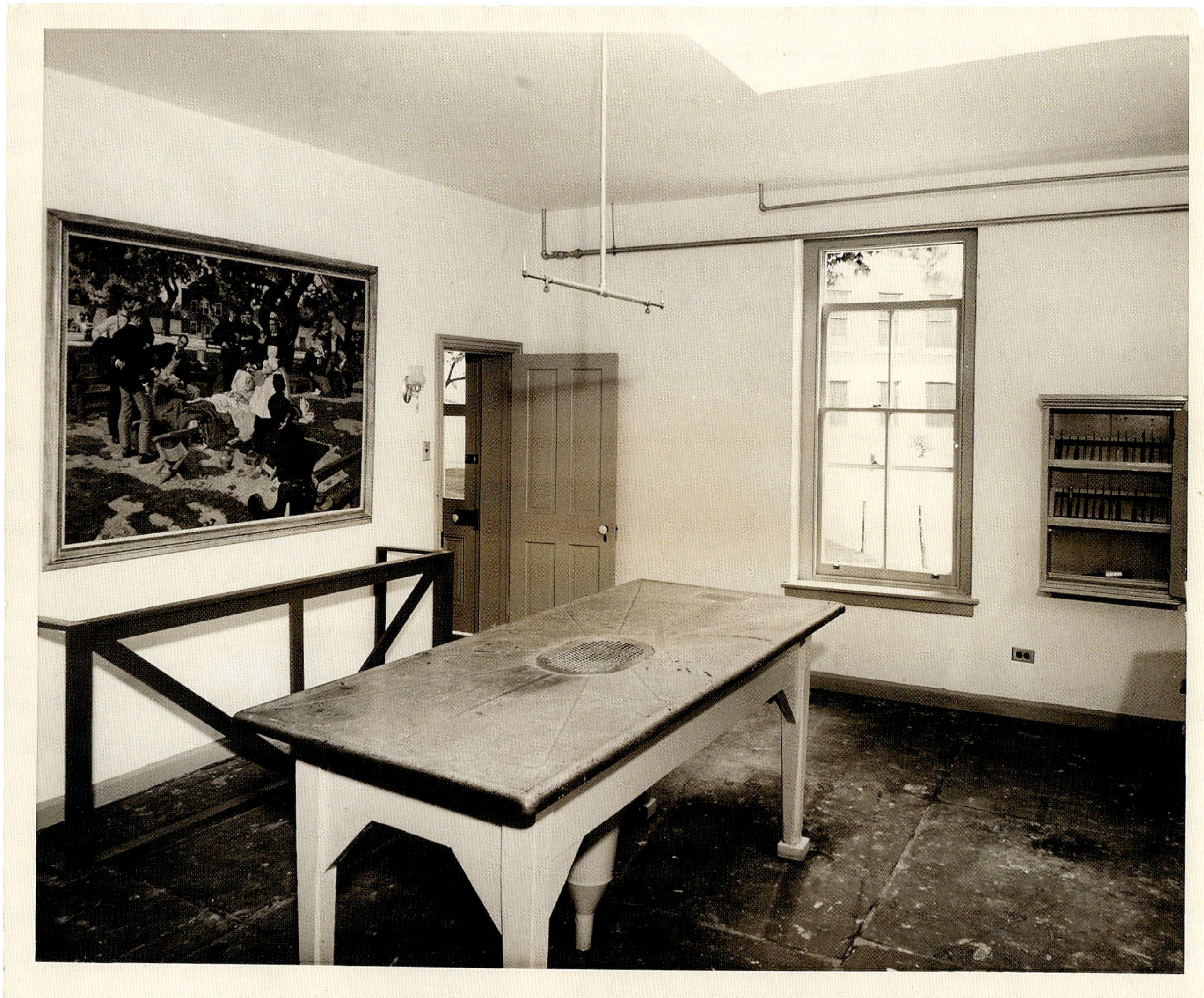

ABOVE AND OPPOSITE: Osler Memorial Building of the Philadelphia General Hospital, restored autopsy room, with autopsy table, cabinet of autopsy tools (opposite), desk, etc., all used by Dr. William Osler (1849–1919), known as one of the most influential physicians in history. Canadian-born Osler came to Philadelphia in 1884 and was a professor in the Department of Medicine at the University of Pennsylvania until 1889, when he became physician-in-chief of Johns Hopkins Hospital and one of four founding members of the Johns Hopkins School of Medicine. He revolutionized medical teaching in the United States and Canada, emphasizing close and frequent contact with patients. His first book, *The Principles and Practice of Medicine* (1892), remained the standard authority on clinical medicine for forty years. Photographer and date unidentified.

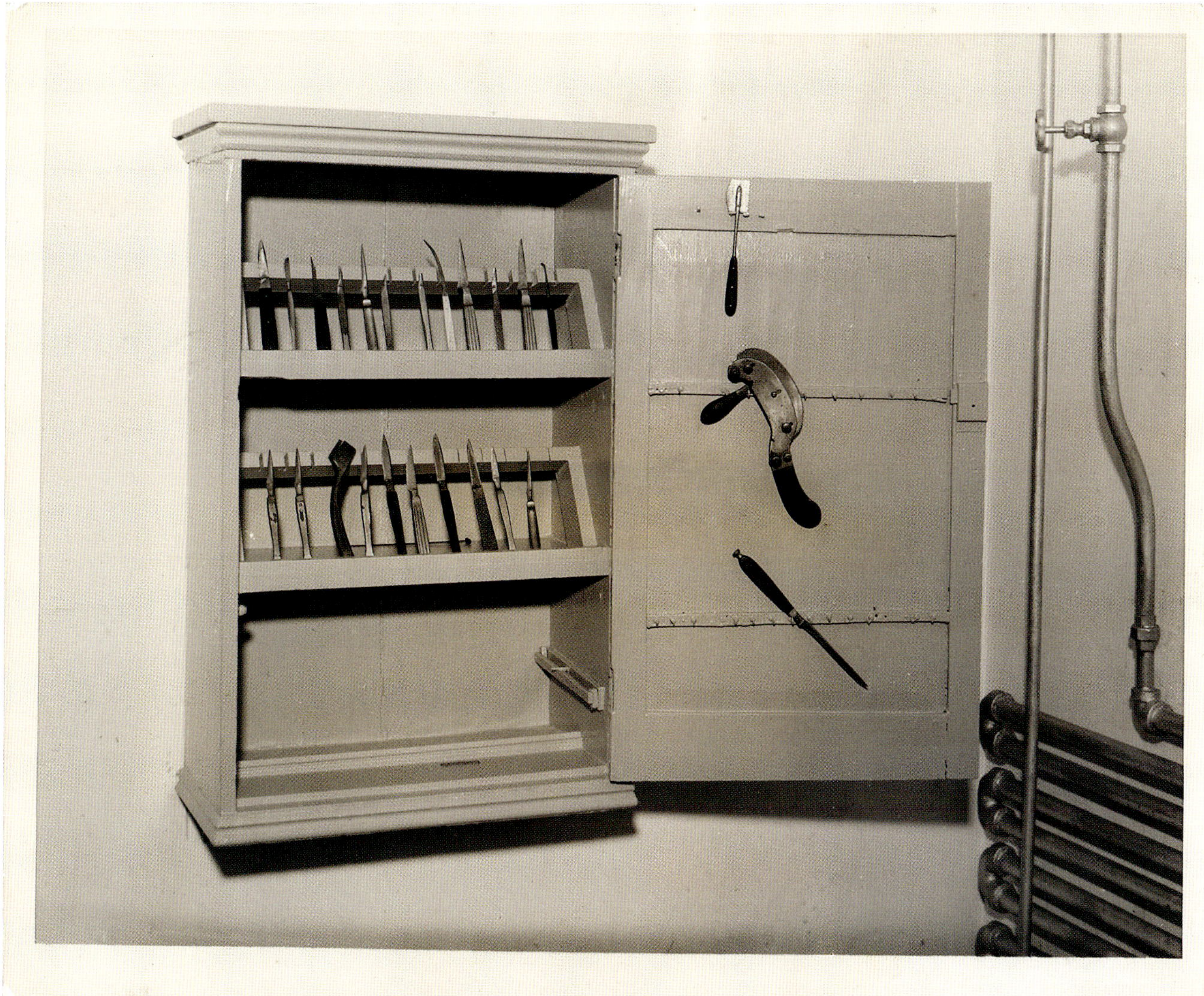

Dr. William Osler (1849–1919), seated at the front of the tables in top hat, and students in the autopsy room, Philadelphia General Hospital, 1884. Photographer unidentified.

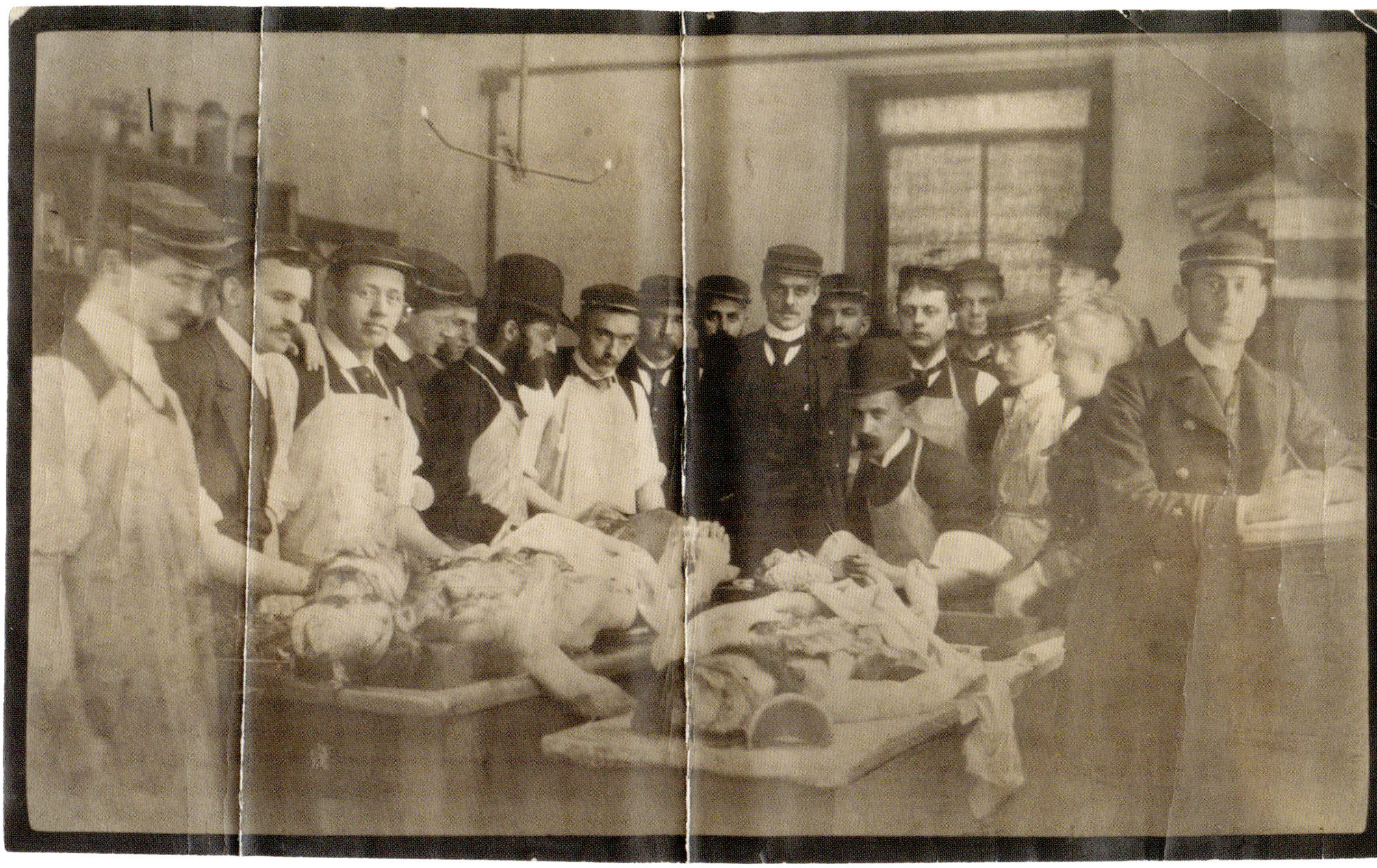

INDEX

Page numbers in *italics* refer to photographs.